Diet and Nutrition

Diet and Nutrition

A guide for students and practitioners

Brenda Piper

Stanley Thornes (Publishers) Ltd

First published in 1996 by Chapman & Hall

Reprinted in 2000 by:
Stanley Thornes (Publishers) Ltd
Delta Place
27 Bath Road
CHELTENHAM
GL53 7TH
United Kingdom

00 01 02 03 / 10 9 8 7 6 5 4 3 2

A catalogue record for this book is available from the British Library.
ISBN 0 7487 5325 7

Typeset by Photoprint, Torquay, Devon
Printed and bound in Great Britain by Athenæum Press Ltd, Gateshead, Tyne & Wear

Contents

Acknowledgements

Many people have helped me in the preparation of this text. I am grateful to former colleagues from the Manchester Metropolitan University: Paul Ainsworth, Jan Carton, Barbara Densem, Heulwen Hall, Jan Mock and George Wilson. Gerry Gee and Myra Woodcock have also advised me.

Elinor Pepper, formerly Head of Home Economics at the City of Manchester College has given a great deal of help with Chapter 21.

Other people who have helped me are: Patsy Carey of the Barlow Moor Medical Centre and Louise and Ian Wright on infant feeding, Mike Wanless on dental health, Chris Reeves and my friends and neighbours, John Elliott and Charles Kinniburgh, who have taught me some computing skills.

Finally, I am indebted to Dominic Recaldin of Chapman & Hall, for an enormous amount of help and encouragement. And I am grateful to my husband, Don, for his customary tolerance and support.

Preface

applications. A less ambitious, but very useful volume, is *Nutrition Matters for Practice Nurses* (edited by A. Leeds, P. Judd and B. Lewis).

There is some overlap between parts of the book. This is intentional to allow busy users to get most of the information they need from a single chapter. Few will want or need to read the book right through.

The section on foods and recipes has been included because of the importance of practical advice. The health visitors to whom I lectured once said, 'it's recipes we need', and so I have included them.

Notes: (i) Dietary energy is measured in Kilojoules (kJ, the SI unit) and Kilocalories (kcal cal). The latter is so firmly embedded in popular use that both units are used.

1 kJ   = 0.239 cal
1 kcal = 4.184 kJ

(ii) The references given are of three types. In some cases they refer to the original research, in others to more advanced textbooks which offer more detail and further references, and some to texts for further study.

Part One
Physiological nutrition

Nutrition, diet and health 1

Introduction

The aim of this section is to establish a general context for the material which will be covered in the book and to outline some of the physiological phenomena which determine and influence nutritional requirements.

Nutrition, diet and health

Everyone knows that a good diet is essential for life and health. In the style of a well-known toy shop, 'Food is me'. Food supplies the raw materials for the *growth* from a single cell to a full-grown adult and to *maintain* the body: there is no other source of the substances we need.

All the cells of the body need a supply of chemical energy (in the form of glucose or fatty acids) which comes ultimately from food. Structural proteins, fats and mineral compounds (as in bone) are formed from the raw materials provided by the diet. Enzymes and their cofactors contain vitamins and mineral elements.

Today, although *life expectancy* in this country is greater than ever before (Figure 1.1), many people are anxious and confused about what they should eat and, judging from the media, one would think our diet is very poor.

What has happened is that, during this century, we have moved from a position where many were under-nourished to a state of general over-nutrition. Today most of us eat enough to supply all the protein, minerals and vitamins we need, but many eat *too much* in relation to energy used and we consume a diet high in fats and sugar. The 'old' problems of rickets, poor growth in children, iron-deficiency anaemia have largely gone but they have been replaced with disability or premature death from coronary heart disease, stroke and cancers (Figure 1.2). In all these, diet plays a role. Thus, the major causes of death have changed dramatically. There are many reasons for this and nutrition is one of them.

The results of nutrient deficiency, like scurvy and iron-deficiency anaemia, can be quickly and dramatically reversed by improving the

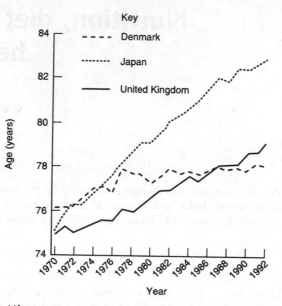

Figure 1.1 Life expectancy at birth, females, 1970–1982. Life expectancy in these countries is greater than ever before. (Redrawn from *Health Trends*, **26**, 1994.)

diet. This is not the case for coronary heart disease and high blood pressure. Diet is implicated in these conditions and in some cancers, but it is not the sole cause. It is reckoned that diet accounts for about 30% of the risk of coronary heart disease. In spite of huge amounts of research, we are much less *certain* about the role of diet in these conditions than in the case of vitamin deficiency, for example. Every week some new dietary hazard or benefit seems to appear, from the dangers of too much coffee to the advantage of raw carrots before transatlantic flights. These reports are usually of *correlations* rather than of cause and effect. This text aims to give the facts as we know them today so that sensible advice can be given and anxiety alleviated.

The study of nutrient deficiencies dominated nutrition for a long time. In the 19th and early 20th centuries under-nutrition was rife among the poor in industrial countries and still is in the developing countries. The classic observations of Rowntree and others showed the devastating effects of under-nutrition on the health of the poor of England (Burnett, 1989).

Although malnutrition of this kind is rare in the industrialized world, today we face the problem in reverse – the effects of dietary excess. As people become more affluent they choose different foods and conse-

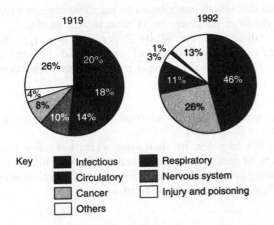

Figure 1.2 Major causes of death, England and Wales, 1919 and 1992. Environmental changes, which include diet, and scientific advances have produced great changes in the causes of death. Note: the key reflects 1919 data rankings; some individual disease groups, categorized as 'others' in 1992 may therefore be greater than those shown individually. (Redrawn from *Health Trends*, **26**, 1994.)

quently their nutrient intakes change. Compared with the early part of the 20th century, people now eat more sugar and less starch, more fat and less fibre, more meat and less vegetable protein and more alcohol, and often more food energy than they use up. These changes occur in all societies as they become more prosperous. Such a diet, in which 60% of food energy may come from fat and sugar, along with a sedentary life-style, appears to be less healthy than a more plain diet and contributes to the development of obesity, coronary (ischaemic) heart disease, hypertension and stroke, dental caries and some kinds of cancers.

DIETARY GOALS AND GUIDELINES

Diet is a recurring theme in the UK Government White Paper, *The Health of the Nation* (1992; see also Bingham, 1991), in *Scotland's Health: A Challenge to Us All* (1993), and in the *Health for All in Wales* produced for Wales (Health Promotion Wales, 1990). This is not surprising. The incidence of coronary heart disease (CHD) in the UK is among the highest in the world and is a major cause of premature death, particularly in males. Alcohol consumption, obesity, high salt intake and other factors (Bingham, 1991) are symptomatic of an unbalanced diet which contributes to the development of hypertension, a crucial factor in coronary heart disease and stroke.

The overall aim of the White Paper (see Box 1.1), based on the recommendations for Europe of the World Health Organization (WHO), is to improve the general health of the population of England by:

- *adding years to life*, by increasing life expectancy and reducing premature death, and
- *adding life to years*, by increasing years lived free from ill-health, reducing or minimizing the adverse effects of illness and disability, promoting healthy life-styles, physical and social environments and, overall, improving the quality of life.

BOX 1.1

THE HEALTH OF THE NATION

The White Paper advised immediate action in key areas of health:

- coronary heart disease (CHD);
- stroke;
- cancers;
- mental health;
- HIV/AIDS;
- accidents.

These areas were chosen because they are all major causes of premature or avoidable ill-health, they can be reduced by effective intervention, and because it should be possible to set objectives and targets and to monitor progress towards them.

A Nutrition Task Force (now disbanded) was set up to prepare an action programme aimed at achieving certain dietary targets to reduce CHD, stroke and some types of cancer (Department of Health, 1994a). The targets were to reduce the percentage of energy coming from saturated and total fat and to reduce obesity (Box 1.2).

These three targets are not the only ways in which we are advised to change our diet. Recommendations for salt, dietary fibre (non-starch polysaccharides) and other carbohydrates have been made by COMA 41 (Committee on Medical Aspects of Food Policy, Department of Health, 1991) and other committees and these will be discussed later.

BOX 1.2

NUTRITION TARGETS

The nutrition targets are:

- to reduce the average percentage of food energy derived by the population from saturated fatty acids by at least 35% by the year 2005 (from 17% in 1990 to no more than 11%);
- to reduce the average percentage of food energy derived by the population from total fat by at least 12% by 2005 (from about 40% in 1990 to no more than 35%);
- to reduce the proportion of men and women aged 16–64 who are obese by at least one-quarter and one-third respectively by 2005 (from 8% for men and 12% for women in 1986/87 to no more than 6% and 8% respectively).

BOX 1.3

DIETARY FIBRE AND NON-STARCH POLYSACCHARIDES

Non-starch polysaccharides (NSP) is the term suggested to replace dietary fibre. These terms can be used synonymously, although they have slightly different definitions (see page 50).

PUBLIC AND INDIVIDUAL HEALTH

These nutritional goals are for *populations* and they give aims for *average* intakes of nutrients. This *nutrition policy* must then be translated into *diets*, and there are innumerable ways of doing this.

The goals are supported by most nutritionists, but there have been criticisms. Some feel they are too precise, given that the evidence on which they are based is incomplete (Skrabanek, 1994).

Certainly there is a difference between advising an individual and considering policies for the nation. Dietary advice to an individual with high blood cholesterol (a known risk factor for coronary heart disease), will depend on the presence or absence of other risk factors, on the person's age and whether there are any observable changes in cardiovascular function. If it is the only risk factor for an otherwise healthy person, then the decision might be made to advise only modest dietary change.

Nevertheless, the vast majority of experts would agree that a general lowering of blood cholesterol levels *in the population as a whole* would be beneficial and would reduce the incidence of coronary heart disease.

HOW BAD *IS* OUR DIET?

A common view today is that we, in the most affluent countries, are ill-fed. How true is this? As we have already said, life expectancy, although showing some variation between countries, is higher than it has ever been in the developed countries. The National Food Survey of the UK carried out each year by the Ministry of Agriculture, Food and Fisheries (MAFF) on a random sample of the population, shows that the estimated requirements are achieved for most nutrients. But we also eat more fat than is desirable, more salt and less fibre and more calories, since the incidence of obesity is rising.

There are also people who, for one reason or another, are at risk of *nutritional deficiency*. Both smoking and high alcohol consumption reduce nutritional status by increasing nutrient requirements through changes in intestinal absorption and/or metabolism. The eating patterns of smokers and drinkers are also usually worse than average. Any state which increases nutrient requirements, like pregnancy, lactation, growth, illness, increases vulnerability to poor nutrition. Poverty is a major factor in determining diet.

HOW TO CHOOSE?

There is an enormous variety of food available today and changes in life-style have tended to alter eating habits. Many people prefer a series of small meals or snacks instead of set traditional meal patterns. Eating out has become more frequent and the 'chippy' and take-away more popular.

The question is, how are we to choose a good diet from this range of palatable foods, without the earlier accepted pattern of meals for guidance and with the commercial pressures of advertising and so on? Ideally we should reverse many of the changes in our eating habits which result from our relative affluence, although it is equally important to prevent under-nutrition due to poverty, excessive slimming or unbalanced diets. In these matters, the health professional has a vital role by offering individually tailored advice. In sickness, diet becomes even more important than in health and the diet of hospital patients is a very significant factor in recovery.

Important definitions and concepts   The terms and concepts described underlie the science of nutrition.

DIET

The term **diet** usually refers to the total food eaten. The whole range of foods eaten and their relative amounts is what is important in determining nutrient intake. In achieving the Health of the Nation targets a change in *patterns* of food consumption is required and a *whole-diet approach* is crucial. The aim is to *modify* dietary patterns, so that we eat more vegetables (thereby increasing non-starch polysaccharides, vitamins and mineral intakes), more starch and less fat, rather than simply adding bran and fruit juice to a poor diet.

FOOD AND NUTRIENTS

Food is any substance which is eaten and which contains nutrients.

Nutrients are chemical substances which are necessary for the proper functioning of the body. There are over 50 known nutrients. The **macronutrients** are carbohydrates, fats and proteins, which form the major part of the diet. These provide energy and major structural compounds. The **micronutrients** are required in much smaller amounts (mg or μg) and are vitamins and mineral elements. **Trace elements** are minerals required in extremely small amounts.

HOMEOSTASIS

Blood and tissue fluid surrounding the cells is kept, in health, remarkably constant in composition and temperature. **Homeostasis** is the term used to describe this constancy. It is a characteristic of humans and the higher animals. This constancy of the internal environment exists in spite of the many changes which may occur in the external environment in which we live: changes in temperature, food and water supply and so on (Figure 1.3).

The body compensates for these changes by a series of homeostatic mechanisms, which frequently work on the same principle as a thermostat, that is, by a negative feedback control.

Food supplies all those substances needed by the body to maintain homeostasis, as well as those needed for growth. With optimal nutrition, homeostasis is maintained and nutrient stores in the body are high but not excessive (for example in the case of fat stores an excessive amount is harmful to health).When diet is very poor, it is not possible to maintain homeostasis and ill-effects occur. Where the homeostatic controls are less efficient (as in old age), diet becomes even more important.

Like the central heating thermostat, a particular homeostatic mechanism will have a 'setting'. There is evidence that events in early life may influence this setting and thus affect long-term health. This subject is dealt with more fully in Chapters 10 and 12. It is one of the many factors which makes research into nutrition so complex.

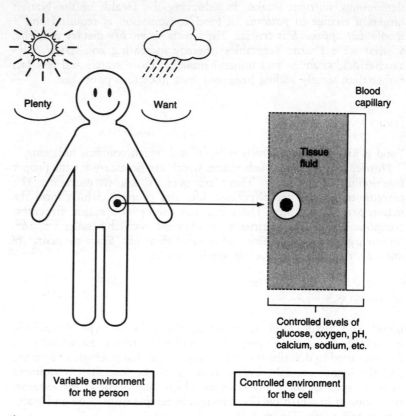

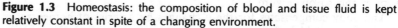

Figure 1.3 Homeostasis: the composition of blood and tissue fluid is kept relatively constant in spite of a changing environment.

ADAPTATION

Human beings **adapt** to all kinds of change. If a person's diet changes and the intake of one or more nutrients is decreased, the body can, to some extent, adapt. A diet habitually low in calcium causes the gut to absorb more calcium and the kidney to excrete less. Semi-starvation, caused by a deficiency of dietary energy, will eventually cause changes in behaviour, like greatly reduced activity, which reduces the calories required.

Humans eat a great variety of diets, both in the types of food chosen and also in the amounts eaten. We have been described as *opportunistic omnivores* because of the way we eat all sorts of plants and animals as food. This range of diets leads to a wide range of nutrient intakes. These differences are compatible with health partly because of *adaptation* to the level of nutrient supply.

Because of this adaptation a person's dietary requirements reflect to some extent their previous diet. Nonetheless, there are obviously limits to adaptation and when these have been reached, symptoms of *nutrient deficiency* will occur.

TURNOVER OF THE BODY'S CONSTITUENTS

All tissues of the body are constantly being broken down and rebuilt. Blood is a good example. Red blood cells have a life span of about 120 days and so are replaced at the rate of 1% a day with an entirely new population every 3 months. Most of the protein and iron from the old cells is reused but some is lost and this must be replaced by the diet.

The same principle applies to bone, body fat (adipose tissue) and the rest of the body, so that diet is *always* important in the maintenance of body structures.

An adolescent who has had a good diet and plenty of exercise will have strong bones, with a high density of calcium. But this is not static; if the dietary calcium falls, then calcium may be drawn from the bones to maintain blood levels and the bone density will fall (see Chapter 7 for more detail).This can happen to young people living alone, when eating properly may not be their first priority.

While a well-nourished body is able to withstand some degree of under-nutrition without harm, too long a period will weaken even the fittest.

NUTRITIONAL BALANCE

The term **balance** is often used in nutrition, as in *energy balance* or *balance studies*. (Note that this is also referred to in later chapters.) It refers to the relationship between loss or utilization of a nutrient and its gain from the diet (Figure 1.4).

For energy balance it refers to the calories (kjoules) eaten and the energy used by the body. If these are equal, the body's energy stores of fat remain constant. If it is negative, with higher expenditure than intake, fat stores will be used up and weight lost. The reverse will occur in positive energy balance.

For protein, the term **nitrogen balance** is used, protein being the major source of nitrogen in the diet. In a well-fed adult, nitrogen intake from dietary protein will equal nitrogen loss from tissue breakdown plus any dietary surplus. In a growing child, nitrogen balance will be positive, intake being greater than loss, as protein is used to form new tissue. A patient with burns, on the other hand, would have a negative nitrogen balance, with increased tissue breakdown unmatched by

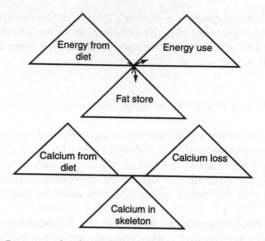

Figure 1.4 Energy and calcium balance: a balance occurs when absorption from dietary intake is equal to expenditure or loss.

dietary intake. Finding the amount of a nutrient required to balance loss is one of the techniques used in estimating nutrient requirements.

Nutrient requirements: Dietary Reference Values

We often want to know how much food or nutrients are required, but the question, 'How much?' is very difficult to answer.

Appetite and hunger drive us to eat so that, usually, we eat enough, in that the energy from food matches energy expenditure. But human beings appear to have no innate sense to choose foods which will supply nutrients missing from their diet, nor to avoid poisonous substances, except for a dislike of bitter tastes and an almost universal liking for sweet and salty-tasting foods. We do learn which substances to avoid, of course, and if we eat something which makes us ill we probably won't touch it again.

Our present knowledge of nutrient requirements is summarized in the *Dietary Reference Values for Food Energy and Nutrients for the United Kingdom* (Report on Health and Social Subjects 41; Department of Health, 1991). This replaces the *Recommended Daily Amounts (RDA) of Nutrients* of 1979 which are still in use in food labelling and in older texts. The WHO also produce estimates of nutrient requirements and many countries produce their own figures.

FACTORS WHICH DETERMINE NUTRIENT REQUIREMENTS

There are a number of factors which determine an individual's nutrient requirements.

Size and age

The bigger the body, the larger is the amount of nutrients needed to maintain the cells. The amount of *metabolically active tissue* determines the demand for nutrients so that *lean body mass* is more important than actual body weight, which may include a large proportion of the less active adipose tissue. If growth is occurring, then relatively more food is needed. The heavier the body, the more energy is needed to move it about.

There are metabolic changes with aging which affect nutrient requirements. In childhood, growth is occurring and later, changes in the utilization of nutrients may occur.

To take these facts into account, the Dietary Reference Values (DRVs) are given for various age groups and for each a standard weight is given. The oldest group, 50+ years, covers a large age range because of the scarcity of data on the particular requirements of the elderly (defined as those over retirement age). More research is needed both for the elderly and for children.

Gender

There are differences in body composition between men and women, women, on average, being shorter and lighter and having a higher proportion of fat. Menstruation also increases the iron requirement of women. Energy requirements are given separately for the sexes from birth and for nutrients from the age of 11 years.

Standard age groups and weights (Table 1.1)

Table 1.1   Age groups and weights used for the Dietary Reference Values

Children		Males		Females	
Age	Weight (kg)	Age (years)	Weight (kg)	Age (years)	Weight (kg)
0–3 months (formula-fed)	5.9	11–14	43.1	11–14	43.8
4–6 months	7.7	15–18	64.5	15–18	55.5
7–9 months	8.9	19–50	74.0	19–50	60.0
10–12 months	9.8	50+	71.0	50+	62.0
1–3 years	12.6				
4–6 years	17.8			Pregnancy	
7–10 years	28.3			Lactation:	
				0–4 months	
				4+ months	

From COMA 41 (Department of Health, 1991). Crown copyright is reproduced with the permission of the Controller of HMSO.

Activity

Activity increases energy requirements.

Variations in the absorption, metabolism and excretion of nutrients

There are large individual variations in the absorption, metabolism and excretion of nutrients and this affects nutrient requirements.

Because of this, within each of the population groups shown here there will be a *range* of requirements. Although detailed evidence is lacking, all the data available suggest that this variation in a group usually shows a **normal** or **Gaussian distribution**, like any other measurable biological characteristic.

This variation between individuals is sometimes called *nutritional individuality* and any nutritional advice or evaluation must take this into account.

BOX 1.4

EXAMPLES OF INDIVIDUAL VARIATION

Experiments have shown a range of 525–1200 mg/day in the vitamin A required for dark adaptation, a range in the breakdown of the body pool of vitamin C per day of 2.6% to 4.1% and a variation in the percentage of iron absorbed from bread from 1% to 40%.

Therefore **three** DRVs are given for most nutrients, for those who need least, for the average and for those with the largest requirements (Figure 1.5). These are:

1. **Estimated Average Requirement (EAR)**: this name is self-explanatory and such an intake would be enough for 50% of a population and insufficient for the other half. This value is given for protein, vitamins and minerals and is the only value given for energy requirements.
2. **Reference Nutrient Intake (RNI)**: this is the intake at which the requirement of 97.5% of a population is met. It equates with the 1979 Recommended Daily Amounts. For most people, it would be enough or more than enough.
3. **Lower Reference Nutrient Intake (LRNI)**: this is the point at the lower end of the curve and represents an intake sufficient for only

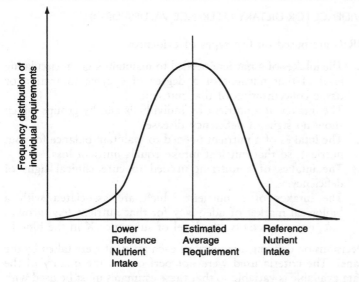

Figure 1.5 The three Dietary Reference Values. (Redrawn from Department of Health (1991), COMA Report 41. *Dietary Reference Values for Food, Energy and Nutrients for the UK*, HMSO, London, 1991). Crown copyright is reproduced with the permission of the Controller of HMSO.

the 2.5% of the population with the lowest requirements. Intakes below this would obviously be inadequate for nearly everyone.

It has not been possible to estimate these three values for all nutrients. For non-starch polysaccharides (NSPs; dietary fibre) a single figure for the adult population is given. For some nutrients (pantothenic acid, biotin, vitamins E and K, manganese, molybdenum, chromium, fluoride) where there is even less data available, values for **safe intakes** are given. This is a level or range of intake at which there is no risk of deficiency, but which is below that where there is a risk of undesirable effects.

USING DRVs TO ASSESS THE DIETS OF GROUPS OR OF INDIVIDUALS

Uses of DRVs

First, whether for a group or an individual, a record of the diet is required. Its nutrient content can then be estimated using food tables and the totals compared with the appropriate DRVs. Caution is required in the interpretation of such dietary analysis data for the following reasons:

BOX 1.5

EVIDENCE FOR DIETARY REFERENCE VALUES (DRVs)

DRVs are based on five types of evidence:

1. The intakes of a nutrient needed to maintain a given circulating level of that nutrient or a degree of enzyme saturation or tissue concentration of that nutrient.
2. The intakes of a nutrient by individuals and by groups which show no signs of deficiency disease.
3. The intakes of a nutrient needed to maintain balance for that nutrient, so that nutrient intake equals nutrient loss.
4. The intakes of a nutrient needed to cure clinical signs of deficiency.
5. The intakes of a nutrient which are associated with a biological marker of adequacy for that nutrient (e.g. growth rate, enzyme activity, the level of substance X in the blood).

Decisions on defining adequacy of each nutrient were taken by the panel. The criteria used were not perfect and the quality of the data available is variable so that these estimates must be used with some caution. They are usually revised every 10 years.

BOX 1.6

When using DRVs remember that:

- they are *statistical* estimates based on present knowledge;
- they apply to *groups* of people (although they are often used for individuals);
- they apply to *healthy* people, since illness and drugs may both alter requirements;
- the DRV for any nutrient presupposes that *requirements for energy and all other nutrients are met*.

- It is very difficult to obtain an accurate record of an individual person's habitual food intake. Total food consumption of a group is sometimes easier to obtain. For individuals there are various methods ranging from the weighing of all food eaten (very time-consuming and laborious) to the 24-hour recall technique, in which the subject is asked to remember everything eaten in the previous 24 hours and to estimate the amounts. The weaknesses of the latter method (an atypical day, faulty memory, inaccurate estimations of quantities) will be apparent. Bingham (1987) has shown that self-reporting of diets nearly always underestimated intake, especially in women.

- Inaccuracies arising from using food tables. Food tables are compiled from laboratory analysis of samples of the foods. Since samples vary, the results will not be accurate for every sample of the food. In general the figures for **macronutrients** (fat, carbohydrate and protein and hence energy) are accurate, especially for dry foods. Values will be less accurate for foods with variable amounts of water and/or fat. For **micronutrients**, the vitamins and minerals, there is a much greater variation between samples of foods according to their variety (the type of potato, for example), methods of production, storage, and processing, so that the figures available may be an *indication* of the amount of nutrient likely to be present rather than an accurate figure.

- Finally, for individuals there is no way of knowing whether their requirement is at the top, middle or bottom of the normal range and, therefore, which DRV is most appropriate.

If you now conclude that the whole process is useless, note that the following assumptions can be made:

1. If the calculated intake is **above** the RNI, then almost certainly it is *sufficient*.
2. If it is **below** the LRNI, then it is very likely to be *less than required* for normal function.
3. Between these two values there is an area of uncertainty, but obviously the lower the intake, the higher the risk of insufficiency.

In assessing the diet for groups, the position is simpler. If the group is large enough, there will be a normal distribution of requirements and the Estimated Average Requirements should be adequate for the group. The use of DRVs to assess the diet of groups is more valid than it is for individuals.

USING DRVs FOR PRESCRIBING DIETS OR FOR THE PROVISION OF FOOD SUPPLIES

DRVs can be used to calculate the nutrients and hence the foods needed for a group for an expedition, for example. If the Reference Nutrient Intakes are supplied then there will be sufficient, or more than sufficient, for everyone. For energy, only the EAR is available; this amount should be adequate for a large group, where the big-eaters will be balanced by small ones.

For an individual, a common use is in the prescription of a therapeutic diet, which should be adequate in all respects apart from the particular therapeutic modification. To be sure of this, the RNI should be provided for all nutrients. Individual requirements for *energy* vary so much that for this appetite must normally be the guide.

USING DRVs FOR FOOD LABELLING

At the time of writing, Recommended Daily Amounts (RDAs) are used for food labelling rather than DRVs. A single value is used rather than a different one for each group. RDAs for use in labelling in the European Community have been produced by *Codex Alimentarius*.

It has been proposed that the use of the EAR for food labelling would prevent unnecessary attempts to reach the RNI, which is an extravagant standard at which to aim.

To sum up, there are many factors which determine an individual's nutrient requirements and even within a homogeneous group there are big variations. The proof of the pudding really is in the eating. If a person is fit and healthy, if a child is growing normally then it is likely that their diet is good. There are estimated nutrient requirements, the DRVs, which are useful *guidelines* for planning or assessing diets. But, when writing about nutrition, there are a lot of ifs, buts and maybes.

Assessing nutritional status of individuals

While **nutrition** is a **process**, the corresponding **state** is termed **nutritional status** or **nutriture**.

Nearly everyone is interested in how well fed they are. In illness, nutritional status will have an important bearing on recovery. A well-nourished person will show no signs of malnutrition and will have good nutrient stores. A less well-fed individual may be in very good health but have low or no nutrient stores.

Does the level of body stores of nutrients matter? Is there any important difference between the first two states in Table 1.2? If there is a good diet and there is no prolonged interruption, the answer is no. But nutrient stores may be needed in times of illness, or in early pregnancy where there may be a prolonged spell of nausea and vomiting. If stores are low and *then* diet is impaired, signs of deficiency will become apparent. At first these are non-specific (fatigue for example) and easily reversed, but the progression indicated in the table below will occur if dietary inadequacy is prolonged (Walker, 1990).

How long will nutrient stores last? For some vitamins good body stores are adequate for years. A well-nourished person has about two

Table 1.2 The relationship between diet and nutritional status

Dietary measurement	Biochemical assessment	Clinical examination
Adequate diet	Full body stores	Good health
Reduced diet	Reduced stores	Good health
Inadequate diet	No stores	?
Very low or no intake	Impairment of function	Clinical signs of disease
	Damage of tissues	Severe clinical signs
	Irreversible damage	

Modified from Walker, A.F. (1990).

years' supply of vitamin A and so a reduction of these stores by 50% or more would not matter. But this does not apply to all nutrients and for some there would only be stores for a matter of weeks.

The health professional often needs to have some idea of an individual's nutritional status. There are various methods which can be used singly or in combination, according to the particular situation.

CLINICAL EXAMINATION

This is the observation of outward signs of malnutrition, changes in the skin, hair, and so on. WHO has produced definitive tests and criteria for assessment (Jeliffe, 1966). These are invaluable where the level of nutrition is poor, as it may be in developing countries.

BIOCHEMICAL TESTS

These estimate the quantity of nutrients or their metabolites in blood or urine, or the activity of an enzyme in which the nutrient is a co-factor. Being more specific (and more expensive) than clinical examination, these tests can show reduced stores as well as impaired function. Examples are urinary nitrogen and plasma albumin for protein and haemoglobin, packed cell volume (PCV) and blood smear for iron.

ANTHROPOMETRIC MEASUREMENTS

These are usually of height and weight, and are quick and easy to carry out. Weight-for-height will, when compared with standard charts and coupled with visual inspection, reveal *obesity* or *wasting*; height-for-age will indicate *total growth* in children (see Chapter 11) and this can be compared with reference charts of height-for-age.

DIETARY ASSESSMENT

Some methods of dietary assessment have already been referred to (weighing all food, 24-hour recall, food diary). What is more often needed are quick and easy methods of dietary assessment which are reasonably accurate. A very simple way is to look at the number of different foods which are eaten. The greater the variety of foods eaten the less likelihood there is of a nutritional deficiency. On the other hand, diets heavily dependent on very few foods (like tea, toast and biscuits) are often deficient.

The use of a check list which also covers money available for food, and other social and cultural factors is often useful. These are covered in the relevant chapters.

Research in nutrition   The study of nutrition encompasses the supply and utilization of the chemicals required for the growth, maintenance and functioning of the body. It is a wide field covering:

- social nutrition: those societal factors which affect the choice and availability of food, and to some extent requirements
- physiology and biochemistry: the functions of nutrients, their absorption and metabolism
- clinical nutrition: the effects of malnutrition, which includes both under- and over-nutrition.

Finally, we eat *food* and therefore need to know about its quality in terms of nutrient content and palatability, understand the effects of processing, storage and cooking on its nutrient content, and appreciate the various traditions which influence food choice. The goals for dietary change are usually expressed in terms of *nutrients*, but this must be interpreted into foods to have any meaning for the general public.

The tools of research into this wide area are diverse, ranging from sociological techniques such as questionnaires to biochemical estimations of enzyme activity.

In broad terms, research can be divided into two main types: observational and experimental. Dietary surveys and much epidemiological work are observational. Experimentation entails making some change, for example comparing a group whose diet is changed in some way with a control group whose diet is left unaltered.

A classic example of nutrition research is the story of vitamin C. During long sea voyages in the 16th and 17th centuries, young sailors often became severely ill with scurvy after a diet of ship's biscuit and other non-perishable foods. Lind (1753) planned an experiment on 12 men, all with a similar degree of the disease. Two were given cider daily, two others 'elixir vitriol' (sulphuric acid), another couple two spoonfuls of vinegar, another sea water and finally, two lucky pairs had two oranges or one lemon daily.

Those two given oranges and lemons were cured within days while the others got worse. In this way, a dietary cure and prevention of scurvy were found, although there was no knowledge of what was in oranges and lemons to bring about such dramatic effects (Walker, 1990).To a certain extent, this happens today, when dietary recommendations are made without complete scientific proof for them.

Eventually vitamin C was identified, its chemical structure elucidated, and its distribution in the body and several of its functions discovered. The distribution of vitamin C in food is known as well as the effects on it of cooking, preservation and storage. Experiments on human volunteers and on guinea pigs (which like humans cannot synthesize vitamin C themselves and therefore depend on a dietary supply) have provided information about requirements and it can be synthesized.

Similar types of investigation have given us a large but still incomplete body of knowledge about the 50 nutrients we need, and this forms the basis of estimations of nutrient requirements. Such work often originated from the effects of nutrient deficiency: the effects are usually clear-cut and rapidly reversed by supplying the deficient nutrient.

Over-nutrition is harder to investigate. Diet is involved in some chronic diseases, such as coronary heart disease (CHD) and essential hypertension (that is, hypertension with no known cause) but the role of diet is difficult to unravel. For one thing, these conditions often develop very gradually and are not always easily reversed. A clear-cut experiment like Lind's is not possible.

EPIDEMIOLOGICAL STUDIES

For many of these so-called diseases of affluence (which ironically are most prevalent among the least affluent of affluent societies) the first links between diet and disease were shown by **epidemiology**. This is the study of the pattern of disease of human populations and can be used to reveal geographical and social class differences among others. It can also be used to understand the causes of disease and to identify high-risk groups. The correlations which are shown can then be tested by further studies.

BOX 1.7

AETIOLOGY

The aetiology of a disease is its cause or causes.

There are three types of epidemiological studies of the **aetiology** of disease. These are descriptive, analytic and experimental.

Descriptive studies

These show the distribution of the disease in different populations and may show the relationships with age, sex and health-related behaviour. They may show geographical variations, the effects of migration and changes with the passage of time.

Such studies therefore reveal correlations between the disease and age, or between the disease and certain behaviours. The resultant hypotheses can then be tested by analytic and experimental studies.

Analytic studies

There are two types. **Retrospective** studies, in which the past histories of persons suffering from the disease are analysed for selected factors and compared with data from a healthy control group and **prospective studies** which look at the experiences of a healthy group and compare the data of those who remain healthy with those who become ill. Retrospective studies are notoriously difficult (who can remember accurately what they ate 10 years ago?) but prospective studies are much easier to control. Both are expensive.

Experimental studies

These are designed to test whether a group of people protected from a suspected causal agent (saturated fat for coronary heart disease for example) shows a lower incidence of the disease than a similar but unprotected group.

CORRELATION AND CAUSALITY

All the studies mentioned above will show correlations which may or may not be causal. Evidence pointing to a causal relationship includes:

- consistency: the same association is found between and within populations (for example between the populations of France, the UK, and so on *and* between groups or individuals within one of these countries).
- dose–response relationship: the incidence of the disease correlates with the amount of exposure to the suspected agent.
- relationship with time: exposure to the suspected agent must precede the onset of the disease and a change in exposure of a population with time should be followed by a similar change in the incidence of the disease.

Finally, **physiological and biochemical research** may elucidate the mechanisms by which the disease is produced. Until this happens, our understanding of some areas of nutrition is very much on the lines of the 'black box' model. We know what goes in (foods and nutrients), and the end result (morbidity and mortality), but the in-between events are shrouded in mystery.

META-ANALYSIS

The study of many of our present nutritional problems began with epidemiological work. There are a number of difficulties in this method of investigation. The most important is the validity of measurements of food intake. It is extremely difficult to measure the diet of free-living people accurately. Second, the conversion of food intake into nutrient intake using food tables introduces inaccuracies, especially for vitamins and minerals.

Some studies are not well designed and the result has been that for coronary heart disease, for example, a huge number (over 200) of risk factors have been found by different workers.

A recent approach is to use the statistical technique known as meta-analysis. This pools the data from separate studies. If the effect of, say, salt on blood pressure is fairly small, it may not show up in 25 studies with 300 people in each but in a larger study of 6000 people it should give a statistically significant result, that is, more than a 95% probability that the result is due to salt intake and not to chance. So meta-analysis avoids organizing another new, large and expensive study by re-analysing all well-planned existing studies. This has, in fact, been done for salt and has revealed a stronger relationship between salt intake and blood pressure than before.

Meta-analysis has its critics, who note that it is only valid if the individual studies were valid and that if it takes large numbers of subjects to show a significant benefit of a procedure, then the real benefit for any individual must be relatively unimportant (Skrabanek, 1994).

RESEARCH BY HEALTH PROFESSIONALS

A recent publication on the core nutrition curriculum for health professionals notes that research may be carried out by health professionals working in academic institutions and within their everyday work (Department of Health, 1994). The demonstration of the beneficial effects of dietary supplementation on the recovery of patients from leg fractures (Chapter 18) is an example of the value of such research. There are many questions in nutrition which remain to be answered and useful publications to help in this (Kern and Booth, 1992; Bell, 1994; Carey and Hawkes, 1994; Miles and Huberman, 1994).

Key points

1. Adequate nutrition is essential for the maintenance of homeostasis and therefore of health and life.
2. Nutrient requirements vary with age, gender and size, but even within an homogeneous group there is a wide range of nutrient requirements, sometimes called 'nutritional individuality'.
3. Requirement for a particular nutrient by an individual is not set at one point; adaptation to a limited range of intakes occurs.
4. Dietary Reference Values (DRVs) are available for many nutrients. Used with caution, they are valuable in dietary assessment and prescription and in food labelling. The values available are the Estimated Average Requirement (EAR), the Reference Nutrient Intake (RNI) and the Lower Reference Nutrient Intake (LRNI). For some nutrients, only Safe Intakes are known.
5. Assessment of the nutritional status of an individual is not easy. A variety of methods are available.
6. Research in nutrition uses many different methods. Elucidation of the effects of deficiency is usually easier than the investigation of the long-term effects of excess, where epidemiological methods are often the starting point.

Digestion, absorption and metabolism 2

The aim of this chapter is to give an outline of the digestion, absorption and metabolism of food to underpin the chapters which follow, and to describe common digestive problems.

Digestion enables nutrients to be absorbed, absorption into the blood enables them to be utilized and metabolism refers to all the chemical changes which take place in the body. Individual characteristics in these three processes are the cause of some of the variation in nutrient requirements between individuals.

Digestion

Food normally enters the body through the gastrointestinal tract and this is known as *enteral feeding*.

Digestion is simply the breakdown of large molecules into smaller water-soluble ones and it occurs in the gastrointestinal tract through the action of enzymes and other substances like bile and hydrochloric acid.

The gastrointestinal tract (Figure 2.1) is a muscular tube of varying diameter, beginning at the mouth and ending at the anus. The smooth muscles in its wall mix the food with the digestive secretions, move the food along the gut by an action called **peristalsis** and, by means of sphincters, partition the tract.

The complex muscular movements of the gastrointestinal tract are controlled by nerve plexuses in the walls of the gut (intrinsic nerve plexuses), by the sympathetic and parasympathetic nervous systems and by hormones (locally released regulatory peptides and others) (see Box 2.1).

Mucus, produced by the cells lining the tract, lubricates the passage of food through the gut.

Food is chewed in the mouth and so broken up into small pieces. The extent of chewing is probably not very important in digestion. Saliva is produced continually but the rate increases by as much as 15 times

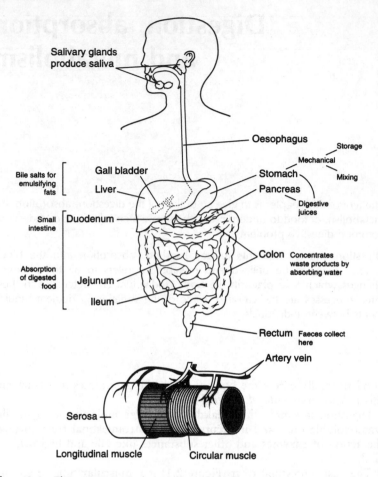

Figure 2.1   The gastrointestinal tract. The inset diagram shows the four layers of the gut wall. The blood vessels into which the digested food is absorbed lie in the mucosa. (Redrawn from Lamb, J.F., Ingram, C.G., Johnston, I.A. and Pitman, R.M. (1991) *Essentials of Physiology*, 3rd edn, Blackwell Scientific Publications, London.)

when food is in the mouth. Saliva dilutes the food and allows water-soluble constituents to dissolve and be tasted, it contains alpha-amylase which digests starch and it keeps the mouth moist and healthy.

Swallowing is a complex action in which food is directed into the **oesophagus** and prevented from entering the trachea. If food does enter the trachea, choking occurs and coughing usually ejects the food.

The oesophagus is simply a muscular tube, with a smooth mucus-lubricated lining, which carries food to the stomach. The main role of

BOX 2.1

REGULATORY PEPTIDES

Peptide	Main action
Gastrin	Stimulates gastric acid secretion
Secretin	Stimulates secretion of bicarbonate from pancreas, neutralizes stomach acid
Cholecystokinin	Contraction of gall bladder so bile enters gut; secretion of pancreatic enzymes
Gastric inhibitory peptide (GIP)	Stimulates insulin release, inhibits gastric acid, stimulates motility
Motilin	Stimulates motility
Vasoactive intestinal peptide (VIP)	Vasodilation, muscle relaxation, secretion
Somatostatin	Antagonizes peptide release
Substance P	Transmitter for sensory nerves, vasodilation, muscle contraction
Bombesin	Releases peptides, anti-somatostatin, trophic agent
Neurotensin	Vasodilation

the stomach is to act as a temporary store of food, passing the mixture of food and gastric secretion, called chyme into the small intestine at a regulated rate. Gastric juice contains hydrochloric acid and enzymes called pepsins, which together digest protein to smaller molecules, peptides. The characteristics increase the surface area for absorption enormously to about 200 m^2.

BOX 2.2

GLOSSARY

Mucosa: inner lining of the gut

Vasodilation: widening or dilation of blood vessels, causing increased blood supply

Motility: muscular movement of gut

Steatorrhoea: large amounts of fat in stools

Insulin: hormone controlling blood sugar. Causes uptake of glucose by cells and therefore fall in blood glucose

Glucagon: hormone controlling blood sugar. Acts in opposite way from insulin

Sphincter: a circular band of muscle, which when contracted closes the tract. Sphincters occur between oesophagus and stomach, stomach and duodenum, and at the anus stomach is able to enlarge as food enters it without an increase in pressure. As a consequence, large meals can be eaten. A long period of semi-starvation reduces this expansive capacity and during the recovery period frequent small meals are necessary to prevent discomfort. This is one of the problems in treating sufferers of anorexia nervosa.

The **small intestine**, consisting of the *duodenum*, the *jejunum* and the *ileum* is where most of the digestion and absorption of food occurs. The internal surface of the small intestine, the mucosa, is folded into finger-like projections, called villi (singular, villus) and then the inner surface of every cell is folded in microvilli (Figure 2.2). Together these

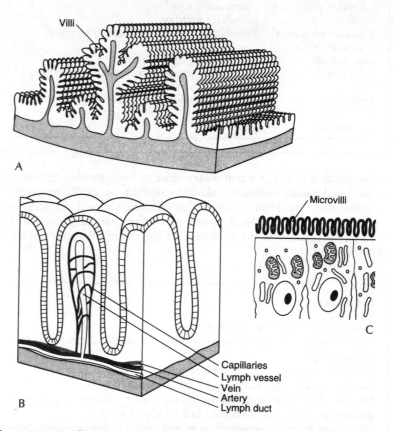

Figure 2.2   Small intestinal villi, showing the enormous surface available for the absorption of nutrients. A: five folds in the small intestine wall, each covered with villi. B: each villus is made up of several hundred cells. C: three cells of a single villus; each cell is coated with microvilli. (Redrawn with permission from Whitney, E.N., Cataldo, C.B. and Rolfes, S.R. (1993) *Understanding Normal and Clinical Nutrition*; West Publishing Company, St Paul.)

The **liver** produces bile, which is stored in the gall bladder and enters the gut after meals. Bile is essential in the digestion and absorption of fats. It is also the vehicle for excreting cholesterol and the bile pigments (which are produced from the breakdown of red blood cells) in the faeces. When bile is not secreted, as in hepatitis, fat is not digested but instead is excreted in the faeces (steatorrhoea) while the bile pigments remain in the body and cause jaundice.

The **pancreas** contains two types of tissue. One, the islets of Langerhans, produces insulin and glucagon and so has an endocrine function. The rest produces enzymes which enter the small intestine through a duct. These pancreatic enzymes digest fat, starch, protein, elastin and collagen (in meat and fish), and RNA and DNA (Box 2.3). The pancreatic secretion is therefore vital for digestion.

In the small intestine proteins are digested to small molecules of two or three amino acids, fats to fatty acids and monoglycerides, and starches to two- and three-unit sugars.

Digestion of these molecules is completed by enzymes produced by the cells of the small intestine itself (**enterocytes**).

BOX 2.3

PANCREATIC ENZYMES		
Enzyme	*Substrate*	*Digestive products*
Trypsin	Protein	To smaller fragments
Chymotrypsin	Protein	To smaller fragments
Carboxypeptidases	Protein	To smaller fragments
Pancreatic lipase	Fats	Fatty acids, monoglycerides
Phospholipases	Lecithin and related compounds	Free fatty acids
Alpha-amylase	Starch	To smaller fragments
Ribonuclease	RNA	
Deoxynuclease	DNA	
Collagenase	Connective tissue	
Elastase	Elastin	

Box 2.1 and 2.3 are reproduced with permission from Lamb *et al.*, 1991, *Essentials of Physiology 3rd ed*, published by Blackwell Science Ltd.

In the **large intestine** the longitudinal muscle is arranged in bands, giving it its typical sacculated appearance. Water is absorbed to produce solid faeces. There is a heavy bacterial flora in the large intestine. Some of the bacteria break down carbohydrates, like non-starch polysaccharides (fibre), and proteins which may be present. The

BOX 2.4

GLOSSARY

Hiatus: literally means gap and in the case of hiatus hernia, refers to the gap in the diaphragm which allows the oesophagus to pass through
Hernia: the passage of an organ through the structures by which it is normally contained

colour of the faeces comes from bile pigments. In their absence, they are greyish-white. Blood and medicinal iron compounds cause a dark colour.

Absorption

Absorption is the passage of foods from the gut into the blood stream. It occurs mainly in the small intestine; some substances are absorbed by active transport (that is, by the expenditure of energy by the cells of the gut), others by passive diffusion.

Over 90% of protein, fats, sugars and starches are absorbed. In the new-born but not in the adult, proteins can be absorbed intact. This allows the absorption of antibodies from breast milk.

Fat-soluble vitamins are absorbed along with fat, water-soluble vitamins by diffusion.

The proportion of minerals and the process by which they are absorbed varies. Some, like sodium, are fully absorbed and the body content is controlled by variable excretion. Others, like copper, iron, calcium and zinc are only partly absorbed. The proportion absorbed and available for use or storage is termed the **bioavailability**. Some dietary substances hinder the absorption of iron, calcium, zinc and copper. These are phytates, oxalates and NSP (all found in plant foods), all of which bind these minerals as insoluble compounds which therefore cannot be absorbed. As well as these factors, the absorption of non-haem iron is controlled by the body's iron status and the absorption of calcium by vitamin D.

Common digestive problems

CHOKING

Choking is when some food has entered the trachea (the windpipe or air passage). If the person cannot make any sound, it means that the air-flow is cut off completely.

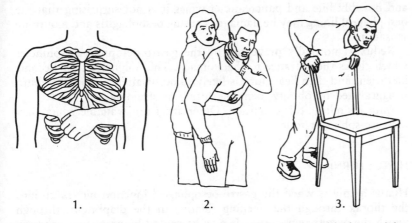

Figure 2.3   The Heimlich manoeuvre, used to dislodge food blockage of the trachea. 1. The rescuer positions one fist directly against the victim's abdomen, as shown and then grasps this fist with the other hand and presses into the abdomen with a **quick, upward thrust**. 2. (i) The rescuer stands behind the victim and wraps their arms around the victim's waist. (ii) The rescuer then makes a fist with one hand and places the thumb-side of the fist against the victim's abdomen, slightly above the navel and below the rib cage. (iii) The rescuer grasps the fist with the other hand and presses into the victim's abdomen with a **quick upward thrust**. (iv) The rescuer repeats the thrust several times as necessary. 3. The victim may attempt self-administration of the standard Heimlich technique. Alternatively, the victim positions himself/herself over the edge of a fixed, horizontal object, such as a chair back, railing, or table edge, and presses the abdomen into the edge with a quick movement. The movement should be repeated several times as necessary. (Redrawn from Whitney, E.N., Cataldo, C.B. and Rolfes, S.R. (1993) *Understanding Normal and Clinical Nutrition*; West Publishing Company, St Paul.)

The Heimlich manoeuvre (Figure 2.3) should be used to dislodge the particle, which will cause death if it is not removed. Choking can be a serious problem in stroke patients and in those with motor neurone disease.

DYSPEPSIA OR INDIGESTION

Dyspepsia (or indigestion) simply means discomfort on eating and has many causes.

HEARTBURN

Heartburn occurs when the lower end of the oesophagus is damaged by reflux of the stomach's contents. Since the reflux contains acid, pepsins, and possibly bile and pancreatic enzymes it is not surprising that the oesophageal lining may be damaged causing oesophagitis and a burning sensation.

Reflux is normally prevented by the gastro-oesophageal sphincter which closes the entrance to the stomach. This sphincter may become inefficient and then heartburn is likely to occur after meals. Heartburn is aggravated by obesity, bending, lifting or straining.

Antacids relieve this condition. Other drugs are available which may increase sphincter tone.

HIATUS HERNIA

Hiatus hernia is when the gastro-oesophageal junction moves up into the thorax through the opening (hiatus) in the diaphragm through which the oesophagus passes. It may be caused by pregnancy, obesity, chronic coughing or constipation.

Sufferers of either or both heartburn and hiatus hernia should lose weight if necessary, eat small, frequent meals, sit upright after a meal and prop the bed-head up by about 4 inches (10 cm). They should avoid smoking and wearing tight-fitting waist bands.

VOMITING

Vomiting occurs when the usual sequence of muscular contractions is reversed, causing an explosive ejection of the stomach's contents. If severe, bile may be vomited. It is caused by various infections and after eating poisons or irritants when it protects the body from their harmful effects.

Vomiting can result in the loss of large amounts of salts and water which must be replaced with saline and glucose.

In an infant, vomiting (as opposed to possetting small amounts) is especially serious.

In bulimia (self-induced vomiting after bingeing), in addition to salt and fluid imbalances, the repeated vomiting causes irritation and possible infection of the pharynx, oesophagus and salivary glands, while the gastric acid may erode tooth enamel.

Projectile vomiting, when the force of ejection is very great, requires immediate medical attention.

DIARRHOEA

The frequent, loose, watery stools of diarrhoea indicate that the passage of intestinal contents has been so fast that normal water absorption has not occurred. Dehydration results. Replacement with water to which salt and glucose has been added rehydrates effectively. There are many possible causes.

CONSTIPATION

Constipation is a marked reduction in an individual's customary frequency of defaecation and hard stools are passed with difficulty.

There are many causes including habitually suppressing the desire to defaecate, a change in life-style, and too little activity. A diet high in NSP (non-starch polysaccharides, dietary fibre) will add faecal bulk and decrease transit time (see page 53). For those who cannot or will not adapt their diet, there are bulk-forming preparations (for example, methyl cellulose). Other types of laxatives act by softening the faeces, by retaining water through osmotic pressure, or by stimulating motility. Adequate fluid intake is essential.

ULCERS

Ulcers may occur in the stomach (gastric ulcer) and in the duodenum (duodenal ulcer). Together they are referred to as peptic ulcers.

An ulcer is an area of erosion. In the stomach the presence of a hydrochloric acid and protein-digesting enzymes (pepsins) prevents healing. In health the gastric mucosa is protected by a thick layer of mucus.

Dietary advice has varied. Generally small, frequent and regular meals, avoiding extremes of temperature and spiciness of food are advised. Smokers should stop and paracetamol rather than aspirin should be used for pain relief.

Drugs used in treatment include antacids. Anticholinergic drugs and H^2 receptor antagonists reduce the secretion of acid. Histamine is produced by some gastric cells and promotes acid secretion. H^2 receptor antagonists block its action.

Complications are haemorrhage, perforation and obstruction of the gut (pyloric stenosis).

GASTRITIS

Gastritis is the inflammation of the gastric mucosa (the lining). It may be acute or chronic. Heavy smokers and drinkers are at risk.

The symptoms are nausea, pain and vomiting. Iron and vitamin B12 deficiencies may occur because of repeated bleeding and reduced production of the intrinsic factor respectively.

PANCREATITIS

The pancreas produces so many digestive enzymes that pancreatitis has a great effect on digestion and absorption. Nutritional therapy is therefore very important and supervision by a dietician is essential.

CYSTIC FIBROSIS

In this hereditary condition there is widespread dysfunction of the exocrine glands (that is, glands which deliver their secretions through ducts rather than directly into the blood stream like endocrine glands). Sufferers have severe nutritional problems because of pancreatic insufficiency and low energy intake. This is a situation where the currently proposed healthy diet, low in fat and sugar, is not suitable. An energy-dense diet is required. Supervision by a dietician is essential.

DIVERTICULOSIS

Diverticulosis is a common condition where small pockets form in the wall of the large bowel (Figure 2.4). It is characteristic of a low-fibre diet. It may be asymptomatic or cause diarrhoea.

Metabolism The term metabolism means the sum of all the chemical reactions which occur in the body. These include the synthesis of glycogen, fat and proteins: this is **anabolism**. It also covers the breakdown of substances either in normal turnover or to provide energy: this is **catabolism**.

The first need of the cells is energy. Amino acids (from proteins), fatty acids (from fats) and monosaccharides (from starch and sugars) can all be used by the cells for energy or converted to fat and stored in adipose tissue (Figure 2.5).

These different molecules are broken down to smaller molecules and finally all the pathways end in a two-carbon molecule called acetyl coenzyme A. Acetyl coenzyme A enters a cycle of enzymic reactions called the citric acid cycle (also called Kreb's cycle after Hans Kreb who

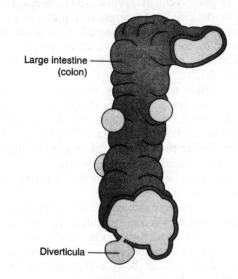

Large intestine
(colon)

Diverticula

Figure 2.4   Diverticula: the pockets of intestinal linings which may form in the weakened bowel wall.

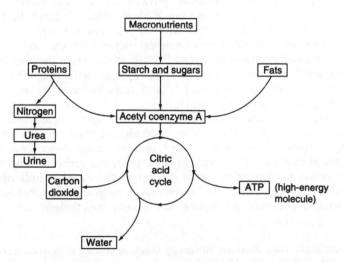

Macronutrients

Proteins   Starch and sugars   Fats

Nitrogen

Acetyl coenzyme A

Urea

Urine

Citric
acid
cycle

Carbon
dioxide

ATP   (high-energy
molecule)

Water

Figure 2.5   A simplified scheme indicating the release of food energy. The citric acid cycle takes place in the mitochondria of every cell in the body.

discovered it). In this cycle of events, acetyl coenzyme A is broken down to carbon dioxide and water and high-energy molecules of adenosine triphosphate (ATP) are formed. ATP is the 'unit' in which energy is produced by the body. Any reaction which needs energy (like the synthesis of protein, the contraction of muscles or a nerve impulse) requires and uses ATP.

After a meal, when the blood is flooded with the products of digestion, amino acids, fats and sugars are taken up by the cells. This is under hormonal control; insulin is released. It causes cells to take in glucose and amino acids and stimulates glycogen, fat and protein synthesis in them. Under the influence of **insulin**, the breakdown of fat is decreased and glucose utilization promoted.

Insulin is sometimes called the 'hormone of feasting' and it produces a state of anabolism or synthesis.

Between meals, the reverse occurs. There is no longer a supply of energy-producing molecules from the gut. Glycogen, stored mainly in the liver, and fat stores are now broken down and used for cellular energy supplies. (During a prolonged fast, body protein would also be used for energy.) Most of the body cells now use fat as a form of energy, leaving glucose for the use of the nervous system, since nerve cells can metabolize only glucose. Glucagon (a hormone produced by the pancreas), growth hormone and adrenaline control metabolism during fasting.

Protein synthesis, from amino acids in the blood, is required to maintain the cells of the body, to make hormones and new tissue. Therefore in pregnancy, lactation, growth and healing there is an increased need for protein. These are anabolic states. A catabolic state is where there is loss of body tissue, as in starvation, fever.

Total metabolic demand will therefore depend on the size of the body, on its composition (muscle cells are more active metabolically than fat cells) and on its state (for example growth, pregnancy, or recovery from injury). Proteins, fats and carbohydrates are the substrates for this metabolic demand.

Vitamins and minerals from the diet function mainly as cofactors for enzymes or form part of the enzyme molecule. Enzymes are substances, usually proteins, which, in very small amounts bring about metabolic or chemical changes. This explains why proteins, carbohydrates and fats are called macronutrients (macro = large) and form the bulk of the diet and vitamins and minerals are known as micronutrients, needed in much smaller amounts but of vital importance nonetheless.

Key points   1.   Nutrients from food are normally taken in from the gastrointestinal tract; this is **enteral** nutrition.
2.   Digestion is the breakdown, mainly by the action of enzymes, of

large molecules of proteins, fats and carbohydrates to smaller, water-soluble molecules.

3. Absorption is the passage of these small molecules into the blood stream, by active transport and/or diffusion.

4. The gastrointestinal tract (gut) is a muscular tube of varying dimensions, the activity of the muscle mixing its contents and moving them along. The tract is divided into sections by sphincters.

5. Food is chewed in the mouth and diluted with saliva, which contains amylase, an enzyme which digests starch.

6. The oesophagus is merely a tube, conveying food to the stomach. Heartburn and oesophagitis, due to gastric reflux, and hiatus hernia are common problems.

7. The stomach expands on eating without the pressure of its contents increasing. Gastric secretions contain hydrochloric acid and pepsins and these begin the digestion of proteins.

8. The small intestine, which has a very large surface area, is the main site of digestion and absorption. Bile (which emulsifies fat), pancreatic enzymes and finally enzymes within the enterocytes (cells lining the small intestine) complete digestion and absorption then takes place here.

9. In the large intestine water is absorbed to produce solid faeces. The bacterial flora breaks down any proteins and some non-starch polysaccharides (fibre).

10. Metabolism, the sum of the many chemical reactions which occur in the body, includes both synthesis or anabolism, and breakdown or catabolism. Energy is the first requirement of cells and can be provided by amino acids, fatty acids or monosaccharides.

11. Common digestive disorders are described, namely choking, heartburn, oesophagitis and hiatus hernia, vomiting, diarrhoea, constipation, ulcers, gastritis, cystic fibrosis, pancreatitis, and diverticulosis.

3 Carbohydrates

The aim of this chapter is to outline briefly the necessary chemistry and physiology of sugars, starches and non-starch polysaccharides and to discuss the present view of their dietary roles in the context of the average UK diet.

The term 'carbohydrates' (Box 3.1) includes sugars, starches and non-starch polysaccharides (the term which is used now instead of dietary fibre). Sugars are the simplest carbohydrates. Joined in long and sometimes complex chains, sugars form starch and non-starch polysaccharides; these two are sometimes grouped under the title complex carbohydrates.

Sugars and starch are one of the main sources of energy supply for the body. They supply essential fuel for the cells (although not an energetic feeling) or they are converted to fat and stored in adipose tissue.

Sugars

Sugars are soluble carbohydrates, usually sweet-tasting, which occur naturally in some foods (like berries and fruits) or can be added as refined sugar.

AVAILABILITY CLASSIFICATION OF SUGARS

From a dietary point of view classifying sugars according to *where they come from* is more useful than the usual chemical classification. The scheme in Table 3.1 was proposed by the Panel on Dietary Sugars and Human Disease (Department of Health, 1989).

It is the *non-milk extrinsic sugars* (NMES), sometimes called 'added' sugars, which are the focus of concern for health.

METABOLISM OF SUGARS

Digestion

Sugars are absorbed into the blood stream as simple sugars or monosaccharides. The disaccharides are digested in the small intestine.

Table 3.1 Classification of sugars

Intrinsic	*Extrinsic*	
Form integral part of certain unprocessed foodstuffs (fruits, vegetables)	Not located within cells	
	Non-milk extrinsic or added sugars	Milk sugars
	Table sugars (fruit juices, honey, sucrose)	Recipe sugars

BOX 3.1

SOME CHEMISTRY

Carbohydrates are a group of compounds whose molecules consist of carbon, hydrogen and oxygen.

The chemical names of sugars have the ending -ose. Sugar molecules may have five or six carbon atoms, the group names being pentoses (5C) or hexoses (6C). The nutritionally important sugars are all hexoses. Sugars may be simple sugars, consisting of single sugar unit, the monosaccharides, or more complex, with each molecule having two units, the disaccharides.

CHEMICAL CLASSIFICATION OF THE MAIN DIETARY SUGARS

Monosaccharides:	glucose
	fructose (fruit sugar)
	galactose
Disaccharides:	sucrose = glucose + fructose
	lactose (milk sugar) = glucose + galactose
	maltose = glucose + glucose

The enzymes sucrase, maltase and lactase are present in the inner edge (called the brush border or the microvilli) of the cells lining the gut, the enterocytes. These enzymes break down sucrose, maltose and lactose to their constituent monosaccharides, glucose, galactose and fructose.

Lactose intolerance

Lactose intolerance is caused by a deficiency of lactase. It is not uncommon, especially in Asians. The unabsorbed lactose causes diarrhoea and therefore lactose intake must be reduced, although a small amount can usually be tolerated.

Sucrose intolerance and galactosaemia are rare conditions.

Absorption of sugars

This occurs both by passive diffusion and by active transport facilitated by sodium (hence the use of salt and glucose in water in the treatment of diarrhoea).

Digestion and absorption of sugars is quick. There is no advantage in giving glucose rather than sucrose in cases of low blood sugar as the digestive products of sucrose enter the blood stream just as fast as glucose.

UTILIZATION OF SUGARS

Glucose, carried to cells by the blood, is a source of cellular energy. The cells of the brain and nervous system and the red blood cells are entirely dependent on blood glucose as an energy source: unlike other cells they cannot use fatty acids and so a fall in glucose concentration will result in signs of brain malfunction, for example confusion and loss of judgement.

The concentration of glucose in the blood is 3.0–5.0 mmol/litre when fasting and in health it is kept within narrow limits by a homeostatic control mechanism involving the hormones insulin, glucagon, cortisol and growth hormone.

If it rises too high (hyperglycaemia) then some of the glucose will be excreted in the urine, causing the typical polyuria (increased production of urine) and thirst of diabetes mellitus.

DIETARY SOURCES AND CURRENT INTAKE OF SUGARS

Sugar is highly palatable and is appreciated from early infancy. Sugar, mainly as sucrose, is important in cooking and food technology because it increases palatability (as a sweetener and also as a flavour enhancer) and the tenderness of cakes and biscuits. In jams it is used as a preservative.

In the UK sugars provide 10–20% of total food energy with an average supply of 69 g non-milk extrinsic sugars per head per day in 1993. We have the highest confectionery consumption in Europe, around 34 g per person per day. There are, not surprisingly, big differences between individuals.

The main sources of added sugars are soft drinks, table sugar, confectionery and cakes, biscuits and puddings. Jams and breakfast cereals provide small amounts only.

RECOMMENDATIONS FOR SUGARS INTAKE

No DRVs for sugars have been given, but the following statements and recommendations were made in COMA Report 41 (Department of Health, 1991).

- There is no evidence that intrinsic sugars (in fruit and vegetables) or lactose in milk or milk products have any adverse effect on health.
- Extrinsic sugars, mainly sucrose, should be reduced to reduce dental caries.
- Extreme intakes of sucrose (more than 200 g/day) should be avoided, since they may be associated with raised blood cholesterol, blood glucose and insulin levels.

ADDED (NON-MILK EXTRINSIC) SUGAR AND HEALTH

It is easy to eat a great many sugary foods and a high sugars intake has been linked with dental caries (decay), diabetes mellitus, cardiovascular disease, obesity and behavioural problems in children. While there is unquestionable evidence linking sugar with dental caries, the evidence for the remainder is not convincing.

Dental caries (tooth decay)

The health of the teeth depends crucially on the diet, in particular on the sugar-containing foods eaten, their consistency and frequency. Caries has been a major health problem in the UK, the incidence peaking in childhood, but in the past 10 years there have been dramatic falls in the prevalence of dental caries, so that by the age of 15 years, 40% of children were free from tooth decay in 1993, compared with only 8% in 1983 (Todd and Dodd, 1994). On the other hand, half the children in England still had some dental decay by the time they were teenagers and there are marked regional inequalities. There is a much higher level of dental caries in Scotland and Northern Ireland than in the rest of the UK. Incidence of dental caries increases again in old age.

According to WHO, caries and periodontal disease are the third highest cause of morbidity in the world and for patients with serious disease, streptococcal septicity linked to active caries may be a major hazard (Department of Health, 1989).

The cause of caries is *acid*, produced from sugar by bacteria present in the plaque on the teeth (Figure 3.1; Box 3.2). Acid causes destruction

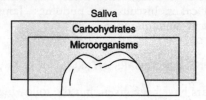

Figure 3.1 Schematic representation of the factors which interact in the development of dental caries. (Redrawn from Rugg-Gunn, A.J. (ed.) (1993) *Sugarless – the Way Forward*; Elsevier Science Publishers Ltd., London.)

BOX 3.2

BACTERIA INVOLVED IN DENTAL CARIES

Streptococcus mutans is usually the primary initiator of decay while *Lactobacillus acidophilus* continues the process.

BOX 3.3

GLOSSARY

Caries: decay
Cariogenic: something which causes tooth decay
Galactosaemia: presence of galactose in the blood

---

of the tooth enamel. The enamel can be repaired naturally in the early stages of the decay by redeposition of calcium and phosphate.

A rough time-scale for these reactions is as follows. Demineralization of the tooth enamel begins seconds after eating sugary foods: within 20–40 minutes the acid is dissipated and a slow repair starts, continuing until more sugar was eaten.

Saliva has an important protective role by removing food debris, inhibiting bacterial activity through salivary enzymes and immuno-globulins, and by buffering or neutralizing acid, since saliva is alkaline.

Cariogenic foods

Epidemiological surveys and animal experiments have established the relationship between sugars and caries. The precise relationship depends on several factors:

- the sugar eaten – while sucrose and glucose are cariogenic, xylitol and sugar alcohols are not;
- the quantity of sugar intake;
- the concentration of sugar in foods eaten;
- the frequency of eating sugar;
- the consistency of the food, foods that are sucked being more cariogenic than those which are chewed;
- the time of eating – salivary secretion and its protective effect are low between meals and when sleeping, so that extrinsic sugar should not be eaten before bedtime or between meals.

Sugary drinks, cakes, biscuits, confectionery and dried fruit are all cariogenic. Although fruit is not cariogenic, fruit juices are. On the other hand, fruit juice drunk quickly is much less cariogenic than if it is sipped slowly, and sweets eaten all at once less than those eaten one by one throughout the day.

Prevention of dental caries

Prevention may be achieved by:

- strengthening the enamel by fluoridization (see page 143);
- good dental hygiene;
- controlling the sugars intake.

Fluoride strengthens the enamel against decay and reduces caries dramatically. It is added to the public water supply in some areas. Some people argue against such addition, on the ground that it removes individual choice.

Children are most at risk of dental caries and therefore sugary foods (apart from fresh fruit and vegetables) should be eaten only as part of meals or three times a day, with three hours or so between, so giving time for repair. Between-meal snacks should be free of *added* sugar. Fruit or vegetables (carrot, celery, pepper sticks) or cheese or savoury snacks are suitable. Drinks between meals should also be sugar-free, such as water, milk, Marmite, or the diet version of soft drinks. This is easier said than done since sweets are readily available at swimming, gym tots and supermarkets. An alternative course is to make some meals sugar-free, by omitting a sweet course and substituting it with soup or by serving bread with the main course.

Children need not be denied the pleasure of sweets but they should not be given as rewards or pacifiers; they should be eaten either straight after a meal or in a glorious weekly splurge. Infants should not be given sugar-sweetened drinks in bottles or reservoir feeders. The slow drip of a sugary solution results in almost continuous enamel demineralization. A similar intake of acid fruit drinks will do the same, because of their acidity (Health Education Authority, 1990; Rugg-Gunn, 1993).

The Oral Health Strategy, setting out objectives for health authorities in England was published in 1994 (Department of Health, 1994a) and there are similar strategies for Scotland and Wales.

SUGARS, ENERGY INTAKE AND OBESITY

Because sugary foods are, for most people, highly palatable, it is possible for them to be eaten in amounts which increase total energy intake above requirement, so causing obesity. This is the obverse of the argument that an NSP-rich diet may prevent obesity. Both hypotheses are difficult to prove.

There is no evidence from psychological studies that obese people have a stronger preference for sugars than normal weight persons. The COMA committee conclude that 'dietary sugars may contribute to the general excess food energy consumption responsible for the development of obesity' but that 'Omission of sugars ... is not usually sufficient as a weight-reducing regimen' (Department of Health, 1989). But of course it may be for someone who eats a lot of sweets and biscuits.

THE EFFECT OF HIGH SUGARS INTAKE ON THE NUTRIENT CONTENT OF THE DIET

Refined sucrose, the main sugar added to food, is a pure food in the sense that it contains no other nutrients, such as minerals and vitamins. Sometimes described as providing 'empty calories', a large intake might cause a reduction in other, more nutritionally valuable foods and lead to inadequate intakes of some nutrients.

While theoretically this may be so, we do not know much about the diets of people eating different amounts of sugar. In one piece of quantitative work the diets of over 200 men and women were analysed by Nelson (1983), using intakes of zinc, magnesium, iron, calcium, thiamin and vitamin C as indicators of the nutritional quality. In nearly all cases intakes of micronutrients were adequate when compared with the Recommended Daily Amounts (in use at that time). Nelson showed that micronutrient density (the quantity of a nutrient per unit of food energy) did not vary much with energy consumption and therefore the *total energy eaten had the greatest effect on total micronutrient intake*. He also found, not surprisingly, that micronutrient density was lowest where added sugars gave the highest proportion of energy.

So, the results showed that the most important determinant of total nutrient intake was total food intake, though mean micronutrient intake was lowest for women with low energy intakes who also ate a lot of sugar.

The COMA report also notes that *sugars provide an acceptable way of contributing to the very high energy needs of some individuals*, which will include not only the very active but also those recovering from illness or malnutrition. For this group there are proprietary drinks and supplements based on glucose or glucose polymers which are useful (Caloreen, Hycal, Maxijul and others) (Thomas, 1994).

It is important that a low sugar diet does not become a high fat one. Nelson (1983) showed that people eating the least sugar had a correspondingly high fat intake.

CARDIOVASCULAR DISEASE

There have been claims that dietary sucrose is causally related to coronary heart disease, but the correlations between sugar intake and disease incidence are weak and clinical and experimental work has not supported this hypothesis. This conclusion has been reached by a number of expert committees (Department of Health, 1989, 1991).

DIABETES MELLITUS

High sugars consumption does not appear to be a dominant factor in *causation* of either insulin-dependent diabetes mellitus or non-insulin-dependent diabetes mellitus (which usually occurs in middle-age or later and is associated with obesity) (Department of Health, 1989).

In the dietetic management of diabetes, it is now recommended that carbohydrate be a major source of food energy (50–55%) so that fat may be reduced to 35% or less of total energy. Unrefined cereals and vegetables are recommended as sources of carbohydrate (Department of Health, 1989, 1991) but sucrose, up to 50 g daily, often improves the palatability of meals and appears to have no detrimental effect on blood sugar control (Peterson *et al.*, 1986).

EFFECT OF SUGARS INTAKE ON MOOD

It has been claimed that a high sugars intake may result in disturbances of mood and behaviour in susceptible adults and children. A possible mechanism for this would be a rebound fall in blood sugar following the surge of insulin secreted in response to a rapid flow of mono-saccharides into the blood. As an investigative area this is fraught with difficulties, the principal one being to quantify hyperactivity in children and mood changes in adults. There is a good deal of anecdotal evidence but little from well-controlled studies, so that the conclusion of the COMA panel and most other experts is that these claims cannot, at the moment, be considered valid (Rapp, 1978; Schauss, 1980).

If the behaviour of children is thought to be affected by high sugars intake, then it is sensible to reduce it unobtrusively. The energy requirement must be made up by other foods, preferably starchy ones. A banana would be a sensible substitute for a bag of sweets.

To sum up, there is no evidence of any deleterious effects from intrinsic sugar (fruits and vegetables) or from lactose from milk and its products. It is usually unwise to eat large quantities of added (non-milk extrinsic) sugar because of its effect on dental health and overall dietary quality. This message is most important for the *young*, who are susceptible to dental caries, and for *small-eaters* whose intake of all nutrients is low. For some people, with high energy requirements, sugar is a useful food. In dietary surveys, a high sugars intake is usually found with a low fat intake.

People often have incorrect views about sugar in foods. Dried fruits – cariogenic because of their stickiness and high sugar content – are often seen as healthy whereas the small amount of sugar in useful foods like baked beans and sweet corn is deemed harmful. Similarly there is little difference between sugar-coated breakfast cereals and the non-sugar version if eaten with added sugar.

SUGARS IN FOODS

Sucrose

This is 'sugar' in ordinary conversation. Granulated and caster sugar are pure sucrose and it is the main sweetener in many foods, like cakes, biscuits, sugar-coated breakfast cereals, ice-cream, preserves, confectionery, drinking chocolate powder, chocolate, condensed milk, many puddings and ripe bananas. Small amounts are added to many foods, such as sauces, yoghurts, processed vegetables and soups, and small quantities occur naturally in cereals, grains and flours, fruit and vegetables.

Glucose

Glucose is present in honey, sugar confectionery, some alcoholic drinks, breakfast cereals, some cakes and biscuits, soft drinks (except low-calorie versions), fruit and fruit juices, sauces, soups, ice-cream, sweetened yoghurts and vegetables. It is about half as sweet as sucrose but has no special nutritional properties.

Fructose

This is mainly present in fruit and fruit products, and in honey. It is intensely sweet.

Lactose

Lactose, the least sweet-tasting sugar, is mainly present in milk and milk products. Where milk, cream, milk powder and whey are added to food products, lactose will be present. Breast-fed infants receive about 40% of their energy intake from lactose.

Maltose

Small amounts are present in some biscuits and breakfast cereals and it is present in foods made with glucose syrups (sugar confectionery and some infant formulas).

Less common sugars which may be found in foods are arabinose and xylose, which may be in white wine and galactose which is in fermented milk products. Mannose is present in fruit.

Glucose syrup

Glucose syrup is a mixture of glucose, maltose and some longer chain carbohydrates.

SUGARLESS SWEETENERS

These are non-sugars which have a sweet taste. There are two types: *bulk sweeteners* which can replace sugars weight for weight; and *intense sweeteners* which are used in very small amounts. Thousands are known but only 20 are permitted to be used in food.

Intense sweeteners

Saccharine

About 300 times sweeter than sucrose, widely used, not metabolized but excreted mainly in the urine.

Cyclamates

Now used in food again after a ban for suspected safety reasons.

Aspartame (Nutrasweet, Canderel)

A good flavour but unstable to heat therefore cannot be used in cooking. *Not recommended in phenylketonuria.*

Acelfame K and thaumatinare

These are also used in the UK.

All the intense sweeteners are non-cariogenic and calorie-free.

Bulk sweeteners

Erythritol, xylitol, sorbitol, mannitol, palatinose, maltitol, palatinit, lycasin, fructo-oligosaccharides are bulk sweeteners.

These sweeteners are non-cariogenic. They are more slowly absorbed from the gut than common dietary sugars and therefore may have a laxative effect. Experimentally, 60 g/day of sorbitol or 40 g/day of maltitol caused watery diarrhoea within 1 hour. Their energy value is very difficult to determine though the Dutch Nutrition Council (1987) has proposed values. Sorbitol is used in soft drinks, jams and confectionery for diabetics.

Starches   Starches are polysaccharides (see Box 3.4). *Resistant starch* is a form of starch which is partially resistant to digestion by amylase (see below).

Dextrins are breakdown products of starch in which the glucose chains have been broken down to smaller units. They are soluble in water and have no sweet taste.

BOX 3.4

SOME MORE CHEMISTRY

The chemical name for starch is alpha-glucan polysaccharide.

It consists of large molecules which are polymers of glucose. There are two main types of starch polymer: amylose and amylopectin. Their relative proportion affects the properties of food starches but is not important nutritionally.

METABOLISM OF STARCH

Digestion

Starches exist in food in many different forms which are digested at different rates. The enzyme alpha-amylase digests starch to maltose. It is present in saliva and in pancreatic juice. Freshly cooked starchy food is rapidly digested in the small intestine.

Resistant starch, present in raw potato and banana, and in most cooked starchy foods after cooling, is only partly digested in the small

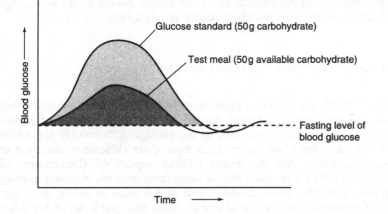

Glucose standard (50 g carbohydrate)

Test meal (50 g available carbohydrate)

Fasting level of blood glucose

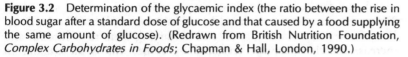

Figure 3.2   Determination of the glycaemic index (the ratio between the rise in blood sugar after a standard dose of glucose and that caused by a food supplying the same amount of glucose). (Redrawn from British Nutrition Foundation, *Complex Carbohydrates in Foods*; Chapman & Hall, London, 1990.)

intestine and some passes into the large intestine where it is fermented by bacteria, so it behaves like non-starch polysaccharides. It causes bulking of the stools – this is an important factor in diets which depend heavily on rice and pasta.

The main difference between eating starch and sugar, apart from the additional nutrients which starchy foods may add to the diet, is in the rate of absorption of glucose.

Glycaemic index

This is the ratio between the rise in blood sugar occurring after a standard dose (50 g) of glucose and that caused by a food or meal also supplying 50 g carbohydrate (Figure 3.2).

While glucose has a glycaemic index of 100, bread scores 70–80, and beans 40–50. This has some practical application to the diet of diabetics, for whom foods with a low glycaemic index are good. Unfortunately, few studies have been done on meals as opposed to single foods (Trowell *et al.*, 1985; British Nutrition Foundation, 1991; Thomas, 1994).

INTAKE OF STARCHES

Healthy diets may have very little, as in the traditional Eskimo diet, or a great deal, up to 80% of energy in parts of the developing world.

There is comparatively little information on starch intake in the UK. The Dietary and Nutritional Survey of British Adults found an average of 24% energy from starch (Gregory *et al.*, 1990).

RECOMMENDATIONS FOR CONSUMPTION OF STARCHES

The COMA report 41 (Department of Health, 1991) suggests that starches and 'natural' sugars should be the main sources of carbohydrate food energy, contributing on average 37% energy for adults and children over two years. Such figures are difficult to interpret in practical terms, but the recent COMA report 46 (Department of Health, 1994b) attempted this in suggesting that the *national average intake* of starchy foods should consist of 4.5 slices of bread, three egg-sized potatoes, one serving of rice or pasta and one bowl of breakfast cereal per day. Obviously some people will eat more and some less. These amounts were calculated by taking the results of the National Food Survey as a starting point and modifying them to reduce fat and increase starch. Although criticized by some, this *is* an attempt to translate nutritional advice into foods. As is shown on page 321, bread and potatoes are excellent foods for all ages.

It is difficult to get an estimate of the amount of starch in foods from food tables and food labels because all carbohydrates are often grouped to give a single total, their equivalent as monosaccharides.

Non-starch polysaccharides (NSP, dietary fibre) Interest in dietary fibre, formerly called 'roughage' and now redefined as non-starch polysaccharides (NSP), has increased enormously over the past 20 years.

DEFINITION

The term non-starch polysaccharides (Table 3.2), which is now proposed instead of dietary fibre, is defined by Cummings and Englyst (1981) as 'comprised of the cellulose, hemicellulose and pectic substances in plant foods' (British Nutrition Foundation, 1990). Dietary fibre is still, however, in common use and is the term used on food labels. It includes all the substances included in NSP, as well as some others, such as lignin.

So, both terms – dietary fibre and NSP – refer to groups of substances. NSP is more useful scientifically since it is confined to the

Table 3.2 Non-starch polysaccharides

Cellulose	Non-cellulosic polysaccharides
Leafy vegetables, peas, beans, rhubarb – insoluble	Pectins (fruit, vegetables – soluble)
	Glucans (oats, barley, rye – soluble)
	Arabino-galactans, arabino-oxylans
	(wheat, rye, barley – partly soluble)
	Gums (additives – soluble)
	Fungal: (mushrooms – insoluble)

Modified from COMA 41 (Department of Health, 1991). Crown copyright is reproduced with the permission of the Controller of HMSO.

specified group of substances given above which can be measured accurately by the Englyst method of analysis.

There are other methods of estimation which have been in use; they measured different groups of substances and so gave varying values. The figures given on food labels should be those from the Englyst method or other methods which give similar results.

The situation at the moment is that the term dietary fibre is in *general* use and most of the figures given are for fibre. NSP is be used in academic work and increasingly elsewhere. *Figures for fibre content of foods are about one-third higher than for NSP.* This is why, in this chapter, when referring to research findings, both terms, NSP and dietary fibre, may be used, according to the method of analysis.

RELATIONSHIP BETWEEN DIETARY NSP AND HEALTH

The intense interest in NSP arose largely from the observations of Burkitt and Cleave who, working in rural Africa, were struck by the rarity of a number of diseases common in developed countries. These different disease patterns must be caused by environmental factors, since migration from a rural to an urban area is followed by a changed disease incidence. Diet is one of the environmental factors and within diet, the NSP intakes show great variation, being much higher in most diets in the developing world than in industrialized countries (Table 3.3).

NSP has profound effects on the gut. The issue which must be considered is whether it is *NSP per se* which is desirable in the diet or whether it is the selection of NSP-rich foods (which additionally usually have low energy density, low fat content and are often good sources of micronutrients) which is beneficial. The evidence, as well as common sense, points to the latter. The pioneers in this field did not advocate that we *add* NSP to our food but that we *stop removing it by refining.*

Table 3.3 Average intakes of dietary fibre

Country	Native	Intake (g/day)
Africa	Masai, male	0
	Masai, female	25
	Kikuyu	130
	Buganda	150
UK		20

NSP has a proven laxative effect; it has also been proposed that a diet high in NSP protects against, among others, obesity, hiatus hernia, varicose veins and CHD (Trowell *et al.*, 1985).

Appetite, satiety and obesity

The proposed hypothesis is that NSP-rich foods produce a higher degree of satiety than refined foods and so help to prevent obesity by reducing energy intake. This is very difficult to *prove*. NSP-rich foods are cereals, beans, fruits and vegetables and they are low in fat. Some are eaten raw when they are bulky and need chewing. So, a diet with a preponderance of such foods would be bulkier, chewier and less energy-dense than one rich in refined and animal foods. It certainly takes longer to eat the equivalent of 200 kcal (8.40 kJ) as raw apples than as Mars bars. In an experiment in which students were given equi-caloric portions of either raw apple, apple purée or apple juice it was found that the effect of physically macerating (as in purée) or removing (as in apple juice) NSP was to reduce satiety and increase blood glucose and insulin levels after eating (British Nutrition Foundation, 1990).

Although similar unequivocal results for *whole diets* are lacking, it is true that a diet with plenty of NSP-rich foods will be more satisfying than a refined diet, as well as being less energy-dense, and thus helpful in controlling energy intake. (See how full you feel after a lentil lasagne compared with a meat-based one!)

The converse is also true; some diets may be too bulky for the small stomachs of children or for the elderly.

NSP does provide some energy, from the products of its bacterial breakdown in the large intestine. The value is about 2 kcal (8.4 kJ)/g.

The effects of NSP on the large intestine

NSP have a laxative effect, increasing stool weight and decreasing transit time (the time from eating of food to the excretion of its residue). The effects of different types of NSP on stool weight vary, those from cereal foods having a greater effect than those from fruit and vegetables. The pectins from fruit and vegetables are digested by the bacteria of the large bowel and much of the increase in stool weight is due to the evacuation of these bacteria. However, in healthy people an increase in any NSP leads to some increase in stool weight.

With NSP-free diets, stool weights fall very low (30–60 g/day) and constipation is common. Constipation can be described as an infrequent bowel habit (less than three times per week), with a long transit time of five days or more and a low stool weight (less than 50 g). It is common in the UK, affecting around 10% of adults and 20% of the elderly (British Nutrition Foundation, 1990). It can be relieved by an increase in dietary NSP although *there is a wide individual variation in response.*

It has been found that in 16 normal subjects eating *identical* diets, stool weight varied from 65 to 194 g per day and transit time from 31 to 117 hours. The laxative effect of increased fibre was greatest in those subjects which had the fastest transit time initially. This, and other experiments, show that NSP is not the only determinant of transit time and stool weight. Hormone secretion and stress are among other factors which affect bowel habit.

It has been claimed that a high NSP intake protects against **diverticular disease** (where pouches develop in the wall of the large bowel), appendicitis and haemorrhoids, because of the laxative effect of NSP and the consequent reduction in intra-abdominal and gut pressures during defaecation. These claims are unproven, although they are supported by epidemiological studies.

NSP has also been cited as protective against large bowel cancer, through the dilution of carcinogens in the larger stool and other factors. This is supported by epidemiological studies which show stool weights below 150 g per day are associated with increased risks of bowel cancer and diverticular disease.

It is on the basis of stool weight therefore that the DRVs for NSP have been set. At 18 g per day, it is higher than most people eat, but a *sudden* large increase in NSP intake is unwise; it may cause discomfort and flatulence, as well as reduced absorption of some minerals.

Insulin secretion

The sugars and starch in NSP-rich foods are digested and absorbed more slowly than from refined foods. This reduces the peak rise in blood sugar and therefore the necessary insulin response.

There are several properties of carbohydrate foods which influence the rise in blood sugar after eating; these include texture and particle size, intact or disrupted cell walls, the type of starch, the presence of fat and the type of NSP present.

For single meals with very large amounts of soluble NSP there is clear evidence of reduced insulin response; the viscosity of soluble NSP slows absorption. Trials of high-NSP diets with diabetic subjects, who would benefit from reduced insulin requirement, are difficult to design and to interpret, but a high intake of complex polysaccharides is currently advised.

The conclusion must be that diets rich in whole cereals, fruit and vegetables will probably elicit smaller rises in blood sugar and insulin secretion than refined diets.

Plasma lipids and cardiovascular disease

It has also been suggested that dietary NSP may modify plasma lipids to reduce plasma cholesterol and hence the risk of cardiovascular disease. Again it is unproven, in no small part because of the difficulty of designing a well-controlled trial.

Effect of dietary NSP on the absorption of minerals

The possibility of NSP binding mineral elements such as calcium, iron, copper and zinc and thus reducing their absorption from the gut has been investigated and this mineral-binding effect has been demon- strated *in vitro* (that is, in test-tube experiments).

Studies on humans have not shown a significant reduction in mineral absorption except where phytate (high in unrefined and unleavened cereals) and oxalate (in plant foods, strawberries) intakes are also high. It may be seen in people eating macrobiotic diets where 50% of energy comes from brown rice; in this group there is a high incidence of rickets and anaemia.

Other populations who habitually eat high-NSP diets, such as vegetarians, do not show deficiencies of these minerals. Recent work suggests that the bacterial breakdown of NSP in the gut reduces the binding effect. Once again, the evidence is difficult to interpret because of the many variables. However, in dietary change caution should be exercised particularly for the elderly and growing children.

DIETARY REFERENCE VALUES

The panel on DRVs felt that there was a basis for values for non-starch polysaccharides in the UK diet (Department of Health, 1991). Because the best evidence for the function of NSP relates to bowel habit, this was used as the basis for the recommendation for an average adult intake of *18 g per day NSP from a variety of foods whose constituents contain it as a naturally integrated component.* The present average intake is 13 g per day. An increase to 18 g should reduce the number of people with stool weights of less than 100 g per day and thus the incidence of constipation and probably of diverticulosis and large bowel cancers. (*Note*: if these figures seem low, remember that they are for NSP and not dietary fibre.)

The recommendation is not applicable to **children**: too fibrous a diet may be too bulky for their small stomachs. The 'muesli belt syndrome', where children are given diets low in fat and sugar and high in NSP-rich foods, may result in inadequate energy consumption. Children's intake of NSP should be in line with their energy intake.

NSP CONTENT OF SOME COMMON FOODS

Foods very rich in NSP	Foods with useful amounts of NSP	Foods with no NSP
All-Bran	Peas	Sugar
Shredded Wheat	Baked beans	Milk
Weetabix	Dahl	Butter
	Cabbage	Other fats
	Cauliflower	
	Potatoes	
	Carrots	
	Apple	
	Banana	
	Dried fruit	
	Bread, white	
	Bread, wholemeal	
	Peanuts	

Modified from Davies, J. and Dickerson, J. (1991).

Examples of two dietary levels of NSP

Level A
Breakfast: wholemeal toast, All-Bran
Mid-morning: apple
Midday: quiche, salad
Evening: steak, jacket potato, peas, cauliflower, banana

Level B
Breakfast: white toast, Rice Krispies
Mid-morning: Penguin chocolate biscuit
Midday: ham sandwich, crisps
Evening: steak, mashed potato, ice-cream.

Meal	Food A	Dietary fibre content (g)	Food B	Dietary fibre content (g)
Breakfast	Wholemeal toast – two slices	5.2	White toast – two slices	2.9
	All-Bran (45 g)	13.5	Rice-Krispies (35 g)	0.4
Mid-morning	Apple (120 g, one)	1.7	Penguin chocolate biscuit – one	0.7
Midday	Quiche, cheese (90 g, one slice)	0.6	Ham sandwich (two slices bread)	2.9
	Lettuce (30 g)	0.4		
	Tomato (75 g, one)	10	Crisps, one packet	3.1
	Cucumber (30 g)	0.1		
Evening meal	Steak, beef (155 g)	0	Steak, beef (155 g)	0
	Potato, jacket (140 g, one)	3.2	Potato, mashed (170 g)	1.4
	Peas, frozen, boiled (75 g)	8.1	Ice-cream (75 g)	0
	Cauliflower (100 g)	1.6		
	Banana (135 g, one)	2.4		
Totals	Dietary fibre	37.8	Dietary fibre	11.4
DRV (adults)	Dietary fibre	30	Dietary fibre	30

Note: the analysis for dietary fibre is given: this is about 30% higher than the values for NSP.

Key points

1. There are three main groups of carbohydrates, namely sugars, starches and non-starch polysaccharides (NSP, formerly called dietary fibre).

2. **Sugars** can be classified according to their chemical make-up and according to their distribution in foods. In foods, intrinsic sugars are those within the cells as in fruit and vegetables and extrinsic sugars are milk sugar and added sugar. It is the added sugar (also called non-milk extrinsic sugar, NMES) which is the focus of dietary concern.

3. Sugars are digested to monosaccharides which enter the blood and are either used by the tissues for energy or converted to fat. The level of blood glucose is homeostatically controlled.

4. Main dietary sources of added sugars are soft drinks, table sugar, confectionery and cakes, biscuits and puddings.

5. There is no evidence that intrinsic sugars or lactose have adverse effects on health. Added sugars cause dental caries (decay) and therefore it is suggested that their intake be reduced.

6. The amount, frequency and texture of sucrose-containing foods affect the incidence of dental caries. Added sugars should be eaten

at mealtimes only and not in between, to allow time for repair of dental enamel.

7. There is no conclusive proof that added sugars are a cause of obesity, cardiovascular disease, diabetes mellitus, hyperactivity in children or mood swings in adults.

8. Although a high intake of sugars reduces the intake of some micronutrients compared with a lower intake, the main determinant of micronutrient intake appears to be total energy intake. A high sugars intake has a serious effect in reducing micronutrient intake, however, in those whose total energy intake is low.

9. **Starches** are polymers of glucose units. Food starches vary in composition.

10. Starch is digested by amylase to maltose, but some resistant starches (for example cooled, cooked starchy foods, banana) are digested only very slowly and some enter the large intestine where they are fermented (digested) by bacteria, thus acting like NSP.

11. COMA Report 46 (Department of Health, 1994b) makes quantitative suggestions for increasing the national average intake of starchy foods, in terms of bread, potatoes, pasta and other cereals.

12. **Non-starch polysaccharides** (NSP), the new term for fibre, form a group of substances from plants, including insoluble cellulose and soluble pectins and glucans.

13. NSP-rich foods have a laxative effect, increasing stool bulk and decreasing transit time, though with considerable individual variation. There is also evidence of a protective effect against large bowel cancer.

14. NSP-rich foods have a smaller glycaemic effect (rise in blood sugar) than sugary foods and so are useful in diabetic diets.

15. There is no *proof* of protection against cardiovascular disease nor obesity although this may be due to the difficulty of such investigations.

16. The absorption of some minerals (iron, zinc, calcium) may be reduced by NSP. There is strong evidence for mineral-binding by NSP *in vitro* but much less evidence of mineral deficiencies in groups eating a diet high in NSP.

17. COMA Report 41 (Department of Health, 1991) recommends an increase in average NSP intake to 18 g per day, based on its effects on the large bowel.

4 Proteins

The aim of this chapter is to outline the chemical composition of proteins and their physiological functions and metabolism. The quality of food proteins is discussed, along with the DRVs, average dietary intake in the UK, and food sources.

The molecules of proteins are large and are made up of **amino acids** which are linked together. It is the amino acids which are absorbed by the body which are important nutritionally.

Metabolism and functions of protein

DIGESTION OF PROTEIN

Food proteins are digested into single amino acids in the gut by the enzymes pepsin (from the stomach), trypsin and others (from the pancreas) and finally by enzymes in the brush border of the enterocytes (the cells lining the small intestine). The amino acids pass first to the liver and then, in the blood, to the cells for protein synthesis.

The **digestibility** of proteins is the percentage of dietary protein which is absorbed. Proteins from eggs, meat and other animal sources have a higher digestibility than vegetable proteins, with a range of values from 78% for a diet of rice and beans, to 96% for a typical meat-based diet.

PROTEIN SYNTHESIS

It is amino acids rather than proteins that are essential to the body and *all body proteins are made from them*. Humans, unlike plants, cannot make amino acids from simpler substances such as nitrates and so they must be supplied in the diet.

To synthesize a particular protein a cell requires the correct array of amino acids. The body is able to convert some amino acids to others (glycine into alanine for example) and such amino acids are called *non-essential* (Box 4.1).

Eight others cannot be produced in this way and *must be supplied by the diet*. These are called **indispensable** and **essential** amino acids.

BOX 4.1

Non-essential amino acids are alanine, arginine, aspartic acid, cysteine, glutamic acid, glycine, proline, serine, tyrosine

BOX 4.2

Indispensable (essential) amino acids are isoleucine, leucine, lysine, methionine, phenylalanine, threonine, tryptophan and valine

For children an additional two amino acids (histidine and arginine) are indispensable. In fact the dividing line between the two groups is less clear-cut than this, with some amino acids being classified as semi-essential, but this classification is adequate for all practical purposes (Garrow and James, 1993).

PROTEIN TURNOVER

Body proteins are constantly being broken down and renewed. Most of the amino acids from tissue breakdown enter the blood and form part of the **free amino acid pool**. Some of the amino acids are broken down and finally are excreted as urea in urine. These must be replaced by amino acids from food.

The amino acid pool is the source of amino acids for cellular protein synthesis.

The rate of protein turnover is hormonally controlled. Insulin and growth hormone stimulate synthesis and glucagon, cortisol and cytokines (recently identified peptides) have the reverse effect.

Not surprisingly the rate of synthesis varies at the different stages of life, being on average 17.4 g/kg body weight per day for premature new-borns, 6.9 g/kg per day for infants, 3.0 g/kg per day for young adults and falling to 1.9 g/kg per day for the elderly.

Injury, infection, burns and cancer result in increased breakdown and a loss of body protein. This may be small after minor surgery, but great enough to be life-threatening after severe burns, when the increase in protein requirement is too great to be treated by diet and intravenous feeding must be used (Thomas, 1994).

NITROGEN BALANCE

If no protein is present in the diet then, as tissues are broken down and not replaced, nitrogen (and protein) is lost from the body. This condition, where body tissue is lost, is called a *negative nitrogen balance*. A deficiency of dietary protein will cause growth or repair to cease.

Some or all of dietary protein is retained and used for the synthesis of new tissue; any surplus amino acids are deaminated (that is, the amino group removed) and used as an energy source or stored as fat. If the loss of nitrogen from tissue breakdown is balanced by retention of dietary nitrogen there is **nitrogen balance**.

In growth or wound repair, providing the diet is adequate in protein and energy, there is a *positive nitrogen balance* as new additional tissue is formed and there is a net gain of protein.

PROTEIN AS AN ENERGY SOURCE

A secondary function for protein is as a source of energy. Its calorific value is the same as carbohydrates, 4 kcal or 17 kJ/g, and the nitrogen part of the molecule is excreted as urea.

If there is a dietary deficit of energy, protein will be used *first* as an energy source rather than for repair and growth, which will diminish or cease. Adding carbohydrate to such a diet will 'spare' the protein for protein synthesis and the term, the protein-sparing action of carbohydrate, is sometimes used. This is one of the reasons why, when food is in short supply, the first priority is to get adequate energy supplies.

Effects of protein deficiency

A deficiency of protein may occur in two ways: through a *low intake of protein* or through a *low energy intake*. In the latter case, the dietary protein, although present in amounts which are ordinarily adequate, is used for energy as explained above.

Some degree of **adaptation** to reduced intakes does occur. With very severe protein deficiency, the concentration of the plasma proteins falls and this causes generalized oedema (sometimes called hunger oedema).

Prolonged deficiency of protein and energy in children causes protein-energy malnutrition, in the forms of marasmus or kwashiorkor, which occur in some developing countries.

PROTEIN RESTRICTION

Special low-protein diets are sometimes necessary, principally in liver or kidney disease, and these require supervision by dieticians (Thomas, 1994).

There has been some concern about the health risks of an excessive intake of protein because it may cause demineralization of the bone.

Effects of excessive intake of protein

It has also been noted that populations eating vegetarian diets, with *lower* average protein intakes than omnivores, have *lower* average blood pressures.

These facts, along with the effect of dietary protein of increasing glomerular filtration rate in the kidney, caused COMA report 41 (Department of Health, 1991) to conclude that 'it was prudent for adults to avoid protein intakes of more than twice the RNI'. Most people would be unlikely to eat such amounts, with the exception of those with very high energy intakes or athletes taking protein supplements.

COMMERCIAL SUPPLEMENTS

Individual amino acids, such as tryptophan, and mixtures of amino acids are available commercially. Little is known about their possible toxic effects.There is normally no need for such supplements.

PROTEIN SUPPLEMENT FOR SPECIAL CASES

This is required in some illnesses and is easily achieved by giving extra protein foods like eggs, meat and so on, or by adding skimmed milk powder to suitable foods.

Food proteins are classified nutritionally according to the number and proportion of essential amino acids they contain. The **biological value** of a protein refers to its ability, *when it is the sole dietary source of protein*, to support protein synthesis and therefore body maintenance and growth (Table 4.1). On this scale, egg and the proteins of breast milk have the highest value of 1.0. All animal proteins except gelatin are

Food protein quality

Table 4.1 The biological value of some food proteins

Food	Biological value
Egg or human milk	1.0
Skimmed milk	0.85
RHM myco-protein	0.84
Meat, fish protein	0.75
Wheat protein	0.50
Peanut	0.40
Gelatin	0.00

(Reproduced with permission from Robinson, Food Biochemistry and Nutritional Value, published by Addison Wesley Longman, 1987.)

complete (that is, contain all the essential amino acids) and so have *high* biological value. Occasionally the old term first-class protein is used for them. Most vegetable proteins, except soya, are *incomplete*, having a *lower* biological value and used to be called second-class.

Because proteins are digested to amino acids, which are then absorbed, what matters is the *mixture of amino acids* which come from the foods which are eaten. So, if a protein of poor biological value, lacking amino acid X but having Y, is eaten with another low value protein, rich in X but not Y, the two together will give a very good mix of amino acids, equal to a high biological value protein. This is known as the **complementation** of proteins. Dietetically this is very important. Most traditional diets show a very good mix of proteins, in which the essential acids missing from one food are supplied by another. Examples are bread and milk, bread and cheese, beans on toast, rice and lentils, spaghetti and cheese.

So, does the quality of dietary proteins matter? It matters very much in the milk-fed infant, where there is rapid growth and only one food given, and it matters in diets which are very low in protein-containing foods, as in parts of the developing world: however, it matters hardly at all for people in industrialized countries where the main sources of protein are meat, milk, bread and other cereals and where most meals contain a mixture of different proteins (from potato, meat or cheese, beans, milk and bread, say). Wheat protein with a biological value of 50 can support life as the only protein source, but twice as much would have to be eaten compared with egg protein. The surplus amino acids would be used for energy and their nitrogen excreted as urea in urine.

In the infant the consumption of a lower biological value protein than breast milk (as in most infant formulas) means there is a higher protein intake, a greater excretion of urea from surplus amino acids and more chance of a sore bottom, when this urea is converted to ammonia on the nappy.

Intake in the UK   Surveys of British adults (Gregory *et al.*, 1990) show high average intakes of protein of 84 g per day for men and 64 g per day for women. There is no evidence of protein deficiency due to dietary causes, though it may occur in chronic alcoholics eating grossly inadequate diets. It might also arise in patients with kidney disease or those with severe injuries.

DRVs for protein   These estimated requirements (Table 4.2) (WHO, 1985; Department of Health, 1991) are based on the recommendations in the Report of the

Table 4.2 Dietary Reference Values for protein. (From COMA 41; Department of Health, 1991). Crown copyright is reproduced with the permission of the Controller of HMSO.

Age	Weight (kg)	Estimated Average Requirement (g/day)	Reference Nutrient Intake (g/day)
Children			
0–3 months	5.9	–	12.5
4–6 months	7.7	10.6	12.7
7–9 months	8.8	11.0	13.7
10–12 months	9.7	11.2	14.9
1–3 years	12.5	11.7	14.5
4–6 years	17.8	14.8	19.7
7–10 years	28.3	22.8	28.3
Males			
11–14 years	43.0	33.8	42.1
15–18 years	64.5	46.1	55.2
19–50 years	74.0	44.4	55.5
50+ years	71.0	42.6	53.3
Females			
11–14 years	43.8	33.1	41.2
15–18 years	55.5	37.1	45.4
19–50 years	60.0	36.0	45.0
50+ years	62.0	37.2	46.5
Pregnancy			+6
Lactation			
0–6 months			+11
6+ months	+8		

FAO/WHO/UNU expert consultation. They are estimates of the amounts of high-quality egg or milk protein required for maintenance and growth (WHO, 1985). Not all dietary proteins are of such high quality, of course, but for adults eating a typical mixed diet in industrialized countries, including vegetarians, there is no need for concern about the amino acid composition. Vegan children, however, may be at risk of deficiency. There is still need for more research into amino acid requirements of children and adults.

Food sources of protein

Meat, fish, eggs, cheese, milk and soya products are all good sources of high-quality protein. Beans and wheat products are good sources of vegetable proteins. Meat is one of the more expensive foods, but it is possible to get enough protein from a small amount of meat (or none) with a mixture of bread, milk and pulses. Fruit and vegetables, other than pulses, contain very little protein.

PROTEIN CONTENT OF FOODS PER AVERAGE PORTION SIZE

Food	Amount (weight in g)	Protein content (g)
Bread, white and wholemeal	Two slices of large, medium sliced loaf	6.3–6.4
Chapattis	One (70)	5.1–5.7
Naan	One (170)	15.1
Cornflakes	25	2.0
Cheddar cheese	40	10.2
Cottage cheese	45	6.2
Egg	One, size 2	7.5
Cod, grilled	Two steaks (130)	27.0
Pilchards in tomato sauce (canned)	105	19.7
Beef, pork, lean	85	17.5–22.5
Sausages, beef, grilled	Two (90)	11.7
Ham	Two slices (55)	10.1
Milk, whole, semi–skimmed, skimmed	⅓ pint (190 ml)	6.2–6.4
Peanuts	30	7.3
Baked beans	200	10.2
Dahl, lentil	155	7.6

From Davies, J. and Dickerson, J. (1991).

Table 4.4 Foods giving the Reference Nutrient Intake (RNI) for males, aged 15–18 years (55.2 g/day)

Food	Amount	Protein content (g)
Bread	Six slices	18.9
Egg	One, size 2	7.5
Baked beans	200 g	10.2
Milk	½ pt (280 ml)	9.0
Sausages	Two	11.7
Total		57.3

As you can see, it is not difficult to achieve this level and in general, in the UK the supply of dietary protein is not a problem.

Key points   1. Food proteins supply the body with amino acids which are essential for the synthesis of protein and therefore for growth and maintenance of the body structure, since protein is a vital component of every cell. Hormones and enzymes are also usually proteins.

2. Amino acids are classified, nutritionally, as indispensable (essential) or non-essential. Protein quality is calculated on the basis of the amino acid profile of the particular protein.
3. The amount of protein in the average UK diet is normally more than sufficient although there may be a minority (alcoholics, patients after surgery, burns) who may be deficient.
4. Excessive amounts (of the order of twice the RNI) are undesirable.

5 Fats

This chapter looks at the average fat intake in the UK and the implications for health, giving the necessary chemistry and metabolism of fat. Current recommendations for fat consumption and their interpretation in terms of foods are given.

Fats, oils and lipids

Fats and oils are similar chemically, both belonging to the chemical group **triglycerides** (Box 5.1). The term **lipids** includes fats and oils but covers a wider group of substances which are fatty in nature (for example, they do not dissolve in or mix with water). Cholesterol is a lipid although it is not a fat.

Current intake of fats

Fat provides just under 40% of energy in the average UK diet. Of that 40%, most comes from meat and meat products (25% of the total), cereal products (which include cakes and biscuits, 20%), fat spreads (15%), and milk and milk products (15%) (Gregory et al., 1990). The current dietary goal for industrial countries is that the total amount of dietary fat should be reduced and the relative amounts of different types of fats altered.

Functions of fats and lipids in the body

- Fat is a major component of cell and intracellular membranes which, typically, are made up of a double layer of phospholipid (molecules of glycerol, two fatty acids and a phosphate group). Cholesterol is also an essential component of such membranes.
- The fats in adipose tissue (Box 5.2), mainly triglycerides, are the main *energy store* of the body.
- Some hormones are lipids.

BOX 5.1

SOME CHEMISTRY

Fats and oils are triglycerides; triacylglycerols is the newer term but triglycerides is used in most medical literature. Triglyceride molecules consist of glycerol with three molecules of fatty acids.

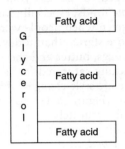

FATS AND OILS

They are both triglycerides but because of the different fatty acids in the molecules, fats are solid at room temperature and oils which are liquid at room temperature.

BOX 5.2

ADIPOSE TISSUE

Adipose tissue is a specialized tissue for the storage of fat. The cells are capable of holding large amounts of fat, from 0.2 μg per cell in a lean person to 0.9 μg per cell in the obese.

Its distribution, under the skin and around some organs, is determined by gender. There is no limit to the amount which can be stored.

Dietary fats and health

The amount of fat eaten by different cultures varies enormously, from 80% of energy intake by some Eskimo groups to 2% energy by the Ho tribe in India (Sinclair, 1953). In neither case does this appear to cause major health problems.

Why then is fat so important in our diet? All research supports the view that it is mainly the *type* of fat which is important, a high intake of saturated fats contributing to the incidence of CHD and some cancers.

Dietary fat is necessary to supply the essential fatty acids and fat-soluble vitamins. It is a compact form of energy and so is particularly useful for people whose energy requirements are very large, such as building-site workers.

Children used to be urged to 'eat up your fat'. Cream, milk and butter were seen as valuable foods, especially for children and pregnant women. This advice was given when people were more active and ate a much plainer diet, with more starch, than today. The extra calories and other nutrients from milk, eggs, butter and cheese were valuable dietary additions. Today fat, especially saturated fat, is thought to be harmful. Why? The reason lies in the life-style changes which occur with affluence. The level of activity falls (Figure 5.1). For example, when energy expenditure was measured accurately in a group of women, it was found that their average daily activity needed only 550 kcals (2301 kJ) more than if *they stayed in bed all day*.

As people become better off, the proportion of fat in the diet rises. An increase in animal foods, which contain saturated fat is typical. This dietary change, which occurred gradually in the UK, year by year, is in fact dramatic when today's dietary fat levels are compared with earlier intakes in the UK or those of the developing countries.

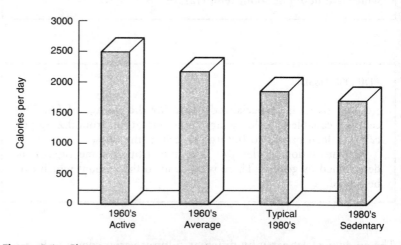

Figure 5.1 Changes in energy expenditure of British women between the 1960s and 1980s, showing the reduction which has occurred. (Redrawn with permission from Pietrzik, K. (ed.), Modern *Lifestyles, Lower Energy Intake and Micronutrient Status*; Springer-Verlag, London, 1991.)

A high fat intake is related to the incidence of obesity, and, a high intake of saturated fat, to coronary heart disease and cancers of the breast and the large intestine.

TYPES OF FAT

Fats vary according to the type of fatty acids they contain. This is important nutritionally because different fatty acids are metabolized differently and influence blood lipoproteins and blood clotting. The following terms are used:

- **Long-chain** and **short-chain** fatty acids vary according to the number of carbon atoms in the molecule (Box 5.3). Long-chain fatty acids have more than short-chain ones.
- **Saturated** or **unsaturated** refers to whether the maximum possible amount of hydrogen is linked to the carbon atoms (when the fatty acid is saturated) or not. Without the maximum complement of hydrogen, there will be one or more *double bonds* between the carbon atoms. One such bond gives a *monounsaturated* fatty acid and more than one, a *polyunsaturated* fatty acid. Fats containing mainly saturated fatty acids are called saturated fats and are usually animal in origin, while unsaturated fats come mostly from plant foods.

The terms *saturates, monounsaturates* and *polyunsaturates* are used in food labelling. *PUFA* is a common shorthand for polyunsaturated fatty acids. The **P/S** ratio is the ratio in the diet of polyunsaturates to saturates and various recommendations have been made for optimal P/S ratios in the diet.

CIS OR TRANS FATTY ACIDS

These terms refer to the arrangement of hydrogen atoms in unsaturated fatty acids (Box 5.4). Nearly all 'natural' fats contain *cis* fatty acids. *Trans* fatty acids, although unsaturated, behave in the body like saturated fatty acids. They are present in some animal fats and dairy products and are formed during processing in margarine. The amounts vary, being between 1–7% in butter fat but up to 35% in some margarines (and their presence is seldom indicated on food labels). For a healthy, lipid-reducing diet, people should choose only those margarines which are labelled high in monounsaturates or polyunsaturates.

Omega-3 or **n-3** and **omega-6** or **n-6** are terms which describe the position of double bonds within the fatty acid molecule. These types of fatty acids are advantageous nutritionally. Linoleic acid, an essential fatty acid, which is present in vegetable oils is an n-6 acid. N-3 fatty

BOX 5.3

SOME MORE CHEMISTRY

(See Garrow and James, 1993.)

Fatty acids consist of carbon, hydrogen and oxygen. The chemical group – COOH is the acidic group and it is attached to a chain of carbon atoms combined with hydrogen as shown below:

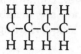

The number of carbon atoms in the chain varies from 12 to 24 for the fatty acids in the diet and they are termed short- or long-chain fatty acids.

A long chain fatty acid

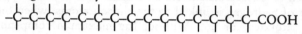

A short-chain fatty acid

—C̶–C̶–C̶–C̶–COOH

TYPES OF FATTY ACID

The type of fatty acids present in fats are important biologically. They also influence the properties of the fats or oils, like melting point.

Saturated fatty acids

Saturated fatty acids (the main type of fatty acid in saturated fats) have carbon atoms which are fully linked with hydrogen, as in the example above. They make fats which are solid and even hard at room temperature and are mainly in animal fats.

Unsaturated fatty acids

Unsaturated fatty acids have less hydrogen and this leaves some 'spare' linkages which form double bonds between carbon atoms. These double bonds are chemically reactive and react with oxygen to form compounds called peroxides. In the body (and in foods) this reaction to harmful peroxides is prevented by various substances including anti-oxidants.

$$\begin{array}{ccc} H & & H \\ | & & | \\ C-C = C-C- \\ | & & | \\ H & & H \end{array}$$

An unsaturated fatty acid (and fats) containing **one** double bond is called **monounsaturated** (present in olive oil in large amounts) and with **two or more, polyunsaturated** (present in corn oil, sunflower oil and others).

PEROXIDATION OF LIPIDS

If the lipids of the cell membranes are oxidized (another way of saying that peroxidation has occurred) their ability to function is impaired. Damage may occur when molecular fragments, called free radicals, are formed. Although free radicals occur naturally to a small extent, they are usually quickly removed and no harm is done. In some states, however, they cause damage. How and when this occurs and what prevents it is discussed on page 90.

acids, present in vegetables and fish oils lower plasma triglycerides and have anti-clotting and anti-inflammatory properties.

CHOLESTEROL

Cholesterol (Figure 5.2) is quite different chemically from fatty acids, and is also *essential* to the body. It is the starting point for the synthesis of many biologically important substances, such as steroid hormones, and it is an essential component of cell membranes, which contain over 90% of the body's cholesterol.

Cholesterol is synthesized by the liver, as well as coming from the diet. The proportion of dietary cholesterol which is absorbed from the gut varies markedly between individuals.

In spite of its unpopular image, cholesterol is harmful only when deposited in the arterial walls or as gallstones.

ESSENTIAL FATTY ACIDS

Fats are necessary in the diet as a source of *essential fatty acids*. There are two essential fatty acids: **linoleic acid**, an n-6 acid, and **alpha-linoleic acid**, an n-3. Both are necessary for the normal composition and function of many biological membranes. Deficiency is rarely seen, but causes skin lesions and decreased efficiency in the use of fatty acids for energy.

Other important fatty acids are formed from these two essential ones. These are arachidonic, eicosapentaenoic and docosahexaenoic

BOX 5.4

CIS AND *TRANS* FATTY ACIDS

These terms refer to the arrangement of the hydrogen atoms in unsaturated fatty acid molecules. This arrangement is important because the *trans* forms of unsaturated fatty acids appear to behave in the body *in the same way as saturated fatty acids*.

The *cis* form has both the hydrogen atoms at the double bond on the same side of the molecule and include most natural fatty acids. In the processing of oils to make margarine, *trans* fatty acids are formed. Instead of being on the same side of the molecule, the hydrogen atoms next to the double bond are on opposite sides.

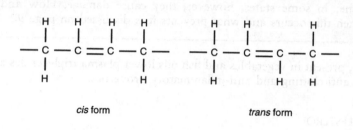

cis form   trans form

OMEGA-3 AND OMEGA-6 FATTY ACIDS

These terms, often written as n-3 and n-6, are a way of denoting the position of the double bond from the free (methyl) end of the fatty acid carbon chain.

N-3 fatty acids have the double bond three carbon atoms from the end. In n-6 fatty acids the double bond is six atoms along.

---

acids. They give rise to a group of substances in the body called *eicosanoids*. These include thromboxanes, prostaglandins, prostacyclins and they have a variety of very powerful actions. For example, prostacyclins inhibit platelet aggregation and lower blood pressure, so have a role in maintaining cardiovascular health.

THE FAT-SOLUBLE VITAMINS

Vitamins A, D, E and K, come from fat in foods although there are alternative sources for vitamin A (plant carotenes) and D (the action of sunlight on skin).

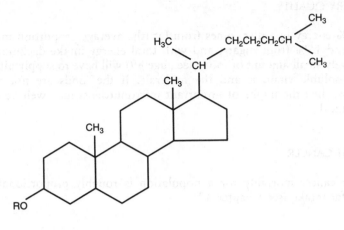

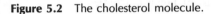

R= hydrocarbon chain

Figure 5.2   The cholesterol molecule.

OBESITY

A high fat intake has been proposed as a cause of obesity. As discussed in the chapter on sugars, *any* form of energy taken *in excess of requirement* will lead to increased stores. There is evidence correlating the amounts of fat eaten to degree of fatness; studies showed that middle-aged men eating high fat diets were more overweight than those who did not (Dreon *et al.*, 1984). And, of course, it is easy for a liking for foods such as chocolate or chips greatly to increase energy intake. It is also true that the energy costs of storage (that is, the conversion of glucose or fat to adipose tissue) are less for fat (a loss of 3%) than for glucose (a loss of 20%), so theoretically a diet in which fat provides excess calories will cause a higher weight gain than a similar high carbohydrate diet.

BOX 5.5

FAT IS A COMPACT FORM OF ENERGY

One Mars bar, weighing 65 g, has 287 kcal (1204 kJ).
This equals the energy of seven apples, or 820 g (nearly 2 lb).

DIETARY QUALITY

If 40% energy in a diet comes from fat (the average proportion in the UK) and 15% from sugars, and with total energy intake declining, a relatively small amount of food (see page 89) will have to supply all the water-soluble vitamins and the minerals. If the foods are not well chosen, then the intake of important micronutrients may well be less than ideal.

BREAST CANCER

Breast cancer mortality for a population is roughly proportional to total fat intake (see Chapter 12).

Health risks related to fatty acid composition   See the Department of Health publication, *Nutritional Aspects of Cardiovascular Diseases* (Department of Health, 1994).

CORONARY HEART DISEASE

Coronary heart disease (CHD) is the narrowing of the lumen of the coronary arteries by atheroma, a deposit which contains cholesterol. The atheroma may then be the site of a blood clot, causing further narrowing and reduction in blood supply. CHD is a multifactorial disease and a number of *risk factors* have been identified, prominent among them being *raised blood cholesterol*. The level of blood cholesterol is influenced by a number of factors and one of them is the percentage of dietary energy from saturated fats (see Chapter 12).

CANCERS

Some cancers are associated with a high fat intake and this is discussed in Chapter 12. The mortality from colon cancer in a population is proportional to its saturated fat intake; mortality from rectal cancer is proportional to the prevailing P/S ratio.

Blood lipids   Dietary fat influences, to a great extent, the relative amounts of the various blood lipids. In contrast to glucose – where the concentration in the blood is controlled within narrow limits – there is a wide variation in the amount of cholesterol present in the blood of different populations. This has important effects on health, which have been summarized above. The digestion and transport of fats explains how these differences occur.

DIGESTION OF FATS

Over 90% of the fat eaten is absorbed from the gut. Being insoluble in water, fat can only be digested by the water-soluble enzymes of the gut at the surface of a globule of fat. This surface, or, more accurately, interface, is enormously increased by the production of a very fine emulsion in the small intestine. Bile (Box 5.6) is essential for this emulsification (Figure 5.3).

BOX 5.6

BILE

Produced by the liver, one of its main functions is to emulsify fat in the gut. In its absence, fat is incompletely digested and much is excreted in the faeces. One of its components is cholesterol. Some of this cholesterol is reabsorbed in the gut and circulated back to the liver. Some is excreted; non-starch polysaccharides (NSP) may increase this loss by binding with cholesterol.

Fat is broken down by the pancreatic enzyme lipase to glycerol, fatty acids and monoglycerides. In the cells lining the small intestine, these digestive products are resynthesized into fat, supplied with a shell of water-soluble protein, and enter the bloodstream as **chylomicrons**. These particles contain cholesterol as well as being rich in triglycerides.

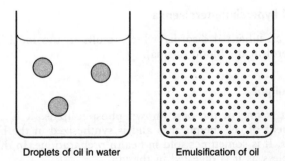

Droplets of oil in water   Emulsification of oil

Figure 5.3 Emulsification of oil.

METABOLISM AND TRANSPORT OF FATS

Like other nutrients cholesterol and fat are carried to the various tissues which need them. The difference is that the lipids are insoluble in water and cannot be carried in solution in the plasma. This difficulty is overcome by the combination of lipids with proteins to form *lipoproteins*. Lipoproteins found in the blood are classified according to their density (Box 5.7).

BOX 5.7

SOME GENERAL POINTS ABOUT LIPOPROTEINS

Classifying lipoproteins by density

Mixtures of substances which are chemically similar but differ in density can be separated according to their *density*. Lipoproteins are an example: when they are centrifuged, they will form layers according to their different densities, allowing them to be easily separated.

Apolipoproteins

You may see the term *apolipoprotein* used. It refers to the protein part of lipoproteins and the letters A, B and C are used to denote different ones.

Macrophages

These are white blood cells which scavenge foreign substances and remove them from the blood.

Familial hypercholesterolaemia

This is an inherited disorder which results in too much (hyper) cholesterol in the blood (aemia).

Phospholipids

Lecithin is one of the best known phospholipids. It is a major constituent of cell membranes and is synthesized in the body by the liver. It is sometimes sold in health preparations. In this form it is useless as it is digested in the gut.

CLASSIFICATION OF LIPOPROTEINS

- **Very low density lipoprotein (VLDL)** – mainly triglyceride
- **Intermediate density lipoprotein (IDL)** – triglyceride/cholesterol
- **Low density lipoprotein (LDL)** – mainly cholesterol
- **High density lipoprotein (HDL)** – phospholipid/cholesterol and the smallest
- **Chylomicrons** – mainly triglyceride, and much the largest particle

After a meal containing fat, *chylomicrons* enter the blood (Figure 5.4). The walls of the blood capillaries in adipose tissue and skeletal muscle contain an enzyme (lipoprotein lipase) which breaks down the fat in the chylomicrons to fatty acids and glycerol. These products are then used by the cells for energy or stored as fat. The chylomicron gradually shrinks and finally chylomicron remnants are left, containing the cholesterol from the diet. These remnants are taken up rapidly by the liver. The amount of cholesterol varies according to the amount in the diet and the proportion of it absorbed.

Between meals, the liver secretes VLDL which supply the tissues with triglycerides. The remnants left from VLDL form IDL and then LDL. LDL is cholesterol-rich, accounting for about 70% of the plasma cholesterol. It is a risk factor for CHD and has been shown to be the source of cholesterol in atheroma.

LDL is removed slowly from the blood. Cells, particularly those of the liver, have LDL-receptors on their surfaces. These receptors allow LDL to enter the cell to supply the cholesterol required and the number of receptors is regulated by the cell's need for cholesterol.

However, there may be more LDL in the blood than is needed by the cells. It seems that if this LDL is modified (oxidized, for example), it enters macrophages (white blood cells) but in an *unregulated* fashion. These LDL-packed cells then become 'foam cells' and, deposited within the arterial wall, begin the development of atherosclerosis.

People with familial hypercholesterolaemia have few LDL receptors. The blood LDL and, therefore, cholesterol level is very high and the risk of premature CHD very great.

HDL transports excess tissue cholesterol to IDL. HDL seems to be protective against CHD.

The blood lipids which are commonly measured are:

	optimal levels
- total serum cholesterol (fasting)	5.2–5.7 mmol/litre
- LDL cholesterol	3.5–4.0 mmol/litre
- total triglyceride	<2.3 mmol/litre
- HDL cholesterol	none recommended

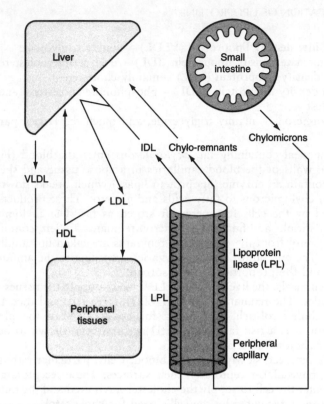

Figure 5.4 Schematic representation illustrating lipid circulation and metabolism. Lipoprotein, a molecule containing lipid + protein, so that lipid becomes water-soluble; VLDL, very low density lipoprotein; LDL, low density lipoprotein; IDL, intermediate density lipoprotein; HDL, high density lipoprotein; LPL, lipoprotein lipase, an enzyme which breaks down lipoproteins. (Redrawn from British Nutrition Foundation, *Complex Carbohydrates in Foods*; Chapman & Hall, London, 1990.)

Dietary fat affects blood lipids and blood clotting in the following ways:

- total plasma cholesterol and LDL are raised by *saturated fatty acids*, carbon length 12 to 16 (present in dairy products, coconut oil, meat fat) and *trans fatty acids* (mainly margarine);
- cholesterol (highest in offal, egg yolk, fish roes, mayonnaise and shell-fish) may raise total blood cholesterol but this effect is very variable and less important than that caused by fatty acids;
- total plasma cholesterol and LDL are *lowered* by *PUFA* of the n-6 series;

- long-chain PUFA of the n-3 series (fish oils) lower plasma triglycerides and have anti-clotting and anti-inflammatory properties.

These facts, derived from epidemiological and experimental studies underlie the recommendations for DRVs which are given below.

Current guidelines for fat intake

[See Department of Health publication, *Reference Values for Food Energy and Nutrition for the UK* (Department of Health, 1991).]

These guidelines propose that:

- total fat intake should average for the population 33% of dietary energy including alcohol or 35% food energy derived from food;
- *cis*-monounsaturated fatty acids should provide about 12% of dietary energy;
- *cis*-polyunsaturated fatty acids should provide on average 6% dietary energy;
- *trans*-fatty acids intake should not increase from the present level of 2% dietary energy.

How can we interpret this in terms of food intake? For most people it means a fall in the amount of fat eaten and the recommendations for total fat are very easily exceeded. To take an example: at a typical energy intake of 2000 kcal (8368 kJ), 35% energy from fat will be 700 kcal (2929 kJ); 11% of the energy from saturated fat would be 220 kcal (920 kJ). A day's meals which included an egg for breakfast, a cheese sandwich for lunch and sausages for the evening meal, butter on bread and two digestive biscuits would give the totals shown in Table 5.1 (Davies and Dickerson, 1991):

Table 5.1 Example of percentage of energy from fat in some foods

Food	Weight	Energy from fat (kcal)	Energy from saturated fat (kcal)
Butter	50 g	370	243
Milk, whole	⅓ pint (190 ml)	68	43
Egg	One, size 2, 60 g	58	17
Sausages, pork, grilled	Two, 90 g	199	77
Biscuits, digestive	Two, 30 g	56	23
Cheese, Cheddar	20 g	62	39
Total		813	399
Recommended		700	263

All other foods would need to be free of fat to hit the target for total fat and the amount of saturates is already exceeded.

Modifications such as semi-skimmed milk, low-fat spread, and cottage cheese (45 g), would make a big difference, giving totals of 537 kcal for total fat and 148 kcal from saturates.

Most people therefore need to reduce their fat intake either by changes in their choice of foods or by modifying their usual foods.

MODIFYING THE USUAL DIET

The modifications made depend on the aim for the individual, and the frequency and amount of fatty foods eaten. Someone who likes butter, say, and enjoys it occasionally has no need to cut it out. On the other hand, someone who eats generously buttered bread at every meal should reduce both amount and frequency of eating. Suggested modifications are to:

- reduce the fat spread on bread, either by spreading more thinly or choosing a low fat spread. Fresh new bread is good enough to eat without using a fat spread. Jam, Marmite, peanut butter, lemon curd (easy to make, delicious, high in vitamin C, some butter but less than using butter only) are spreads that can be used alone. When using butter, make sure it is not too hard to spread thinly. A few seconds in a microwave oven is an easy way to soften it;
- choose skimmed or semi-skimmed milk;
- grill, rather than fry, foods such as bacon, sausages, etc.;
- choose lower fat cheeses such as Edam or cottage cheese, or eating smaller quantities of high fat cheeses (easier if full-flavoured cheeses are used);
- use oven chips or home-made 'baked' chips (for a recipe, see page 392) rather than deep-fat fried chips;
- choose low-fat cakes rather than rich fat ones – usually yeast-raised ones like iced fingers, tea cakes, Chelsea buns;
- remove visible fat from meat;
- alter the proportions of foods in the diet – less meat and more vegetables, including pulses;
- read food labels. For example, one brand of frozen shortcrust pastry contains 28% fat by weight, while a puff pastry, which would be expected to contain much more, actually has less, only 25% by weight and you use less because you roll it thinner.

CHANGING FOOD CHOICE

Possible changes are to:

- substitute fruit or jellies for puddings, ice-cream, etc.;
- have soup as a first course instead of a pudding as a second course or with bread as a snack;

- use some Chinese-style dishes which are low in fat;
- have chips only once a week;
- for home baking, instead of pastry, make up a batch of bread dough (much easier than most people think and enjoyed by young children who can have a bit to knead). Make a pizza, some rolls, add some sugar and sultanas to another bit for a fruit loaf and roll out the last lot to make apple turnovers. All these are low in fat and are delicious (see page 395).

Lower fat foods are less energy dense and therefore more bread and cereals should be eaten to make up the shortfall.

CHANGING THE FATTY ACID PROFILE

Saturated fats are present mainly in animal foods and so the following changes will reduce their intake and increase the intake of PUFA and monounsaturates (see Table 5.2).

- reduce butter intake and use low fat spread or good quality margarine;
- use oil high in PUFA for frying, cake making;
- eat more oily fish (herring, sardines, mackerel, tuna and salmon).
- eat lean meat.

COMA report 46 (Department of Health, 1994) gives weekly intakes of foods which would meet their recommendations. Although this was given a critical press, it can be used as a basis for sensible meal-planning. It was not intended to be used as specific advice for individuals, but to represent national averages. Since it is extremely hard to translate nutrient advice into diets, even for professionals, this attempt is useful.

Food sources of fats and oils

Fats are often classified as visible (as in butter, margarine) and invisible (as in biscuits and cakes). It is true that many people do not realize that biscuits and cakes are high in fat and it is sometimes said that the food industry removes fat from foods where it is obvious and reintroduces it as 'hidden' fat. Food labelling is not always helpful, since 'low fat' means only 'lower than the normal version' and such a food may still be very high in fat, as in low fat spreads. The fatty acid content as well as total fat must be considered. Some data are given in Tables 5.3 and 5.4.

Table 5.2 The fat and saturated fatty acid saving from a variety of dietary substitutions. (The recommendations in this Report imply a reduction in national *per capita* average consumption for total fat of around 15 g per day, and for saturated fatty acids of around 11 g per day) (Department of Health, 1994)

Food swap	Fat saving (g/portion)	Saturated fatty acid saving (g/portion)
One bowl breakfast cereal with whole milk exchanged for one bowl breakfast cereal with semi-skimmed milk	2	1
One bowl breakfast cereal with whole milk exchanged for one bowl breakfast cereal with skimmed milk	4	2
One egg fried in oil exchanged for one egg boiled	3	1
Two rashers grilled bacon and one fried egg exchanged for one bowl breakfast cereal with semi-skimmed milk and two slices toast with low fat spread	28	11
Two slices bread with butter exchanged for two slices bread with low fat spread	11	9
Two slices bread with butter exchanged for two slices bread with polyunsaturated margarine	0	8
Cheddar cheese sandwich with butter exchanged for reduced fat Cheddar type cheese sandwich with low fat spread	19	15
Cheddar cheese sandwich with butter exchanged for Cheddar cheese sandwich without butter	18	11
One thick and creamy fruit yoghurt exchanged for low fat fruit yoghurt	3	1
Two digestive biscuits exchanged for one banana	7	3
One chocolate bar exchanged for one apple	15	9
One packet crisps exchanged for low fat crisps	5	1
Two grilled sausages exchanged for two low fat grilled sausages	13	5
One pork chop, lean and fat grilled exchanged for one pork chop, lean only	19	7
100% beefburger in a bun exchanged for low fat beefburger in bun	5	2
Cheeseburger (100%) beef in bun exchanged for 100% beefburger in bun	5	3
White fish in batter, fried in oil exchanged for white fish, steamed or baked (no added fat)	33	3
Baked potato with butter exchanged for baked potato with low fat spread	18	8
Baked potato with butter exchanged for baked potato with baked beans	15	10
Baked potato with Cheddar cheese exchanged for baked potato with cottage cheese	16	10
One medium portion chips fried in oil exchanged for one medium portion boiled potatoes	12	1
Sponge cake with butter icing exchanged for currant bun with low fat spread	11	3
Pie with two crusts exchanged for pie with one crust	6	2
Egg mayonnaise exchanged for egg with reduced fat mayonnaise	31	4
Four mugs tea/coffee with whole milk exchanged for four mugs tea/coffee with semi-skimmed milk	2	1

Table 5.3   Fatty acid content of some fats and oils

Oils/fats	Total fat (g/100 g)	Saturates (excluding trans) (g/100 g)	Monosaturates (g/100 g)	PUFA (g/100 g)
Corn oil	99.9	10.1	12.6	72.1
Soya oil	99.9	14.0	23.2	56.5
Sunflower oil	99.9	11.9	20.2	63.0
Margarine (good quality)	81.0	16.2	20.6	41.1
Blended oil (good quality)	99.9	6.5	60.2	28.4
Blended oil (poor quality)	99.9	13.8	53.5	23.1
Butter	82.0	54.0	19.8	2.6
Lard	99.0	40.8	43.8	9.6
Olive oil	99.9	14.0	69.7	11.2

Modified with permission from Thomas (ed), *Manual of Dietetic Practice*, Blackwell Science Ltd, Oxford, 1994.

CHOLESTEROL

Although control of dietary cholesterol is not usually important, for some people a high intake may be undesirable.

- *Rich sources* are all offal and pâté, egg yolk, fish roes, mayonnaise, shellfish.
- *Moderately rich sources* are meat fat, cold meats like salami, whole milk, cream, ice-cream, cheese, butter, most commercially made cakes, biscuits and pastries. Crisps and all shop-bought foods made with unspecified oil.
- *Low sources* are all fish, all lean meats and chicken without skin, low fat dairy products, bread, 'low cholesterol' margarines.
- *Cholesterol-free foods* are all vegetables and vegetable oils, egg white, sugar (Thomas, 1994).

Fat substitutes or replacers

Because of the need to reduce fat intake and because of its desirable qualities of mouth-feel, there is a market for fat substitutes. To be acceptable to the consumer these have to be similar to fats in price, functions in food preparation and in mouth-feel.

- *Carbohydrate-based fat substitutes* – these are used in a wide range of foods such as frozen desserts, cheese analogues, confectionery, baked goods and salty snacks. Examples are Paselli SA 2, N-oil, Maltrin, Litesse (a polymer of dextrose with some sorbitol and citric acid) and Nutrifat C (a blend of several hydrolysed starches

Table 5.4   Reference list for fat content of foods

High fat foods (>20 g fat/100 g)	Medium fat foods (10–20 g fat/100 g)	Low fat foods (5–10 g fat/100 g)	Very low fat foods
Fats and oils, butter, margarine, vegetable oils, lard, dripping			
Double, whipping, single and soured cream, milk powder	Full fat yoghurt	Evaporated, condensed milk, gold-top milk	Whole milk, semi-skimmed and skimmed milk, low fat yoghurt
Most hard cheeses, cream cheese, cheese spreads	Feta, Tendale, curd cheese Pizza	Macaroni cheese, cauliflower cheese	Cottage cheese
Eggs and egg products Mayonnaise, salad cream			
Streaky bacon, chops with fat, roast duck with fat, pâté, luncheon meat, pork sausage, sausage roll, pork pie, meat pasties, pies	Lean bacon, fried rump steak, lean lamb and pork chops, roast chicken, liver, corned beef, steaklets, beefburgers, moussaka, Bolognese sauce	Lean ham, grilled rump steak, lean roast beef, lamb, pork, roast chicken without skin, hot pot, shepherd's pie, curry	Turkey breast
Taramasalata, fried whitebait	Cod in batter, canned salmon, sardines, fish-fingers, fried scampi	Pilchards in tomato sauce	All poached and steamed white fish and shellfish
		Soft rolls, Ready Brek, muesli	All bread, except chapattis, soft rolls, pasta, rice, cereal, breakfast cereals
Chips, frozen fried chips	Thick chips		All vegetables cooked without added fat
Chocolate biscuits, filled wafers, custard creams, chocolate digestive, shortbread, Lincoln	Cream crackers, rich tea, oatcakes, ginger nuts, wafers (unfilled)		
Crisps, low-fat crisps, nuts and nut butters, milk chocolate	Mars bars, toffees		All plain sweets
Flaky pastry, shortcrust pastry, Victoria sponge, chocolate éclairs, mince pie, cheesecake	Madeira cake, rock cakes, doughnuts, jam tarts, scones, iced fingers, custard tart, pancakes, sponge pudding, fruit pie	Currant bun, fatless sponge, trifle, fruit tart, bread and butter pudding, ice-cream, apple crumble, egg custard	Meringues, jelly, fresh, canned or frozen fruit, custard or other puddings made with skimmed milk

Modified with permission from Thomas (ed) *Manual of Dietetic Practice*, Blackwell Science Ltd, Oxford, 1994.

which can replace 81% fat in some products). Oatrim, Olestra, Slendid are other examples.

- *Protein-based fat substitutes* – these are generally not heat-stable but can be used in spreads and frozen desserts. Examples are Simplesse, Trailblazer, Nutrifat PC and Nutrilac.

What are the implications for the consumer? Ideally, such substances would bring about a fall in fat consumption, but the *major* sources of fat in the diet are not affected by these substitutes, which reduce the fat in richer products. It is *food consumption patterns* and *food choice* which determine the fat intake of individuals.

Key points

1. Lipids is a term which refers to fat-like substances, which are not soluble in water, for example. Fats and oils are lipids; they are similar chemically and are classed as a sub-group triglycerides.
2. In the UK, fat consumption is high with an average of 40% of energy being eaten as fat.
3. Dietary fat is a compact form of energy and supplies essential fatty acids and fat-soluble vitamins.
4. Dietary cholesterol is not usually important from the point of view of health. It is vital in the body as a component of cell membranes.
5. Dietary fat may affect health. There is evidence that, in industrialized countries, high fat intakes contribute to obesity, and high saturated fat to CHD and cancers of the large intestine and breast.
6. Fat and cholesterol are transported in the blood as lipoproteins. There are several types which are classified on the basis of density. LDL (low density lipoprotein) is a major risk factor for CHD, while HDL (high density lipoprotein) is protective.
7. Current guidelines for fat are that intake should be reduced to 30–35% energy, more than half being in the form of unsaturated fats.
8. Ways of modifying the diet to achieve these changes are suggested.

6 Vitamins

The aim of this chapter is to discuss the general issues relating to vitamins, to describe their properties and functions, to identify groups at risk of deficiency, and to give food sources and the dietary reference values for each. Practical points, important for patients, are highlighted.

Vitamins are organic substances which are needed by the body in very small amounts. They cannot be synthesized in the body (or, at least, not in amounts that are necessary) and therefore *must* be supplied in the diet. They are usually part of enzyme systems, often involved in the metabolism of the major substrates, that is, fats, proteins and carbohydrates. This explains why they are needed in small amounts but are essential to life.

There are 13 vitamins, of which A, D, E and K are fat-soluble and the B vitamins (B1, B2, niacin, B6, folate, B12, pantothenic acid, biotin) and C are water-soluble.

General principles and considerations

REQUIREMENTS

DRVs are available for eight vitamins, namely A, B1 (thiamin), B2 (riboflavin), niacin, B6, B12, folate and C (Table 6.1).

In general, requirements are higher, per kg body weight, for children, pregnant and lactating women and in recovery from illness.

There is very little frank vitamin *deficiency* in the wealthy developed countries and Nelson's study (see Nelson, 1983, in Chapter 3), indicated that, usually, the *more* a person eats in terms of calories, the *greater* their intake of micronutrients, which includes vitamins. The person who only eats a little and *in addition* has a relatively high intake of sugars, fats and/or alcohol is at risk of eating less than the ideal amount.

BODY STORES

If water-soluble vitamins are eaten in amounts greater than are needed and body stores are high, the surplus is excreted in the urine. Low body

Table 6.1   Reference Nutrient Intakes for vitamins. (From COMA 41, Department of Health, 1991)

Age	Thiamin (B1) mg/day	Riboflavin (B2) mg/day	Niacin (nicotinic acid equivalent) mg/day	Vitamin B6 mg/day	Vitamin B12 µg/day	Folate µg/day	Vitamin C mg/day	Vitamin A µg/day	Vitamin D µg/day
Children									
0–3 months	0.2	0.4	3	0.2	0.3	50	25	350	8.5
4–6 months	0.2	0.4	3	0.2	0.3	50	25	350	8.5
7–9 months	0.2	0.4	4	0.3	0.4	50	25	350	7
10–12 months	0.3	0.4	5	0.4	0.4	50	25	350	7
1–3 years	0.5	0.6	8	0.7	0.5	70	30	400	7
4–6 years	0.7	0.8	11	0.9	0.8	100	30	500	–
7–10 years	0.7	1.0	12	1.0	1.0	150	30	500	–
Males									
11–14 years	0.9	1.2	15	1.2	1.2	200	35	600	–
15–18 years	1.1	1.3	18	1.5	1.5	200	40	700	–
19–50 years	1.0	1.3	17	1.4	1.5	200	40	700	–
50+ years	0.9	1.3	16	1.4	1.5	200	40	700	**
Females									
11–14 years	0.7	1.1	12	1.0	1.2	200	34	600	–
15–18 years	0.8	1.1	14	1.2	1.5	200	40	600	–
19–50 years	0.8	1.1	13	1.2	1.5	200	40	600	–
50+ years	0.8	1.1	12	1.2	1.5	200	40	600	**
Pregnancy	+0.1***	+0.3	*	*	*	+100	+10	+100	10
Lactation									
0–4 months	+0.2	+0.5	+2	*	+0.5	+60	+30	+350	10
4+ months	+0.2	+0.5	+2	*	+0.5	+60	+30	+350	10

*No increment; **After age 65 the RNI is 10 µg/day for men and women; ***For last trimeter only +Based on protein providing 14.7% of EAR for energy.

stores are replenished when diet improves. Fat-soluble vitamins cannot be lost through the kidneys and a very high intake of vitamins A, D and K is toxic.

In a well-nourished person it is not essential that the daily requirements for vitamins are met every day. It is the *average* intake that is important. If body stores are high, a low intake would not lead to adverse effects for some time, depending on the particular vitamin. For vitamin C it might be weeks, for the fat-soluble vitamins, months and for B12, years.

FOOD TABLES FOR VITAMINS

The values for vitamin contents in food tables are less reliable than the values for the macronutrients (protein, carbohydrates and fat), because of the considerable variation between different samples of food, and the effects of storage, processing or cooking on vitamin content. Claims for vitamin content on food labels are likely, if anything, to be exceeded by the actual amount present.

LOSSES OF VITAMINS IN PROCESSING AND COOKING

Losses may be considerable. Water-soluble vitamins will be lost into cooking water, especially if the food is chopped. This can be avoided by steaming vegetables rather than boiling them. This is a surprisingly practical method, taking no longer than boiling and enabling a variety of vegetables to be cooked at one time. It is especially practical when cooking for one or two (Figure 6.1).

Vitamins B1, C and folate are also destroyed by heat and oxygen so that badly cooked vegetables (prepared early and soaked in water, cooked in a large amount of water for a long time and then kept hot) may have lost nearly all their vitamin C and folate.

Cooking by microwave has similar effects to traditional methods, except that little water is used, reducing loss. Re-heating by microwave causes little additional breakdown of vitamins.

Bicarbonate of soda should *not* be added to vegetables to keep them green. It destroys all the ascorbic acid.

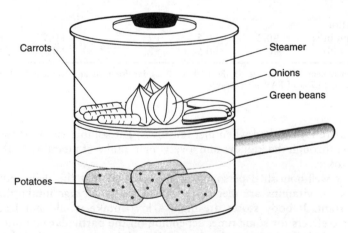

Figure 6.1 Steaming vegetables: an easy way of cooking vegetables which is especially useful when cooking for one or two.

The fat-soluble vitamins are quite stable and losses in cooking are small.

GROUPS AT RISK OF DEFICIENCY OR OF SUB-OPTIMAL INTAKE

Although overt vitamin deficiency is uncommon in the industrialized countries, there is concern that some groups may be eating less than the optimal amount. This stems from some characteristics of our life-style, namely:

* *low levels of activity or slimming diets*, leading to low energy intake and so often a reduced intake of vitamins. For example, an energy intake of 1500 kcal, with 40% from fat and 20% from sugars and alcohol means that virtually all vitamins have to come from the remaining 600 kcal;
* *alcohol consumption* affects both requirements and intake of vitamins. Absorption, activity and storage of thiamin and B6 may be reduced and folate deficiency is a common deficiency in alcoholics. Secretion of bile salts may be low because of liver damage and this may reduce absorption of fat and fat-soluble vitamins. And, of course, the diet is likely to be poor;
* *long-term medication*, common in the elderly, may also affect requirements. Laxatives may affect the absorption of many nutrients, bile acid sequestrants bind fat-soluble vitamins, and antibiotics may affect the absorption of vitamin K and/or retinol. Anticonvulsants can affect folate, vitamin D or thiamin status. Barbiturates may reduce metabolism of vitamin K. There is some evidence of reduced utilization of the B vitamins, and vitamins C and A in contraceptive pill users; in one study changes in pyridoxine metabolism, and falls in folate and riboflavin levels were observed (*Which?*, 1990). In practical terms, it seems that long-term oral contraceptive users may require some B-vitamin supplements or a few helpings of Marmite a week;
* *food faddism*, leading to bizarre or very restricted diets;
* *smoking* – studies comparing the mean levels of circulating vitamins of smokers and non-smokers have shown, in smokers, greatly reduced levels of folate and B12 (though not B6) and a smaller reduction of beta-carotene and vitamin C. Smoking, like alcohol, affects both food selection and nutrient metabolism and, of course, the two habits often go together (Pietrzik, 1991).

VITAMIN SUPPLEMENTS

A lot of people feel that they would be 'better' if they took vitamin supplements. In fact, with a good diet, supplements are not necessary.

It has been claimed that *the intelligence of schoolchildren may* be increased if vitamin supplements are given: well-designed trials have not confirmed this (Nelson *et al.*, 1990).

Groups for whom supplements are useful include:

- those with impaired absorption due to illness;
- those with increased needs due to illness or surgery;
- those with a high alcohol intake;
- women hoping to become pregnant, whose previous diet has been poor;
- women who have had a child with neural tube defect require folate supplement (see Chapter 10);
- infants, children and pregnant women of Asian descent require vitamin D supplements.

Best buys for vitamin supplements

A *Which?* report (1990) found that Sanatogen Multivitamins contained the majority of the essential vitamins and was one of the cheapest. Of the multivitamin and mineral supplements, Boots Plurivite M, was one of the cheapest and did not have excessive amounts of any nutrient.

FREE RADICALS AND DISEASE

The damage which can be caused to the body by free radicals and the importance of vitamins and minerals in protecting against such damage has recently aroused much interest.

Free radicals are molecular fragments which are extremely reactive so that they quickly cause harmful chemical changes. During normal metabolism a small proportion of free radicals are formed but they are immediately rendered harmless or quenched by various substances, including vitamins and some metallo-enzymes.

Free radicals can damage cell membranes. Cell membranes contain lipids, some of them unsaturated (see page 66), and these lipids react with free oxygen radicals to become lipid peroxides, the same reaction as rancidity in fat. The effect on the cell is to damage the barrier between its contents and tissue fluid; this results in mixing compounds which are normally separated and so normal function is disturbed.

If free radicals are not quenched, then a chain reaction can start, which produces extensive damage to tissues.

In some situations the production of free radicals increases and the protective mechanisms fail; examples are smoking (every puff of smoke contains huge numbers of free radicals), ageing, inflammation (for example rheumatoid arthritis), tissue injury following heart attack and certain types of chemical poisoning.

The protective anti-oxidant vitamins are riboflavin, vitamins C and E, and carotenoids. The enzymes include superoxide dismutase, containing copper or manganese (and so fashionable that it is uselessly sold as a supplement) and glutathione peroxidase, which contains selenium.

The advice to eat more fruit and vegetables is based partly on the importance of the anti-oxidant vitamins and their protective effects (Table 6.2).

CHEMISTRY

Vitamin A

There are two types of compounds, *retinol* or *pre-formed vitamin A*, which is present in animal foods, and carotenoids or carotenes which are coloured compounds found in yellow, green and orange vegetables. Some carotenes, notably beta-carotene, are converted into vitamin A in the intestinal mucosa; 6 μg of beta-carotene produce 1 μg of vitamin A.

FUNCTIONS OF VITAMIN A AND CAROTENOIDS

Retinol is part of the molecule of rhodopsin, present in the retina of the eye and used in dim-light vision. So a deficiency of vitamin A causes night blindness, an abnormally slow adjustment to poor lighting.

Retinol plays an important part in many cells, in promoting growth, development and tissue differentiation.

Carotenoids may be important in their own right as protective anti-oxidants, a property which vitamin A lacks. Some epidemiological work has linked high intakes of carotenoids with a lower risk of some cancers, which may be a reason for some of the beneficial effects of eating a lot of vegetables. More research is needed to elucidate this.

DEFICIENCY OF VITAMIN A

The effects are night blindness and xerophthalmia (the cornea of the eye breaks down, a common cause of blindness in the developing world) and formation of plugs of keratin in the skin hair follicles, called hyperfollicular keratosis.

AT-RISK GROUPS

There is little evidence of deficiency in the UK. Average body stores are adequate for 1–2 years before signs of deficiency occur. However, if fat

Table 6.2 Characteristics of dietary vitamins

Vitamin	Functions	Deficiency	Main sources	Loss in cooking	Groups at risk in UK	Toxicity	Incidence of deficiency in UK
A; retinol	Retinal pigment for night vision Cell differentiation	Night blindness Xerophthalmia Some skin changes	Carrots, milk, margarine, butter	Stable Some loss in frying and long storage	None	Yes Vomiting, headaches, liver, bone damage Danger in pregnancy	Negligible
Beta-carotene	Antioxidant ? Protection against some cancers		Yellow, green fruit and vegetables			Not toxic but yellow skin	
D; calciferol	Calcium balance via intestinal absorption and bone calcium	Rickets in children Osteomalacia in adults – muscle weakness, bone pain	Few: fatty fish, eggs, margarine, some breakfast cereals Mainly from sunlight on skin	Stable	Asians, elderly Supplements needed for some children, pregnant, lactating women	Yes Infants most at risk Calcification of soft tissues	Some in at-risk groups
E; tocopherols, tocotrienols	Antioxidant, especially for lipid membranes	Rarely seen, characteristic neuropathology	Vegetable oils, cereals, eggs No DRVs	Stable	If vitamin not absorbed or utilized	Few effects reported	Rare
K; phylloquinone, menaquinone	Synthesis of blood clotting factors, production coagulation inhibitors	Impaired blood clotting, haemorrhagic disease	Vegetables; cabbage, cauliflower, peas, cereals Synthesized by intestinal bacteria No DRVs	Stable	Infants, first months – haemorrhagic disease of new-born or 3–8 weeks, breast-fed	None, but menadione (synthetic) not advised	Rare except in new-born
B1; thiamin	Metabolism of carbohydrate, also fat, alcohol	Beriberi Wernicke–Korsakoff syndrome (CNS lesions)	Bread, cereals potatoes, milk, meat	Unstable Easily lost in cooking water, especially if bi-carbonate added	Alcoholics, narcotic abusers	At continued very high intakes (100 × RNI)	In at-risk groups

	processes						
		mouth, seborrhoeic dermatitis, lesions surface genitalia	fortified cereals, egg	Lost in cooking water, increased by bicarbonate Exposure to light (milk)	Possibly slimmers	Only at very high doses	No
Niacin	Coenzyme component in intermediary metabolism	Pellagra; light-sensitive dermatitis Fatal if untreated	Meat, potatoes, bread, fortified cereals	Lost in cooking water but otherwise stable	None		
B6; pyridoxine pyridoxal pyridoxamine	Amino acid metabolism, steroid hormone actions	Not known	Widely distributed Also synthesized from tryptophan	Lost in cooking water and destroyed by heat	None	Reversible sensory neuropathy	Rare
Folate (folic acid)	Normal formation of blood cells, normal growth	Megaloblastic (large cell) anaemia	Green leafy vegetables, yeast extract, liver	Lost in cooking water and destroyed by heat	Pregnant women, elderly, alcoholics	Little danger	Repeated pregnancies, elderly, alcoholics
B12; cobalamin	Nerve myelination Interacts with folate	Megaloblastic (pernicious) anaemia Nerve damage	Almost all animal products	Little	Vegans, after gastrectomy	Extremely low	Rare
Pantothenic acid	Release of energy from macronutrients	Experimental deficiency only	Widely distributed No DRVs	Lost in cooking water	None	Possible diarrhoea	None
Biotin	Lipogenesis, gluconeogenesis, and breakdown of some amino acids	Dermatitis, hair loss, anorexia, nausea	Widely distributed in foods and synthesized by intestinal flora No DRVs	Lost in cooking water	Prolonged total parenteral nutrition Eating large number of raw eggs	No evidence	Rare
C; ascorbic acid	Collagen synthesis (wound healing) Antioxidant Aids absorption non-haem iron	Scurvy – bruising bleeding gums, fatigue	Potatoes, fruit juice, citrus fruit, green vegetables	Very easily destroyed: in storage, bruising, chopping, cooking water (especially if bi-carbonate added); keeping hot	Elderly, smokers (estimated extra intake – 80 mg/day)	Some risks with *very high* intakes	Occasionally in elderly

absorption is reduced, then the normal absorption (80% of total) of vitamin A will be reduced and this may cause deficiency, as in *coeliac disease, cystic fibrosis* and *chronic liver disease*.

TOXICITY OF VITAMIN A

The main threat is to *pregnant women*, who should eat no more than 330 μg/day. Liver, because of present animal feeding practices, may have a very high content and therefore pregnant women are advised not to eat liver or liver products. Children are more sensitive to toxicity than adults. There is no evidence of toxicity from carotenes, though too much turns the skin yellow.

Table 6.3 Vitamin A content of average servings of foods

Food	Amount/weight (g)	Vitamin A content (μg)
Milk, whole	⅓ pint (190 ml)	109 (skimmed milk, 2)
Cheeses	40 g	57–198 (none in soya cheese)
Butter	8 g	71
Margarine	8 g	72
Low-fat spread	8 g	87
Ice-cream, dairy	75 g	111
Liver (lambs)	90 g	18 549
Mackerel, canned pilchards	Average serving	55–65
Naan bread	One, 170 g	170
Paratha	One, 125 g	175
Ovaltine	Four heaped teaspoons	94
Horlicks	Four heaped teaspoons	125
Egg	One, size 2	34

From Davies, J. and Dickerson, J. (1991).

Table 6.4 Carotene content of average servings of foods

Food	Amount/weight (g)	Carotenes (μg)
Fresh mango	One, 315 g	370
Fresh peach	One, 125 g	91
Fresh apricots	Three whole, 110 g	253
Canned apricots	Five halves, 140 g	234
Carrots (boiled)	75 g	1300
Cabbage (boiled)	75 g	38
Tomato juice (canned)	One glass	166

From Davies, J. and Dickerson, J. (1991).

FOODS FOR VITAMIN A AND CAROTENES

Dietary provision of vitamin A and carotenes (given in average portion sizes) are listed in Tables 6.3 and 6.4, respectively.

CHEMISTRY

Vitamin D

The substance *cholecalciferol* (vitamin D3) is formed in the skin by sunlight. It is also present in some foods. There is a synthetic compound, *ergocalciferol* (D2), which is used for enriching foods and which acts in the body in exactly the same way. Vitamin D is the generic name for both D2 and D3. (There is not a vitamin D1.)

Strictly speaking, vitamin D is not a vitamin, since it is modified first by the liver and then by the kidney, to form the active substance, 1,25-dihydroxycalciferol (also called calcitriol). This substance is classed as a hormone. The production of calcitriol is regulated according to the amount needed to maintain calcium homeostasis.

FUNCTIONS OF 1,25-DIHYDROXYCALCIFEROL (CALCITRIOL)

Calcitriol acts to maintain the level of calcium in the blood constant. Within the cells of the intestinal mucosa it increases the absorption of dietary calcium, which varies from 18–46% of the amount eaten (see page 30).

Calcitriol also acts on the bones, if necessary mobilizing calcium from them to keep up plasma levels or causing the laying down of new bone by different mechanisms.

It is now becoming clear that vitamin D has a number of other functions such as cell proliferation and maturation.

DEFICIENCY OF VITAMIN D

The primary deficiency is lack of exposure to sunlight and therefore lower production of vitamin D in the skin. Seasonal changes in vitamin D status occur in everyone.

Rickets is the deficiency disease of children. The bones lack calcium salts because of poor absorption through lack of vitamin D and so they remain soft. This causes pain on walking and the soft bones may become deformed, producing bow legs or knock knees, pelvic deformities and collapse of the ribcage. Toddlers and adolescents are peak ages of occurrence.

This is not the only form of rickets; vitamin D-resistant rickets is also known.

Osteomalacia is the form of deficiency in adults. The bones lose calcium and soften causing bone pain, especially of the shoulder, spine and hip.

Osteoporosis occurs in post-menopausal women and is due to loss of sex hormones. It is not prevented or cured by vitamin D supplements but the risk is lessened if the peak bone density in youth is high.

AT-RISK GROUPS

Asians living in the UK are at risk and in the 1960s presented the first cases of rickets in this country for two decades. It is caused by low dietary intake of vitamin D in vegetarians (most cases have been among the vegetarian Hindus), the consumption of unleavened bread (poppadoms, chapattis) which is high in phytate and so reduces calcium availability, little exposure to the sun and racially determined requirements. This group has been targeted to receive dietary supplements. Britons from Africa and the West Indies are not at risk.

The *housebound elderly* are at risk due to lack of exposure to the sun and decreased efficiency of production of vitamin D by the skin. They rely more on dietary sources (see also Chapter 13). The lowest vitamin D status is seen in institutionalized elderly in countries like the UK which do not routinely fortify foods with vitamin D.

TOXICITY OF VITAMIN D

Vitamin D is toxic in excess. It causes a raised level of plasma calcium, which can lead to constriction of blood vessels and a raised blood pressure. High vitamin D intake can also cause calcification of soft tissues, like kidney, heart and blood vessels.

In the 1950s, there were some cases of vitamin D poisoning in infants caused by the fortification of infant foods. This is no longer a risk, but overenthusiastic mothers may still believe that if a few vitamin drops are good, then more must be better. The toxic level for infants may start at 50 μg per day. The level for adults is unknown.

SOURCES OF VITAMIN D

Sunlight acting on the skin

Exposure to ultraviolet (UV) light converts 7-dehydrocholesterol, in the dermis, to previtamin D, which is then transformed into cholecalciferol and absorbed into the blood stream. UV light (wavelength 300 nm) is present in the UK only between March and November, between about 11am and 3pm. It is reduced by cloud and dust. It will penetrate thin clothes but absorption is less in pigmented skins.

The value of sunlight in preventing rickets has been known for a long time. Today the link between sunlight and skin cancer must also be taken into consideration. Skin cancer, which is rising, is linked with sunburn and with 'toasting' on the beaches of southern Europe. *Moderate exposure* to sun in the UK is unlikely to produce cancer. But the amount of UV light required to produce vitamin D is very small and the use of skin protection especially for babies is wise; most creams do not block out all the UV light and so some vitamin is formed. The frequency and duration of exposure is crucial in determining the incidence of skin cancer: for example, farmers are at risk of facial skin cancer in this country, cases having been seen from the turn of the century.

The production of vitamin through the skin will never reach toxic amounts in the body.

Dietary sources

Vitamin D is found in only a few foods. These are margarine (a much better source than butter), fatty fish (herring, kipper, salmon, sardines, pilchards), eggs and breakfast cereals. For useful recipes using fatty fish, see page 385.

CHEMISTRY   **Vitamin E**

The term vitamin E refers to two groups of compounds, the tocopherols and the tocotrienols. The one which is most commonly in foods is *alpha-tocopherol*.

FUNCTIONS OF VITAMIN E

Vitamin E is present in the cell membranes where it acts as an anti-oxidant and quenches free oxygen radicals, so protecting the lipids of cell membranes from damage. In doing so it is rendered inactive but is restored by reacting with vitamin C.

Vitamin E protects LDL (low density lipoprotein, the main form of cholesterol in the blood, see page 77) from oxidation, and decreases the damage caused by ischaemia–reperfusion (the restoration of blood flow after a period of cessation, as in a heart attack).

Evidence is accumulating that high vitamin E status decreases the incidence of certain forms of cancer, decreases mortality from coronary (ischaemic) heart disease and also decreases the risk of cataract.

DEFICIENCY OF VITAMIN E

Deficiency causes severe damage of the membranes of nerves and muscle.

AT-RISK GROUPS

Deficiency due to *dietary* lack is unknown, but deficiency does occur in people who *cannot absorb fat* and *fat-soluble vitamins*. *Premature infants* are also at risk because they are born without adequate reserves. This lack affects the membranes of their red blood cells and may lead to haemolytic anaemia. *Smokers* may be at risk because of increased requirements. Tobacco smoke contains large amounts of free radicals and the alveolar fluid of smokers contains less vitamin E than non-smokers.

HIGH DOSES OF VITAMIN E

There is evidence that high doses, for example, 400 i.u. (International Unit, equivalent to 1 mg of synthetic d-alpha-tocopherol acetate) three times daily may decrease the symptoms of neurological disorders, such as tardive dyskinesia, slow the progression of Parkinson's disease and improve the mobility of arthritis sufferers.

TOXICITY OF VITAMIN E

Few effects have been reported.

REQUIREMENTS AND FOODS FOR VITAMIN E

There are no DRVs for vitamin E. The requirement increases with increasing intake of polyunsaturated fatty acids but fortunately foods containing PUFA are also good sources of vitamin E. The inverse relationship between vitamin E intake and mortality from CHD and some cancers, shown by epidemiological work and mentioned above, raises questions about what is the best level of intake. More work is needed.

Most foods contain vitamin E. Good sources are vegetable oils, poultry and fish, fortified breakfast cereals, eggs and whole-grain bread.

CHEMISTRY

Vitamin K includes three compounds, phylloquinone (the normal dietary source), menaquinone (compounds which are formed by intestinal bacteria) and menadione (a synthetic substance which is converted to phylloquinone in the body).

FUNCTIONS OF VITAMIN K

Vitamin K is essential for the formation of prothrombin and several other clotting agents and hence is essential for normal blood clotting.

DEFICIENCY OF VITAMIN K

The effect of deficiency is defective clotting of the blood.

AT-RISK GROUPS

Haemorrhagic disease of the new-born occurs in infants born with very low reserves. Almost all babies born in the UK are given vitamin K soon after birth either by intramuscular injection or orally. The dose given varies between centres.

There is a trend towards oral administration after reports in 1992 of an unexpected association between intramuscular vitamin K and later childhood cancer, although this association is so far unconfirmed.

Warfarin, used clinically as an anticoagulant, is an antagonist to vitamin K and theoretically its effect would be negated by large intakes of vitamin K.

TOXICITY OF VITAMIN K

Vitamin K is toxic in excess causing haemolysis and, in infants, anaemia, hyperbilirubinaemia (high level of bile pigments in the blood) and kernicterus, a condition of the new-born with severe neural symptoms.

FOODS FOR VITAMIN K

There are no DRVs. Although vitamin K is synthesized by bacteria in the gut, a dietary supply is also necessary. Volunteers on a vitamin K-deficient diet have shown prolonged blood clotting time, a symptom of deficiency. It is present in vegetable foods, such as spinach, cabbage, cauliflower, peas (the greener the vegetable, the more vitamin K) and cereals. It is stable to cooking but destroyed by light.

Vitamin B1 (thiamin)

CHEMISTRY

Thiamin is a single substance. In the body it is a coenzyme (a factor necessary for an enzyme to work) which is essential for several metabolic changes, including the breakdown of carbohydrate to produce energy.

DEFICIENCY OF THIAMIN

Beriberi is the disease resulting from long-term deficiency of thiamin but it is rare in the UK. Here the **Wernicke–Korsakoff syndrome** is seen in alcoholics. Symptoms include nystagmus of the eyes, a wide-based walk and confusion. Damage to the central nervous system results in loss of short-term memory and the inability to retain new information.

AT-RISK GROUPS

Alcoholics, in whom absorption from the gut is impaired.

Malnourished patients who are being supplemented with a high carbohydrate intake. Deficiency may be caused by the combination of low status and increased requirements because of the carbohydrate load.

TOXICITY OF THIAMIN

This is seen only at continued very high intakes, around 100 times the RNI.

FOODS FOR THIAMIN

A lot of foods contain small amounts of thiamin. Examples (in average portion sizes) are shown in Table 6.5.

Table 6.5 Thiamin (vitamin B1) content of average servings of foods

Food	Amount/weight (g)	Thiamin content (mg)
Bread (white)	Two slices, large, medium sliced loaf	0.16
Bread (brown)	Two slices, large, medium sliced loaf	0.19
Bread (wholemeal)	Two slices, large, medium sliced loaf	0.24
Rice (white)	165 g	0.02
Rice (brown)	165 g	0.23
Breakfast cereals	Average serving	0.25–0.66
Baked beans	200 g	0.14
Dahl, chickpea	155 g	0.22
Beef (steak)	85 g	0.14
Bacon	85 g	0.23–0.47
Marmite	One teaspoon, 5 g	0.16
Horlicks	Four heaped teaspoons	0.20
Ovaltine	Four heaped teaspoons	0.15

From Davies, J. and Dickerson, J. (1991).

FUNCTIONS OF RIBOFLAVIN

Vitamin B2 (riboflavin)

Riboflavin forms a coenzyme which is necessary for the release of energy from food.

DEFICIENCY OF RIBOFLAVIN

Deficiency is not fatal. The signs are cracking at the corners of the lips (cheilosis), a smooth, sore tongue (glossitis) and skin changes.

AT-RISK GROUPS

Deficiency is rare in the UK but a biochemical test (erythrocyte glutathione reductase coefficient) showed more abnormal results in elderly men than in young adults, suggesting that there may be some deficiency in the elderly. There is a need for more research on the needs of this group and of pregnant women.

TOXICITY OF RIBOFLAVIN

No cases are known.

It is widespread in foods and the main sources in the average British diet are milk, meat, fortified cereal products and egg.

Vitamin B3 (niacin)

CHEMISTRY

Niacin refers to two substances, *nicotinic acid* and *nicotinamide*. **Note:** nicotine from cigarettes has **no** vitamin activity.

FUNCTIONS OF NIACIN

Niacin is also a coenzyme involved in the liberation of energy from food.

DEFICIENCY OF NIACIN

The deficiency disease is pellagra, characterized by dermatitis, diarrhoea and dementia. It is almost unknown in the UK.

AT-RISK GROUPS

None.

TOXICITY OF NIACIN

High doses of nicotinic acid (but not nicotinamide) cause flushing. Very high doses (3–6 g/day) cause reversible liver malfunction.

FOODS FOR NIACIN

It is present in many foods. In the UK we get most of our niacin from meat and meat products, potatoes, bread and fortified breakfast cereals.

Niacin can be formed from the amino acid tryptophan, 60 mg being equivalent to 1 mg niacin. Because of this niacin values for food are expressed in **niacin equivalents** which equal mg niacin plus 1/60 mg tryptophan. The average intakes of tryptophan in this country are more than enough to meet the entire requirement for niacin.

CHEMISTRY

B6 refers to pyridoxal, pyridoxine, pyridoxamine and their 5'-phosphates, which are all converted in the body into the active pyridoxal phosphate.

FUNCTIONS OF B6

B6 is a coenzyme involved in the conversions of one amino acid to another (transamination), the metabolism of glycogen in muscle and liver, and in terminating the activity of steroid hormones, such as oestrogen, androgen and cortisol.

DEFICIENCY OF B6

Convulsions in infants, now extremely rare, result from deficiency.

It has been shown recently that deficiency of B6 results in increased nuclear uptake of steroid hormones and enhanced sensitivity of the target organs to hormone activity. This may be related to the cause and treatment of the hormone-dependent cancers of breast, uterus and prostate.

AT-RISK GROUPS

None. There are contradictory reports in the literature as to the effect of the contraceptive pill. Some experts claim that requirement is increased and that women on marginal dietary intakes may be at risk and others (COMA Report 41, Department of Health, 1991) state that oral contraceptives do not cause deficiency. Similarly conflicting reports exist on whether large (pharmacological) doses may overcome some of the side effects of the contraceptive pill or alleviate the premenstrual syndrome.

TOXICITY OF B6

Reversible peripheral sensory neuropathy has been reported in people taking 50–500 mg/day for several months.

FOODS FOR B6

The requirement depends on protein intake and rises proportionately with it. The main sources in an average diet are meat, potatoes and other vegetables.

Vitamin B12   CHEMISTRY

There are several cobalt-containing compounds which have vitamin B12 activity. These include cyanocobalamin, which is the commercially available form, aquocobalamin and methylcobalamin.

FUNCTIONS OF B12

It is needed for nerve myelination (the myelin sheath is essential for normal transmission of nerve impulses) and interacts with folate coenzymes.

DEFICIENCY OF B12

This causes **pernicious** or **megaloblastic anaemia** in which the normal division of red blood cells is disrupted so that they enter the blood stream at an early stage, when they are bigger and fewer then normal. Prolonged deficiency leads to irreversible neurological damage.

B12 deficiency in pregnancy is a risk factor for neural tube defects in the new-born.

AT-RISK GROUPS

Dietary deficiency is unusual, except in some *vegans*. But groups with very low intakes (0.26–0.4 μg per day) have been reported as showing no symptoms.

For absorption of the vitamin to occur it must bind first to a factor in saliva (salivary haptocorrin) and then to the intrinsic factor, which is secreted by the parietal cells of the stomach. Lack of the intrinsic factor is the common cause of pernicious anaemia, which occurs in the *elderly*, and *after gastrectomy* and in *Crohn's disease*.

TOXICITY OF B12

It has extremely low toxicity.

FOODS FOR B12

B12 is found only in animal foods and the main sources in the diet are offal, meats and milk. It is present in the yeast extract Marmite, at

0.33 μg per 4 g serving, so that two generous servings would give 50% of the adult RNI.

CHEMISTRY

Folic acid (pteroyl glutamic acid) gives rise to a large number of derivatives and these have the collective name of folates; therefore this vitamin may be referred to as folic acid or as folate. Folacin is sometimes used on food labels.

FUNCTIONS OF FOLATE

Folate is involved in a number of chemical reactions in the body, which are closely linked with those of B12. For further details of these metabolic functions see Bender and Bender (1982).

DEFICIENCY OF FOLATE

Rapidly dividing cells are most severely affected and this leads to megaloblastic anaemia (or megaloblastosis). Other effects are large blood platelets, abnormalities of the intestinal mucosa and slowed growth in babies and young children.

AT-RISK GROUPS

There is increased requirement of folate in *pregnancy*. Women who have been on long-term oral contraceptive medication before repeated pregnancies are at risk, as are women with repeated pregnancies.

Neural tube defects (spina bifida, anencephaly) in the new-born are due, in the vast majority of cases, to a block in folate metabolism (see pages 203–4), which can be overcome by high levels of folate before conception.

The *elderly* and *alcoholics* may also be at risk of folate deficiency.

TOXICITY OF FOLATE

There is little danger of toxicity but high intakes may reduce zinc absorption. Folate supplements given to people with B12 deficiency may confuse the diagnosis.

FOODS FOR FOLATE

Folate occurs in small amounts in many foods. Green leafy vegetables, liver and kidney, nuts and whole-grain cereals are good sources. However, there are many people who eat these foods rarely, and folate is easily destroyed in cooking. Normal cooking destroys 80% of the folate in vegetables and with longer cooking and keeping hot there is complete destruction. The increase in take-away food may mean that many people have low intakes. Yeast extracts such as Marmite are a useful source.

Pantothenic acid FUNCTIONS OF PANTOTHENIC ACID

Pantothenic acid forms part of the molecule of coenzyme A which is essential for the liberation of energy from carbohydrates, fats and proteins.

DEFICIENCY OF PANTOTHENIC ACID

There is no good evidence of pantothenic acid deficiency occurring in humans except experimentally, when the symptoms are fatigue, headache, dizziness, muscle weakness and intestinal disturbances.

AT RISK GROUPS

None.

TOXICITY OF PANTOTHENIC ACID

Very large doses (10 g per day) may cause diarrhoea and gastro-intestinal disturbances but no other toxic signs have been noted.

FOODS FOR PANTOTHENIC ACID

It is widely distributed in foods and there are no DRVs. Average intakes in the UK are between 3–7 mg per day and are obviously sufficient to meet requirements.

FUNCTIONS OF BIOTIN

Biotin is important in the formation of adipose tissue (lipogenesis), the production of glucose from other energy sources in the body and in the metabolism of some amino acids.

DEFICIENCY OF BIOTIN

The only cases of deficiency have been in people who eat large amounts of raw egg white (which contains a protein, avidin, which binds biotin and makes it unavailable); they showed a fine scaly dermatitis and hair loss. Experimental studies of depletion have also been conducted, producing additional symptoms of glossitis, anorexia, nausea and mental changes.

AT-RISK GROUPS

Those maintained on total parenteral (intravenous) nutrition for long periods and those consuming very large amounts of raw egg white.

TOXICITY OF BIOTIN

There is no evidence.

FOODS FOR BIOTIN

There are no DRVs and the COMA report 41 (Department of Health, 1991) concluded that intakes of between 10 and 200 µg per day are safe and adequate. It is synthesized in the gut and is in offal, egg yolk, milk and dairy products, cereals, fish, fruit and vegetables.

Vitamin C (ascorbic acid)

CHEMISTRY

Vitamin C, or ascorbic acid, is a sugar which is a powerful anti-oxidant. It is easily destroyed. In fruit and vegetables there is an enzyme, ascorbic acid oxidase, which inactivates vitamin C and which is released by bruising and chopping. Cabbage or a salad, if chopped in advance of use, will lose a lot of vitamin C because of this. The enzyme is inactivated by boiling.

Vitamin C is also lost into cooking water and by keeping hot. Adding bicarbonate of soda, to keep vegetables green, destroys all the vitamin C.

FUNCTIONS OF VITAMIN C

Vitamin C is involved in the formation of collagen and therefore in wound healing. It is an important anti-oxidant, especially in the regeneration of oxidized vitamin E in membranes in the body. In this way it is important in maintaining membrane structure. It aids the absorption of iron from vegetable sources (that is, non-haem iron).

DEFICIENCY OF VITAMIN C

The deficiency disease is **scurvy**. Impaired collagen formation leads to small haemorrhages at base of hair follicles, inflammation and bleeding of the gums, loosening and eventual loss of the teeth and bone pain. Impaired synthesis of adrenaline and noradrenaline causes depression and irritability.

Less severe deficiency, which might be encountered today, presents with extreme fatigue, personality changes and haemorrhages in the lower limbs (Pietrzik, 1991).

Signs of mild deficiency are stated to be lassitude, fatigue, anorexia and greater susceptibility to infection and stress (Pietrzik, 1991).

Vitamin C deficiency is often linked with other nutritional deficiencies.

AT-RISK GROUPS

Vitamin C is found only in fruits and vegetables and is very easily destroyed. The *elderly, young girls* and *athletes* are at-risk groups. Smokers and pregnant and lactating women require high intakes to reach a maximum pool of ascorbic acid and diabetes seems to increase the metabolic turnover. The recognition of early signs of deficiency is important.

TOXICITY OF VITAMIN C

There is no evidence of toxicity.

Table 6.6 Vitamin C content of average serving of foods

Food	Amount/weight	Vitamin C content (mg)
Fresh apple	One	2
Banana	One	8
Orange	One	93
Tangerine	One	21
Guavas, canned	Six halves	315
Grapefruit, canned	Six segments	36
Orange juice, canned	One glass	62–70
Tomatoes	Two	30
Tomatoes (canned)	140 g	25
Lettuce	30 g	5
Peppers	45 g	45
Coleslaw	85 g	27
Potatoes (boiled)	150 g	9–14
Chips	150 g	27
Peas (frozen)	75 g	27
Carrots	65 g	3
Cauliflower	100 g	20
Swede	120 g	20
Mushrooms	55 g	1

From Davies, J. and Dickerson, J. (1991).

FOODS FOR VITAMIN C

The vitamin C content of foods is listed in Table 6.6. Dried fruits, processed peas and jams contain no vitamin C nor do cereals and grains, unless fortified.

VITAMIN C

Pauling (1970) advised the intake of 14 g of ascorbic acid per day. This amount was derived theoretically by extrapolation from the ascorbate production of rats and other mammals. There is no evidence of any obvious benefits. A large proportion of such a dose will be excreted in the urine, increasing the risk of kidney stones by increasing the excretion of oxalic acid and interfering with the dip-stick test for glucose in urine.

There have been repeated reports that large doses (0.5–1 g) reduce the severity of the common cold, but proof is lacking. Such intakes would do no harm.

The Household Food Consumption and Expenditure survey shows average intakes well above the RNI (Table 6.7). This would indicate no

Large (pharmacological) doses of vitamins

Vitamin intake in the UK, 1991–1993

Table 6.7 Average vitamin intakes as a percentage of Reference Nutrient Intake. (National Food Survey figures)*

Vitamin	1991	1992	1993
Thiamin	153	150	149
Riboflavin	144	139	142
Niacin equivalent	182	179	178
B6	132	139	156
B12	360	354	350
Folate	129	130	127
C	144	131	134
A (retinol equivalent)	181	185	179

* A 10% allowance for wastage has been made and meals taken outside the home have been allowed for.

Table 6.8 Vitamin intake, 1993, by income group (as percentage of RNI). (National Food Survey figures)

	Income groups						
	Gross weekly income of head of household						
	Households with one or more earner				Households without an earner		
	£520+ A	£280–520 B	£140–280 C	Less than £140 D	£140+ E1	Less than £140 E2	OAP
Thiamin	152	145	145	150	177	145	156
Riboflavin	146	138	135	133	163	135	143
Niacin equivalent	184	176	174	173	210	172	181
B6	163	154	153	159	179	153	153
B12	366	347	347	345	394	337	349
Folate	137	126	122	126	151	123	125
C	185	141	122	113	179	112	118
A	165	170	178	190	213	171	215

A, B, C, D, E1 and E2 designate socioeconomic classes.
(Table 6.7 and 6.8 are from COMA report, 1993. Crown copyright is reproduced with the permission of the Controller of HMSO.)

cause for concern about the vitamin intake *of most people* (MAFF; annual reports). However, average values may conceal very big variations and it is those with increased need and/or dietary limitations, whether from poverty, unusual food beliefs or just poor cooking, who are at risk. Note the effect of a reducing income on vitamin intake (Table 6.8). A similar effect is seen with increasing household size.

VITAMIN CONTENT OF TWO DIETS

Two diets are given below, one fairly typical of an 'unhealthy' diet (although it is quite possible to eat much worse than this) and the other

one much better balanced. Average portion sizes and food tables have
been used to give estimates of five vitamins.

Diet 1

Breakfast:	Toast (white), margarine, tea
Mid-morning:	Chocolate biscuit, tea
Lunch:	Tuna sandwiches, crisps, tea
Afternoon:	Ginger biscuits, tea
Evening:	Shepherd's pie, doughnut, tea
	Beer
	Toast, tea

Table 6.9 shows that the lack of fruit and vegetables has resulted in a
low intake of vitamins C and A (there are virtually no carotenes in the
diet). However, there is enough of these five vitamins to maintain
health in normal circumstances although stores may be low.

Table 6.9   Diet 1 – vitamin content

Food	Amount/weight (g)	Vitamin A – retinol equivalents (µg)	Thiamin (mg)	Riboflavin (mg)	Niacin equivalents (mg)	Vitamin C (mg)
Toast, white	70g (two slices)	0	0.16	0.05	2.6	0
Margarine	16 g	144	Trace	Trace	Trace	0
Tea		0	Trace	0.02	0.2	0
Tea		0	Trace	0.02	0.2	0
Chocolate biscuit (Penguin)	One, 25 g	Trace	0.01	0.03	0.4	0
Tuna sandwich: margarine	16 g	144	Trace	Trace	Trace	0
Tuna	95 g	Not known	0.04	0.10	16.3	0
Bread	70 g	0	0.16	0.05	2.6	0
Crisps	One packet	0	0.06	0.02	1.8	5
Tea		0	Trace	0.02	0.2	0
Tea		0	Trace	0.02	0.2	0
Biscuits, ginger	20 g	Not known	0.02	0.01	0.4	0
Shepherd's pie	165 g	23	0.07	0.20	5.3	3
Doughnut	70 g	Not known	0.15	0.05	1.8	Not known
Tea		0	Trace	0.02	0.2	0
Beer (bitter)	Two pints	0	0	0.34	6.8	0
Toast, white	70 g	0	0.16	0.05	2.6	0
Butter	16 g	142	Trace	0	0	Trace
Milk in tea	⅓ pint (190 ml)	109	0.06	0.33	1.6	2
Totals		562	0.89	1.33	43.2	10
RNI, male, 19–50 years		700	1.0	1.3	17	40

From Davies, J. and Dickerson, J. (1991)

Diet 2

Breakfast:	Cornflakes, orange juice, toast (wholemeal), marmalade
Mid-morning:	Digestive biscuit, milk
Lunch:	Sardine sandwich, tomato, tea
Afternoon:	Banana, tea
Evening:	Roast chicken, potatoes, carrots, cabbage.
	Rice pudding, tea

Table 6.10 shows that the RNIs are exceeded in all cases and therefore the eater will not only be well-nourished but will have good body stores. Clearly no vitamin supplements are needed if a good diet is eaten.

Table 6.10   Diet 2 – vitamin content

Food	Amount/weight (g)	Vitamin A – retinol equivalents (µg)	Thiamin (mg)	Riboflavin (mg)	Niacin equivalents (mg)	Vitamin C (mg)
Cornflakes	25 g	0	0.25	0.38	4.2	0
Milk	115 g	26	0.05	0.21	1.0	1
Orange juice	200 g	16	0.14	0.04	0.6	62
Bread, wholemeal	70 g	0	0.24	0.06	4.1	0
Marmalade	20 g	2	0	0	0	2
Milk, semi-skimmed	One glass, 195 ml	45	0.08	0.35	1.7	2
Biscuits, digestive	Two, 30 g	0	0.04	0.03	0.7	0
Sardines	70 g	Trace	0.03	0.25	8.8	0
Bread	140 g	0	0.48	0.12	8.2	0
Tomato	One, 75 g	75	0.04	0.03	0.6	15
Tea		0	Trace	0.02	0.2	0
Milk, in tea	35	8	0.01	0.06	0.3	0
Banana	One, 135 g	27	0.03	0.05	0.7	8
Chicken, roast	85 g	0	0.05	0.14	8.9	0
Potatoes, boiled	150 g	0	0.12	0.05	1.7	14
Cabbage	75 g	38	0.02	0.02	0.3	11
Carrots	65 g	1300	0.03	0.03	0.3	3
Rice pudding (semi-skimmed milk)	85 g	20	0.03	0.14	0.9	1
Totals		**1559**	**1.64**	**1.98**	**43.2**	**119**
RNI, male, 19–50 years		700	1.0	1.3	17	40

From Davies, J. and Dickerson, J. (1991).

CASE STUDY

Restoration of a brilliant mind

She was in her 80s, a distinguished elderly academic . . . her general practitioner telephoned me with the sad news that she was 'on the way out', confused, short of breath. . . . Her once brilliant mind was unravelled indeed. Pallid, wild-eyed and breathing with extreme difficulty . . . her calories had come mainly from her substantial stock of good clarets. Her pallor had a lemon tint and her pernicious anaemia was promptly diagnosed and confirmed. A large retrosternal goitre explained . . . respiratory difficulty . . . accompanying hypothyroidism . . . .

More balanced nutrition with liberal vitamins, vitamin B12 by injection, careful thyroxin replacement, and the passage of time saw a miraculous transformation. . . .

(Reproduced with permission from Keen H, British Medical Journal, 307, 1194.)

Key points

1. There are 13 vitamins, four fat-soluble and the rest water-soluble. DRVs have been produced for eight.
2. In general, requirements are higher, per kg body weight, for children, pregnant and lactating women and those recovering from illness or surgery.
3. A well-nourished person has sufficient stores for a period of weeks for most water-soluble vitamins, for months for the fat-soluble and for years for B12 and so it is the *average* rather than the daily intake which is important.
4. Values of vitamins from food tables are *indications* rather than exact amount due to variables including the loss in cooking of water-soluble vitamins. The content on food labels is usually exceeded.
5. Most people eating a good diet have more than adequate intakes of vitamins and do not need supplements. Groups at risk of sub-optimal intakes are those with low energy intake, alcoholics, heavy smokers, those on long-term medication and food faddists. Asians are at risk of vitamin D deficiency and pregnant women have increased needs for folate. Low maternal folate status is related to neural tube defects in the new-born.
6. Best buys for supplements (*Which?*, 1990) are Sanatogen Multi-vitamins and Boots Plurivite M.
7. Vitamin A is seldom deficient except where fat absorption is impaired as in coeliac disease, cystic fibrosis, chronic liver disease. Excess intake is dangerous for pregnant women and they should not eat liver.
8. Vitamin D may be deficient in young and pregnant Asians and the house-bound elderly. The deficiency is usually due to lack of sunlight.
9. Vitamin E is particularly important for smokers and in large doses has useful therapeutic effects in tardive dyskinesia, Parkinson's disease, cataracts and arthritis.

10. Vitamin K is present in many foods. It is given routinely at birth to prevent the haemorrhagic disease of the new-born.
11. Thiamin may be deficient in alcoholics. Malnourished patients, being given carbohydrate supplements, will have increased need. It is easily lost in cooking. Ovaltine and Horlicks are good additional sources.
12. Vitamin B12 is found in animal foods only so vegans may be deficient. It is not absorbed after gastrectomy. Marmite is a useful source.
13. Riboflavin, niacin, B6, pantothenic acid and biotin are unlikely to be deficient.
14. Folate requirements are increased in pregnancy and supplements should be given to women who have had a child with neural tube defects; it reduces the incidence of this defect. Chronic alcoholics may be deficient. It is easily lost in cooking. Marmite is a useful additional source.
15. Vitamin C is present only in vegetables and fruit. It is easily lost in cooking and so those with a poor diet or poorly cooked vegetables may be deficient. There is no proof that very large doses protect against cancer and other diseases and they may interfere with the dip-stick test for glucose in urine.

Mineral elements 7

This chapter gives an outline of the functions of the mineral elements in the body and the effects of deficiency, identifies the groups at risk and the main dietary sources.

Mineral elements, such as calcium, sodium, iron, zinc and copper, are essential in the diet but are needed in small or very small amounts. Those minerals required in small amounts are called *micronutrients* while those needed in very small amounts are often called *trace elements*. The trace elements are chromium, copper, iodine, iron, manganese, molybdenum, selenium, zinc, cobalt and fluoride.

Minerals play a variety of roles in the body. Some, such as calcium, phosphorus and magnesium, are part of the structure of bones and teeth. Others, such as sodium and potassium are present in the blood or the cells, respectively. Yet others, such as zinc, copper and selenium, are part of enzymes, which carry out vital reactions in the body.

Mineral elements are not, like vitamins, destroyed by cooking but the dietary source is not always fully available to the body, or, in scientific terms, the **bioavailability** is often limited (see Box 7.1).

BOX 7.1

Bioavailability is the proportion of the nutrient from the diet which is used in the body. It depends on a number of factors and varies with different nutrients.

Of the mineral and trace elements, calcium, iron, zinc and copper have limited bioavailability. For example, the presence of phytate, oxalate and other substances in foods may bind the minerals and render them unavailable. Other factors are physiological ones, such as age, nutritional status, state of health, and the ability of individuals to adapt to variations in nutrient supply.

Phytate is an organic compound, found in unrefined cereals. It is broken down during the action of yeast in bread, rolls and buns.

Oxalate is an organic acid which is found in rhubarb, strawberries and spinach, for example.

Table 7.1 Reference Nutrient Intakes for Minerals

Age	Calcium (mg/day)	Phosphorus* (mg/day)	Magnesium (mg/day)	Sodium† (mg/day)	Potassium‡ (mg/day)	Chloride§ (mg/day)	Iron (mg/day)	Zinc (mg/day)	Copper (mg/day)	Selenium (µg/day)	Iodine (µg/day)
Children											
0–3 months	525	400	55	210	800	320	1.7	4.0	0.2	10	50
4–6 months	525	400	60	280	850	400	4.3	4.0	0.3	13	60
7–9 months	525	400	75	320	700	500	7.8	5.0	0.3	10	60
10–12 months	525	400	80	350	700	500	7.8	5.0	0.3	10	60
1–3 years	350	270	85	500	800	800	6.9	5.0	0.4	15	70
4–6 years	450	350	120	700	1100	1100	6.1	6.5	0.6	20	100
7–10 years	550	450	200	1200	2000	1800	8.7	7.0	0.7	30	110
Males											
11–14 years	1000	775	280	1600	3100	2500	11.3	9.0	0.8	45	130
15–18 years	1000	775	300	1600	3500	2500	11.3	9.5	1.0	70	140
19–50 years	700	550	300	1600	3500	2500	8.7	9.5	1.2	75	140
50+ years	700	550	300	1600	3500	2500	8.7	9.5	1.2	75	140
Females											
11–14 year	800	625	280	1600	3100	2500	14.8**	9.0	0.8	45	130
15–18 years	800	625	300	1600	3500	2500	14.8**	7.0	1.0	60	140
19–50 years	700	550	270	1600	3500	2500	14.8**	7.0	1.2	60	140
50+ years	700	550	270	1600	3500	2500	8.7	7.0	1.2	60	140
Pregnancy	NI	NI	NI	NI	NI	NI	NI	NI	NI	NI	NI
Lactation											
0–4 months	+550	+440	+50	NI	NI	NI	NI	+6.0	+0.3	+15	NI
4+ months	+550	+440	+50	NI	NI	NI	NI	+2.5	+0.3	+15	NI

* Phosphorus RNI is set equal to calcium in molar terms.
† 1 mmol sodium = 23 mg.
‡ 1 mmol potassium = 39 mg.
§ Corresponds to sodium 1 mmol = 35.5 mg.
** Insufficient for women with high menstrual losses where the most practical way of meeting iron requirements is to take iron supplements.
NI, No increment.

For those eating a varied diet, there is little risk of mineral deficiency in the UK, except for iron (see page 124), though those with a very low energy intake may have some marginal inadequacies.

The main concern is too much dietary sodium, which is linked to the development of *essential hypertension* (raised blood pressure of no known cause).

Mineral supplements are not, generally, advisable. They are not usually needed and a supplement of zinc, say, may reduce the absorption of copper. As for all nutrients, a varied diet is the best solution.

We will now look at the separate minerals in turn, the main characteristics of which are summarized in Tables 7.1 and Table 7.2. Further details for each mineral are included in the text.

There is little evidence of either dietary deficiency or excess in the UK. Bodily deficiency or excess of calcium is usually caused by too little or too much vitamin D (see page 95).

Calcium

IMPORTANCE OF CALCIUM

Some 99% of the body's calcium (about 1.2 kg in an adult) is in the bones and teeth where it contributes to their structure and hardness. Peak bone mass is achieved around the age of 30 and the higher it is, the stronger the bones. It begins to fall a few years later, accelerating in females about five years after the menopause (see Box 7.2).

A number of factors are known to affect *peak bone mass*. These are:

- Genetic – genetic factors are the main determinants of bone mass, accounting for about 80% of the total. Environmental factors affect the other 20%.
- Nutritional – calcium, protein and energy intakes appear to be important.
- Hormonal – growth hormone, sex hormones, parathyroid hormone and calcitonin are involved in calcium metabolism.
- The amount of exercise taken – exercise increases bone mass. In tennis players the bones of the playing arm are thicker and the mineral content is higher than for the other arm.

A small but vital amount of calcium is present in the blood, where it is essential for the normal excitability of nerves and muscles. A fall in blood calcium causes *tetany* (spontaneous contraction of muscles).

Table 7.2 Characteristic of dietary mineral elements

Mineral element	Functions	Deficiency	Excess	Main dietary sources
Calcium	Bones, teeth Nerve excitability	Rickets, osteomalacia, but usually vitamin D lack	No harm	Milk, cheese, bread, green vegetables
Phosphorus	Bones Metabolic compounds	Unknown	Tetany in new-born	Nearly all foods
Magnesium	Skeletal development Nerve, muscle impulses	Weakness, cardiac effects Rare	No toxicity from diet	Widespread
Sodium and chloride	Extracellular fluid volume, nerve, muscle impulses	Cramps, fall in blood pressure	Hypernatraemia in infants, possibly hypertension in adults	Mainly processed foods
Potassium	Main intracellular cation	Muscle weakness, cardiac irregularities	Unlikely from diet	Vegetables, meat, milk
Iron	In haemoglobin, oxygen carrier	Anaemia; fatigue, pallor, breathlessness	Can be lethal	Meat, bread, potatoes, vegetables
Zinc	Enzyme component	Slow growth Skin changes	Nausea, vomiting Prolonged-blood changes	Meat, milk, bread, other cereals
Copper	Enzyme component	Leucopenia, skeletal changes In adults, cardiovascular effects	Toxic but unknown in UK	Meat, bread, other cereals, vegetables
Selenium	Enzyme component	Keshan disease (cardiomyopathy) Unknown in UK	Some toxicity	Cereals, meat, fish

BOX 7.2

Risk factors for **bone loss** include:

- immobility;
- early menopause;
- family history;
- low calcium intake;
- underweight;
- high alcohol consumption;
- smoking.

Calcium is necessary for blood clotting and for the normal action of some hormones.

CALCIUM DEFICIENCY

Calcium deficiency causes *rickets* in children (Box 7.3) and *osteomalacia* in adults (Box 7.4). The deficiency is nearly always because of lack of vitamin D (see page 95). Rickets is still something of a puzzle; a calcium deficiency with adequate vitamin D does *not* cause rickets although growth is slowed.

BOX 7.3

Rickets is a condition of growing children. The bones are softer than normal because of a lack of calcium compounds. Symptoms are:

- bone pain and tenderness;
- deformity: bandy legs, knock knees, swelling at the ends of long bones;
- infants are pale, fretful, slow to crawl and walk.

BOX 7.4

Osteomalacia affects adults. There is loss of bone mass with bone pain or tenderness, particularly in shoulder, hip and spine.

Osteoporosis is a condition in which the bones become lighter or less dense than normal. The bone salts are unchanged but there is less of them. Fractures are more likely.

The incidence has doubled over the past 30 years. Incidence and severity are reduced if the maximum peak bone mass is achieved in youth.

Osteoporosis is not caused directly by diet. For post-menopausal women, hormonal replacement therapy is the most effective treatment. But those at risk may benefit from raised calcium intakes and this is worth trying as there is no risk of toxicity.

EFFECTS OF EXCESS DIETARY CALCIUM

It is almost unknown for dietary calcium to cause a bodily excess, since absorption is controlled. It may occur in cases of vitamin D excess or hormonal imbalance.

CALCIUM REQUIREMENTS

The average calcium intake in the UK in 1993 was 121% of the RNI (Table 7.3) (MAFF, 1995b). This figure from the National Food Survey shows that there is no real cause for concern, even though the average calcium intake has been falling (Figure 7.1). Intake has fallen because people have been eating less bread in total, and more wholemeal, which, unlike white bread, is not fortified with calcium. Milk and cheese, too, are now seen by many people as high fat foods to be avoided rather than foods rich in protein and calcium.

Table 7.3 Dietary Reference Values for calcium (mg/day). (From COMA 41, Department of Health, 1991) Crown copyright is reproduced with the permission of the Controller of HMSO.

Age	Lower Reference Nutrient Intake	Estimated Average Requirement	Reference Nutrient Intake
0–12 months	240	400	525
1–3 years	200	275	350
4–6 years	275	350	450
7–10 years	325	425	550
11–14 years, male	450	750	1000
11–14 years, female	480	625	800
15–18 years, male	450	750	1000
15–18 years, female	480	625	800
19–50 years	400	525	700
50+ years	400	525	700
Pregnancy: no increment	–	–	–
Lactation	–	–	+550

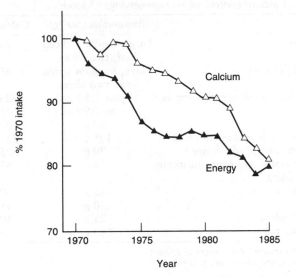

Figure 7.1 Decline in calcium and energy intake in Britain between 1970 and 1985. Data from the British National Food Survey, MAFF 1970–1985. (Redrawn with permission from Pietrzik,.K. (ed.), *Modern Lifestyles, Lower Energy Intake and Micronutrient Status*; Springer-Verlag, London, 1991.)

There is concern that some groups, particularly teenage girls, may not achieve maximum bone density because of the combined effects of a low intake of calcium and an inactive life-style and may therefore be at risk of osteoporosis in later life (Pietrzik, 1991).

BIOAVAILABILITY OF CALCIUM

The absorption of calcium from the gut is controlled by 1,25-dihydroxyvitamin D (calcitriol) according to the needs of the body. Absorption is increased in pregnancy and during growth.

Certain foods, such as rhubarb, strawberries and spinach, are rich in *oxalates* which bind calcium and prevent it being absorbed in the gut. *Phytates*, present in unleavened wholemeal cereals, have the same effect.

This combination of dietary and hormonal factors makes it difficult to predict how much will be absorbed but studies on subjects eating a mixed diet have shown average absorptions of calcium of between 18–46%.

There is adaptation to low intakes, and this is clearly shown in populations who customarily have very low calcium intakes and show no deficiency.

Table 7.4 Calcium content of average servings of foods

Food	Amount/weight (g)	Calcium (mg)
Bread (white)	Large, medium sliced loaf, two slices	83
Bread (wholemeal)	Large, medium sliced loaf, two slices	38
Milk (whole, semi-skimmed, skimmed)	⅓ pint (190 ml)	224–234
Soya milk	⅓ pint (190 ml)	25
Cheese, hard	40 g	220–288
Canned pilchards in tomato sauce	105 g	315
Sardines, canned in oil, drained	70 g	385
Evaporated milk, as cream substitute with pudding	30 g	87
Fromage frais	45 g	40
Peanuts	30 g	18
Cabbage (boiled)	75 g	40
Spinach (boiled)	130 g	780

Plantain and yam are poor sources of calcium.
From Davies, J. and Dickerson, J. (1991).

FOOD SOURCES OF CALCIUM

Calcium is present in milk and milk products in large quantities. It is added to white flour but not to wholemeal flour. Green vegetables are rich in calcium. Hard water may be a useful source.

CALCIUM CONTENT

Typical calcium content for common foods (average portions) are shown in Table 7.4 (Davies and Dickerson, 1991).

The group requiring the most calcium are young males and so we have chosen them as an example to show how their needs can be met from common foods.

EAR for males of 11–18 years	= 750 mg
RNI for males, 11–18 years	= 1000 mg

Example 1

One pint milk	= 660 mg
50 g cheese	= 400 mg
Four slices white bread	= 166 mg
Total	= **1226 mg** (above the RNI)

Example 2

⅓ pint milk	= 234 mg
Two slices wholemeal bread	= 38 mg
Baked beans, 200 g	= 90 mg

Fruit yoghurt, one small carton = 240 mg
Crisps, two packets = 22 mg
Coco Pops, 75 g helping = 24 mg
Mars bar, one = 104 mg
Total = **752 mg** (reaches the EAR but below the RNI)

It has been noted that milk and cheese are very important contributors to calcium intake. What about those who like neither? Milk can be introduced in yoghurts, ice-cream, evaporated milk, and by using dried milk powder in soups, mashed potato, and so on. Milk shakes, made by whisking milk with drinking chocolate powder, are popular with children. Cheese may be often preferred in toasted sandwiches or as soft processed cheese. Alternatively, plenty of green vegetables and oily fish (including kippers and herring) are excellent sources of calcium.

Phosphorus

Phosporus-containing compounds are very important in the body but nutritionally there are no problems of deficiency or excess. Phosphorus is present in all natural foods and in many processed ones, and so rarely arouses the anxiety of nutritionists.

There is nearly as much phosphorus in the body as calcium. It is present in the bones and in all tissues as metabolically important phosphate compounds, such as adenosine triphosphate and glucose-6-phosphate.

The only point of dietetic importance is that for infant feeds the ratio of phosphorus to calcium should not be outside the range of $1.2 : 1$ to $2.2 : 1$, weight-for-weight. This is followed by manufacturers of artificial feeds.

Iron

Iron is present in foods in fairly small amounts with no single common food being a very rich source. In addition, absorption from the gut may be low so that iron deficiency is the most common mineral deficiency. In assessing diets, particularly for women and infants, the supply of iron should always be considered.

FUNCTIONS OF IRON

Most iron, about 4–5 g in an adult, is in the oxygen-carrying pigment, haemoglobin, in the red blood cells. As such it is vital in the transport of adequate supplies of oxygen to the tissues. Smaller amounts of iron are found in the muscles in myoglobin, another oxygen-carrying compound. Iron is also part of important enzyme systems, vital in oxidizing substrates to release energy needed by cells. These enzyme systems act as electron carriers in the cell and as such are important in the use of oxygen to release energy from food.

Free iron is harmful. It acts to catalyse (or promote) oxidation, for example of the unsaturated lipids of cell membranes (see Box 7.5) so that they no longer function as a barrier for the cell. The iron in the body is harmless because it is usually bound to protein and segregated within the cells. It is *transported* in the blood plasma bound to a protein, transferrin.

BOX 7.5

LIPIDS OF CELL MEMBRANES

You'll remember that the cell membranes are composed of a bi-layer of unsaturated fatty acids, and if these are oxidized, as in fats that have gone rancid, they no longer function properly as a barrier.

Iron is *stored* in the liver, the spleen and the bones. The storage compounds are ferritin and haemosiderin. These stores may vary from zero to 1500 mg: they are usually higher in men, rarely being more than 500 mg in women.

IRON DEFICIENCY

Iron deficiency usually develops slowly. There are two stages; the first, iron deficiency and the second, the more severe, iron-deficiency anaemia.

Iron deficiency is characterized by low iron stores, low saturation of transferrin with iron and therefore by a reduced iron supply to the tissues. This reduced supply affects cells with a high turnover most, such as intestinal mucosal cells and red blood cells (Box 7.6). Haemoglobin production falls and the haemoglobin level will fall below the optimum level for the particular individual.

BOX 7.6

TURNOVER OF CELLS

This is their life span and rate of renewal. Red blood cells have a life of about 120 days, one of the shortest of all cells.

There has been a considerable amount of research carried out in iron-deficient animals which suggests that the capacity for physical work is reduced and studies on humans, in spite of methodological difficulties, also indicate that work performance and productivity are reduced. Results from animal experiments show changes in brain composition and metabolism, and iron-deficient rats perform less well in learning and memory tasks. There have been some studies in humans which suggest, but do not prove, that there may be lasting ill-effects of iron deficiency in infancy.

Iron-deficient schoolchildren showed an improvement in their school performance after iron supplements (Pietrzik, 1991; Department of Health, 1994).

Iron is essential for some immunological responses and there have been several studies on this; however, no firm conclusions can yet be made (Pietrzik, 1991).

Iron-deficiency anaemia occurs when the haemoglobin level has fallen below 130 g/l of blood for men and 120 g/l for women. Normal values are 150 g/l and 140 g/l respectively. The most obvious symptoms are those of a reduced oxygen supply to the tissues, breathlessness and lack of energy. Pallor and sometimes amenhorrhoea are characteristic.

BOX 7.7

> **Amenorrhoea** is the absence of menstrual cycles in women of reproductive age.

Vulnerable groups in the UK for iron deficiency are those with high physiological requirements: infants and toddlers, adolescents, pregnant women and women with high menstrual loss (an estimated 5% of menstruating women). Also vulnerable are those with poor absorption (such as the elderly) and those with a high intake of dietary iron inhibitors, such as tannin from tea.

IRON EXCESS

Iron homeostasis is maintained through control of absorption as there are no excretory mechanisms. If the intestinal control is swamped by very large intakes, iron poisoning can occur. Most cases occur in children, mistaking iron tablets for sweets. The acute toxic dose in infants is around 20 mg. For adults, 100 mg is lethal.

Table 7.5 Dietary Reference Values for iron (mg/day). (From COMA 41, Department of Health, 1991)

Age	Lower Reference Nutrient Intake	Estimated Average Requirement	Reference Nutrient Intake
0–3 months	0.9	1.3	1.7
4–6 months	2.3	3.3	4.3
7–9 months	4.2	6.0	7.8
10–12 months	4.2	6.0	7.8
1–3 years	3.7	5.3	6.9
4–6 years	3.3	4.7	6.1
7–10 years	4.7	6.7	8.7
11–14 years, males	6.1	8.7	11.3
11–14 years, females	8.0	11.4	14.8
15–18 years, males	6.1	8.7	11.3
15–18 years, females	8.0	11.4	14.8
19–50 years, males	4.7	6.7	8.7
19–50 years, females	8.0	11.4	14.8
50+ years	4.7	6.7	8.7

REQUIREMENTS OF IRON

DRVs for iron are shown in Table 7.5.

There are no recommended increments for pregnancy or lactation, unless iron stores at the start of pregnancy are low, as may be the case in women who have been slimming or have had a poor diet for one reason or another.

The intake in the UK, from the Household Food Consumption and Expenditure for 1993, ranges from 9.5 mg to 12.5 mg per day, according to income. The lower intakes were for those on low incomes (MAFF).

IRON BIOAVAILABILITY

The absorption of iron from the small intestine is complex. The absorptive mechanisms for haem iron (from meat) and for non-haem iron (the inorganic form, from plant foods) are different.

Haem iron is usually better absorbed (on average, about 25% of the total on average) than non-haem iron and the proportion is not much influenced by iron status. The absorption of non-haem iron (from vegetable sources) *is* affected by iron status, absorption being greatly increased in people with low iron status. Non-haem iron must be changed (in chemical terms, reduced) from the iron $3+$ or ferric state to iron 2+ or ferrous state before absorption. Vitamin C, eaten at the same meal, speeds up this reaction.

A variety of other substances influence non-haem iron absorption:

- *Oxalates and phytates* – these combine with non-haem iron, as with calcium, to form insoluble, non-absorbable compounds (see effect of increasing non-starch polysaccharides, page 54).
- *Phenolic compounds* – like tannin; these are present in tea, coffee and cocoa, in some vegetables (for example, spinach) and some herbs and spices (oregano). They inhibit iron absorption. This inhibition is reduced by eating meat and vitamin C at the same meal.
- *Soya protein* – this causes a reduction in absorption, again counteracted by vitamin C.
- *Dairy products* – these reduce the absorption of both haem and non-haem iron.
- *Meat and fish* – these enhance the absorption of *non-haem* iron.

In practical terms, if vitamin C-containing foods are eaten at most meals, iron absorption will be increased. For example, orange juice or grapefruit at breakfast and vegetables cooked to retain vitamin C at dinner. Tea and milk reduce the absorption of iron and so for vulnerable individuals should be drunk between meals rather than with the main meal.

The total absorption of iron, from a mixed diet, averages 15%. The individual range may be from 5% to 40% (Department of Health, 1994).

FOOD SOURCES OF IRON

The main sources in the average UK diet are meat, bread and other cereals, potatoes and vegetables (Tables 7.6 and 7.7) (MAFF, 1995a).

Sodium and chloride

Sodium and chloride are dealt with together because sodium is often present in the body and in food as sodium chloride (common salt), so that, rather carelessly, the terms sodium and salt are often used interchangeably.

Much interest centres on the role of dietary sodium in the development of **essential hypertension** (which is the term used for hypertension of no apparent cause) in middle age. Potassium may also be important here and the general consensus of opinion, on the available evidence, is that most people in the UK would be wise to reduce their sodium intake and increase their potassium intake.

Table 7.6   Iron content for average servings of some foods

Food	Amount/weight (g)	Iron content (mg)
Bread (white)	Two slices from large, medium sliced loaf	1.2
Bread (wholemeal)	As above	1.9
Chapattis	One, 70 g	1.6
All-Bran	45 g	5.4
Cornflakes	45 g	1.7
Chocolate, milk	50 g	0.8
Egg	Size 2	1.1
Cod steaks	130 g	0.5
Beef or lamb (lean)	85 g	2.4
Pork (lean)	85 g	1.1
Corned beef	Two slices, 60 g	1.7
Liver	90 g	9.0
Sausage (pork)	Two, 90 g	1.4
Chicken, roast	85 g	0.7
Salad vegetables	Average portion	0.2–1.0
Vegetables, cooked	Average portion	0.2–1.3
Liquorice Allsorts	100 g	8.1

From Davies, J. and Dickerson, J. (1991).

Table 7.7   Iron content of a typical diet

Food	Amount/weight (g)	Iron content (mg)
Bread (wholemeal)	Two slices	1.9
Bread (white)	Two slices	1.2
Cornflakes	25 g	1.7
Ham	Two slices	0.7
Chocolate biscuit, Penguin	One	0.4
Chicken joint	190 g	1.0
Peas, frozen, boiled	75 g	1.1
Carrots, boiled	65 g	0.3
Beer, bitter	One pint	0.1
Total		8.3

From Davies, J. and Dickerson, J. (1991).

This shows how easy it is to fall below the highest requirements for teenage girls and women of reproductive age of 14.8 mg/day.

FUNCTIONS OF SODIUM

Sodium is the main element or *cation* (positively charged molecular fragment) in the blood and tissue fluid. The *tonicity* (the concentration of dissolved substances, sometimes called the oncotic pressure) of the blood is controlled within very narrow limits and so the amount of sodium in the body determines the volume of blood and tissue fluid. If total sodium falls, because of, say, heavy sweating and is not replaced, water will be excreted to bring the tonicity of the blood back to normal, giving temporarily a smaller blood volume. If excess sodium is retained, perhaps because of kidney failure or hormonal imbalance, water is also retained, which may eventually cause **oedema** (swelling because of extra tissue fluid).

Sodium is also essential for the transmission of nerve and muscle impulses.

SODIUM BALANCE

Sodium from the diet comes mainly from salt which has been added during processing, cooking or at table, since most fresh foods have a low salt content.

Sodium is fully absorbed from the gut. It is excreted in the urine, the amount controlled by hormones to maintain homeostasis, and it is also lost in sweat. When intake is low, urine may be virtually sodium-free; when intake is high, large amounts of sodium are excreted. The control of sodium excretion, to maintain the volume and oncotic pressure of body fluids, occurs through the complex interaction of many hormones (Box 7.8).

BOX 7.8

CONTROL OF SODIUM EXCRETION

The main hormones involved are the anti-diuretic hormone and aldosterone. There is some evidence for a natriuretic hormone, which increases the loss of sodium in urine.

SODIUM DEFICIENCY

In healthy people, sodium deficiency is very uncommon. It might occur after heavy sweating if sodium is not replaced, but this is unusual.

It does occur in Addison's disease, also rare, when the lack of adrenal cortical hormones leads to sodium loss and therefore to low blood pressure and weakness. However, in general, the human body is very well equipped to conserve sodium and is able to reduce urinary sodium loss to zero.

SODIUM EXCESS

Any physiology textbook will refer to sodium homeostasis, noting that dietary excess will cause a temporary increase in extracellular fluid volume through a salt-induced thirst (well-known to publicans who often sell salty crisps and sandwiches!). This increase in salt and water is gradually corrected over about 24 hours, with urinary excretion of both. This homeostatic response is less effective in the very young and in the elderly.

In developed countries, however, salt intake is *habitually* very much higher than is necessary and blood pressure commonly rises with age. A sizeable minority of adults (5–20%) have high blood pressure and, of these, more than 95% have essential hypertension.

It has been suggested that humans have adapted, through evolutionary experience, to conserve sodium. It is possible, although unproven, that increases in dietary sodium cause, in some susceptible individuals, an expansion of extracellular fluid volume and a resulting increase in blood pressure. Another explanation might be that in these individuals an elevated blood pressure is necessary for the excretion of large amounts of sodium. The evidence stems from:

1. Population studies, which compare average salt intake with average blood pressure in adults.
2. From the effect of reducing dietary salt in hypertensives.
3. From animal experiments which have begun to elucidate possible physiological mechanisms.

Population studies are always difficult, especially those for salt intake and blood pressure. Salt intake is difficult to measure, since a lot may be left on the side of the plate, used in preserving and so on. Twenty-four-hour urinary excretion is the most reliable estimate and, because of daily variation, an 11-day period is needed for accurate results.

Blood pressure also must be measured under standard conditions (the sight of a white medical coat being enough to cause hypertension in some people!).

Law *et al.* (1991) carried out a meta-analysis (Box 7.9) and analysed data from 24 communities, selecting studies with reliable methodology. To minimize the effect of cultural, physical and economic differences

BOX 7.9

META-ANALYSIS

This is the collection of a number of studies of similar methodology and the re-analysis of their results as a whole (see page 23).

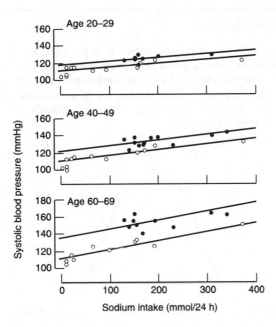

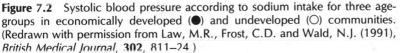

Figure 7.2 Systolic blood pressure according to sodium intake for three age-groups in economically developed (●) and undeveloped (○) communities. (Redrawn with permission from Law, M.R., Frost, C.D. and Wald, N.J. (1991), *British Medical Journal*, **302**, 811–24)

which might affect blood pressure, they classified the communities as (i) economically developed and (ii) undeveloped, and compared them separately (Figure 7.2).

This analysis showed that blood pressure varies according to sodium intake and that the effect on blood pressure of increasing sodium intake is greater with increasing age. This response had a normal distribution (Box 7.10) and seemed to be genetically determined, features already shown in experiments on rats.

Comparison of sodium intake and blood pressure *within* populations as opposed to *between* them has not, in small studies, given clear-cut results. However, another meta-analysis by Law *et al.* on 14 such studies showed, using all the data, similar correlations between sodium intake and blood pressure as were shown between populations.

It has been known for a long time that a *very* low sodium diet will reduce a high blood pressure. (Kempner, in 1948, fed his patients an effective but unpalatable fruit and rice diet.) More recently, studies have been carried out to find the effect of smaller and more acceptable reductions in dietary salt.

BOX 7.10

NORMAL DISTRIBUTION

This is the way a characteristic occurs in a population. There is a typical spread of values, which is shown on the graph below. In this case, a few people would show almost no increase in blood pressure with increased sodium intake, a few would have shown a much greater response than this, and most people would fall between these two extremes.

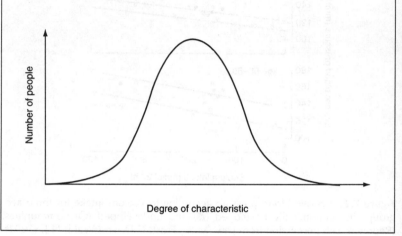

Law *et al.* again looked at all these results. In those studies where the salt reduction was maintained for five weeks or longer, the results showed a fall in blood pressure in hypertensives. In people aged 50–59 years a reduction in daily sodium intake of about 3 g of salt would – after a few weeks – lower systolic blood pressure by an average of 5 mmHg

BOX 7.11

BLOOD PRESSURE

Systolic blood pressure is the peak pressure after contraction of the heart and *diastolic* blood pressure is the low point between heart beats. Normal values in young people at rest are 120 mmHg for systolic and 80 mmHg for diastolic blood pressure.

HYPERTENSION

Blood pressure raised above normal.

and by 7 mmHg in those with high blood pressure (systolic pressure 170 mmHg). They estimate that such a reduction in salt intake in the UK would reduce the incidence of stroke by 26% and of ischaemic heart disease by 15%.

There is a good deal of critical comment about the relationship between salt intake and blood pressure in the literature, often highlighting the lack of agreement shown between some of the studies comparing different populations. It is also true that no increase in blood volume has been recorded in hypertensives and that in health the blood volume is closely controlled over a very wide range of fluid and salt intakes. Whatever the interpretation of the results, it is true that nearly all in the UK eat much more salt than they need, and to reduce it would do no harm and probably much good. In all these discussions it is easy to assume that *only* salt intake affects blood pressure and this is not so. Recent work shows that early life (birth weight and weight at one year, see page 225) has an influence and so does physical activity and alcohol intake.

The physiological mechanisms whereby sodium may affect blood pressure chronically are not fully worked out. Potassium intake is possibly involved (see page 243). Also, the current dietary advice of increasing fruit and vegetables would increase potassium intake.

Who should reduce their salt intake? It is sensible not to produce salt overload in the very young and in the elderly, nor in those with hypertension or with a predisposition to it. Since this last group is, to a large extent unknown, the consensus is that moderate salt reduction is sensible for all.

SODIUM REQUIREMENTS

The COMA report 41 (Department of Health, 1991) does not give EARs for sodium but the LRNIs and RNIs shown below are provided. It is noted that extra salt may be necessary after hard exercise or in hot climates. For the group aged 19–50 years, the LRNI is 575 mg per day and the RNI 1600 mg per day.

Daily sodium intakes in the UK are between 2 and 10 g. It has been estimated that 84–88% comes from processed foods. About 40% of the total comes from bread and breakfast cereals, and about one-third from highly salted foods (bacon and ham for example). Estimates made in Australia show that a diet relying heavily on processed foods could supply up to 6.5 g sodium per day, on take-away foods about 5.1 g sodium per day and a diet containing little of either only 1.6 g sodium per day. Generally, our intake of sodium is above the DRVs. COMA Report 46 (Department of Health, 1994) recommends that the average intake of common salt be reduced by one-third.

HOW TO REDUCE SODIUM INTAKE

- By cooking vegetables in unsalted water or steaming them without added salt.
- By choosing processed foods without added salt, like canned vegetables, baked beans, peanuts, crisps. The biggest reductions here come from baked beans and crisps.
- By avoiding foods high in sodium (see below).
- By changing food choice and eating fewer processed and take-away foods and more home-prepared foods.
- By using other flavourings in cooking like pepper, other spices and herbs, lemon juice.
- By adding salt to part of a meal only. For example, in a meal of rice, chicken and a sauce, add salt only to the sauce. It has been shown that this allows a smaller amount to be used and the meal is more acceptable than if the same amount of salt is spread throughout.
- By eating yeast-raised cakes (currant buns, doughnuts) instead of those using baking powder, which contain sodium compounds.
- By reducing salt added at table. For those who must and will do so, it has been shown that a salt shaker with one hole only (3 mm diameter) reduces the amount used.
- By making bread at home and halving the recommended amount of salt.
- By gradually reducing the salt added in cooking. People adapt to a lower level often without noticing it.
- By avoiding the use of commercial stock cubes for gravy and using home-made stock instead (see page 356).

SODIUM IN FOODS

Typical levels of sodium in foods are shown in Table 7.8 (Davies, J. and Dickerson, J., 1991).

Table 7.8   Sodium content of foods

Food	Amount/weight (g)	Sodium (mg)
Soy sauce	Spoonful, 5 ml	286
Marmite	Spoonful, 5 ml	225*
Cornflakes	45 g	522
Smoked haddock	100 g	1220
Sausages	One, large	350
Bacon	One back rasher	350
Cheese	50 g	300
Bread (white or wholemeal)	One slice	130

* Also high in potassium.

LOW SALT FOODS

The following are low in salt:

- most unprocessed foods;
- fresh or frozen meat or fish;
- breakfast cereals – Shredded Wheat, Puffed Wheat, Sugar Puffs;
- rice, spaghetti, and other pasta;
- all fresh or frozen vegetables;
- all fresh or tinned fruit, but not dried fruit;
- sugars, jams, plain chocolate, boiled sweets, peppermints, marshmallows and marzipan.

Potassium

There is no evidence of potassium deficiency as potassium is widely distributed in foods, but there is some evidence that a high potassium intake affects, beneficially, the metabolism of sodium, aiding the excretion of a sodium load.

The body content of potassium averages 125 g for men and 79 g for women. Dietary potassium is almost completely absorbed from the small intestine. Excretion is regulated through the kidney. Small amounts are lost from the gut and in sweat.

FUNCTIONS OF POTASSIUM

About 95% of body potassium lies inside the cells rather than in the fluid surrounding them. The sodium/potassium differential between cells and their surroundings is maintained by a sodium–potassium 'pump'. This differential is essential for muscle contractility and the passage of nerve impulses.

POTASSIUM DEFICIENCY

As already noted, *dietary* deficiency is very rare but deficiency may occur through diarrhoea, diabetic acidosis, alcohol abuse and medication with diuretics, glucocorticoids and laxatives. Symptoms are muscular weakness, cardiac arrhythmias or arrest, loss of intestinal movement and mental depression and confusion.

POTASSIUM EXCESS

Excess is almost unknown provided that kidney function is normal, but there are vulnerable groups such as the elderly, whose kidney function may be reduced. (See note on salt substitutes below) Liquorice (as in Liquorice Allsorts) is very high in potassium and so it is not the best sweet for great-grandma.

LINK WITH SODIUM INTAKE

Evidence suggests that the intake of potassium affects the metabolism of sodium. In healthy young men a sodium load was more readily excreted by those who had a high potassium intake. This may be relevant to the effect of high sodium intake on blood pressure.

POTASSIUM REQUIREMENTS

The average intakes found in the Dietary and Nutritional Survey of British Adults were well above the LRNI although somewhat below the RNI (MAFF, 1995b). As for sodium, the EAR has not been estimated. For the 19–50-year group the LRNI is 2000 mg per day and the RNI 3500 mg per day.

FOOD SOURCES OF POTASSIUM

The main sources of potassium are vegetables, meat and milk. Instant coffee is a reasonably good source, with about 100 mg per cup so that five cups a day will give one-seventh of the adult RNI; bananas, too, are a good source.

POTASSIUM-RICH SALT SUBSTITUTES

LoSalt contains about 340 mg potassium and 135 mg sodium per gram. If this is used to replace added salt in the diet there would be about a 25% increase in potassium intake. While a healthy person would have no difficulty in excreting this extra potassium, some, such as the elderly, persons with renal impairment and those on drugs such as potassium-sparing diuretics may be at risk of potassium toxicity. In such people near fatal **hyperkalaemia** (raised blood potassium) may result. It is recommended therefore that salt substitutes should be added to food at table only and not used in cooking (Department of Health, 1994).

Magnesium is a vital mineral but there is little evidence of deficiency except for special groups such as alcoholics. Severe deficiency may be lethal.

Magnesium

FUNCTIONS OF MAGNESIUM

The adult human body contains about 25 g magnesium and about 60% of this is in the skeleton. Magnesium is also a cofactor for a large number of enzymes, it is necessary for normal skeletal development and in the maintenance of the excitability of nerve and muscle membranes. Intestinal absorption varies according to intake and excretion is controlled at the kidney.

MAGNESIUM DEFICIENCY

Deficiency may be caused by unsuitable slimming regimes (or starvation), alcoholism, malabsorption syndromes or prolonged vomiting or diarrhoea. There is a wide range of symptoms which include muscular weakness, tachycardia (fast heart rate), ventricular fibrillation, and psychological symptoms such as anxiety and insomnia. Coma and death may occur.

MAGNESIUM EXCESS

In adults with normal renal function there is no evidence of toxic effects from high intake of magnesium from foods.

MAGNESIUM REQUIREMENTS

DRVs of LRNI, EAR and RNI are available. The RNI for men aged 19–50 years is 300 mg per day and for women 270 mg per day. The household diet in the UK provides, on average, sufficient magnesium to meet the RNI.

FOODS FOR MAGNESIUM

Magnesium is widespread in foods, both vegetable and animal. There is no need for concern about dietary intake.

Zinc   Interest in zinc has increased in recent years. It is important in very many biological functions, growth and taste sensitivity among them. Although there is little evidence of frank deficiency in the UK population, marginal deficiency may exist in some groups, such as rapidly growing children, pregnant women, and sufferers of anorexia nervosa.

FUNCTIONS OF ZINC

The average adult body contains only about 2 g of zinc, distributed throughout the body, largely as a component of more than 70 enzymes and as part of other protein molecules. The absorption of zinc by the gut is very variable and depends on dietary and physiological factors and on the requirements of homeostasis.

ZINC DEFICIENCY

In mild deficiency states the symptoms, as with so many nutrients, are non-specific. Growth retardation is one of the earliest signs. Maturation of the sex organs is retarded, there are skeletal changes, skin lesions, wound healing is slower than normal and the immune system may be impaired. Neuropsychiatric signs such as irritability and tremor have been reported. The effect of zinc deficiency in reducing the appetite has been shown in animal experiments and in humans.

AT-RISK GROUPS

Pre-school children of low-income families and persons with a low energy intake (many women, constant dieters, and some elderly people) may be at risk of mild deficiency. Increased urinary zinc excretion occurs in surgery, burns, multiple injuries, diabetes mellitus, protein deprivation and starvation. Liver cirrhosis, nephrotic syndrome (Box 7.12) and sickle cell disease increase excretion. Malabsorption of zinc may occur in patients with type II (non-insulin dependent) diabetes.

BOX 7.12

NEPHROTIC SYNDROME

There is heavy loss of protein in the urine, along with oedema and hypoalbuminaemia. Nephrotic syndrome has various causes, among them diabetes mellitus and systemic lupus erythematosus.

ZINC EXCESS

Toxic effects have been reported (nausea and vomiting after acute excess and anaemia and a lowered white blood cell count after chronically high intakes) but such situations are unlikely to arise. Enthusiastic consumers of dietary supplements could be at risk.

ZINC REQUIREMENTS

The data on which requirements are estimated is far from perfect. The average intakes of British adults have been shown to be well above the RNI at 9–12 mg per day. However, the amount of zinc in different samples of a food vary greatly and there are possibly errors in these figures for intakes.

BIOAVAILABILITY OF ZINC

Like iron and calcium, the absorption of zinc is inhibited by non-starch polysaccharides, oxalates and phytates.

FOODS FOR ZINC

Oysters, wheatgerm, wheatbran and cocoa are the richest sources of zinc, although not the most common. Good sources are lean red meat, bacon, liver, All-Bran, Shredded Wheat, sardines and many kinds of nuts. Fruit and vegetables, fats and oils are, on the whole, poor sources.

FUNCTIONS OF COPPER

Copper

Copper, present in the body in much smaller amounts than zinc (50–120 mg in the adult) is also a component of enzymes. As such, it has an important role in many reactions, including the quenching of free radicals (page 90). Zinc is antagonistic to copper absorption, an example of the importance of *balance* in the diet.

COPPER DEFICIENCY

Leucopenia and neutropenia (falls in numbers of white blood cells and neutrophils respectively) are early indicators of copper deficiency. Anaemia occurs later, and later still, bone demineralization occurs. Ultimately, copper deficiency is fatal. In adults early signs may be defects in cardiovascular function.

Interestingly, in copper-deficient ataxic (staggering movement) lambs' levels of dopamine in the brain are increased by copper supplementation. In Parkinson's disease dopamine levels are similarly low.

AT-RISK GROUPS

Two genetic diseases, Menkes' syndrome and Wilson's disease show low blood copper in spite of adequate dietary intake.

Infants fed a milk diet for too long may be at risk, and so are children with chronic malabsorption syndrome. Kidney dialysis may also be a cause.

COPPER EXCESS

Copper is toxic in excess but no cases have been reported in the UK.

COPPER REQUIREMENTS

Lack of data means that only the RNI has been estimated. This is 1.2 mg per day for adults. Surveys show adequate average intakes in the UK.

FOODS FOR COPPER

The main sources in the diet are meat, bread, other cereals and vegetables. Shell-fish and liver are particularly high in copper.

Selenium   Selenium, like copper and zinc, is another trace element which has aroused a great deal of interest lately. In popular journalism, selenium has been accorded almost magical properties. Deficiency is unknown in the UK, although low blood levels are found in patients with gastrointestinal cancer and in total parenteral nutrition.

FUNCTIONS OF SELENIUM

Selenium is also a component of enzymes (including one called glutathione peroxidase which is involved in the quenching of free radicals) and therefore has a role in the maintenance of the integrity of cell membranes.

Between 55% and 65% is absorbed from the gut and excess selenium is excreted in the urine.

SELENIUM DEFICIENCY

Except in some areas of China, where the soil is low in selenium, deficiency is not known. Signs include muscle pain and weakness.

SELENIUM EXCESS

Selenium is toxic at intakes above 750 μg/day. Selenium preparations are sold in the UK, the labels suggesting daily doses between 10 and 250 μg.

SELENIUM REQUIREMENTS

LRNI and RNI have been estimated. The requirements are minute, the RNI for adult males being 75 μg/day and for females 60 μg/day.

FOODS FOR SELENIUM

Selenium is present in many foods.

Iodine

Deficiency in the UK is rare. Historically, iodine deficiency was common in Derbyshire, where the soil is low in iodine, the resulting goitre being known as 'Derbyshire neck'.

FUNCTIONS OF IODINE

Iodine is part of the thyroid hormones (thyroxine and triiodothyronine), which are necessary for normal growth and development, for cellular metabolism and the integrity of the connective tissue. Iodine is well absorbed from the gut, and excreted in the urine.

DEFICIENCY OF IODINE

A deficiency of iodine means a deficiency of the thyroid hormones along with the development of goitre (swelling of the thyroid gland). The effects are a slowing of the basal metabolic rate, and in children, reduced growth and, if prolonged and severe, a condition called *cretinism*, where growth is reduced and mental deficiency occurs.

IODINE EXCESS

There are reports of toxic effects and, although the risk is slight, the COMA Report 41 recommends a safe upper limit of 17 µg/kg body weight or less than 100 µg/day (Department of Health, 1991).

IODINE REQUIREMENTS

The LRNI and RNI have been estimated. The RNI for adults is 140 µg per day.

FOODS FOR IODINE

Milk is the main dietary source followed by meat and eggs. Seafood is a reliable source. Iodized salt is available.

Fluorine   FUNCTIONS OF FLUORINE

Fluorine, as calcium fluoropatite, produces a dental enamel in teeth which is resistant to decay. Fluorine may be involved in bone mineralization.

FLUORINE DEFICIENCY

Fluorine is not *essential* as are the other mineral elements. The body functions normally in its absence. However, tooth decay is increased in populations with a low intake of fluorine and is reduced by dietary fluorine. *Dietary* fluorine is protective in this way up to the age of about 13 years.

FLUORINE EXCESS

This condition is called *fluorosis* and causes ugly mottling of tooth enamel and bone changes.

REQUIREMENTS OF FLUORINE

No DRVs are available but the COMA Report 41 (Department of Health, 1991) endorsed the recommendation that water supplies be fluoridized to achieve levels of 1 ppm. An upper limit of intake for infants and young children of 0.05 mg/kg body weight is suggested. *Where water is fluoridized supplements for children are not necessary.*

FOODS FOR FLUORINE

Tea is the major source in the diet, providing 70% of the total. Other sources are seafood and fluoridated toothpaste.

Other trace elements

- **Molybdenum** is essential as part of some enzymes and a level of safe intake has been proposed.
- **Manganese** is also essential, but deficiency has never been seen in humans. About half the average UK intake comes from tea. It is not toxic.
- **Chromium** is part of a complex which enhances the action of insulin. It is present in yeast, meat, whole grains but low in highly refined foods.

Key points

1. The mineral elements required in the diet are calcium, phosphorus, sodium, potassium and magnesium. Trace elements, which are required in much smaller amounts, are chromium, copper, iodine, iron, manganese, molybdenum, selenium, zinc, cobalt and fluorine.

None of these is destroyed by cooking, but some have limited bioavailability.

2. Bioavailability (the proportion of dietary intake which is used by the body) may be affected by dietary factors (phytates and oxalates for calcium, iron and zinc) and by physiological factors like age, health, nutritional status and the adaptation to nutrient supply. Low status causes increased bioavailability.

3. In the UK mineral deficiency, except for iron, is not a problem. The focus of concern is the high intake of sodium chloride. Mineral supplements are therefore not generally required, nor are they wise since an increased intake of one mineral may reduce the absorption of another (for example, copper and zinc).

4. Calcium. Most of the body's calcium is in the bones, but a small and vital amount is in the blood. Peak bone mass is important and calcium, protein and energy are the dietary factors which affect it. Deficiency of calcium is usually caused by lack of vitamin D. Dairy products are good sources of calcium.

5. Phosphorus, also present in the bones and in many metabolically active compounds, is not important dietetically.

6. Iron is part of the oxygen-carrying compounds haemoglobin and myoglobin. Some groups (infants, toddlers, adolescents, pregnant women and those with high menstrual loss) are at risk of iron deficiency, which may develop into anaemia. Iron deficiency affects work output and possibly mental function. Iron from animal sources is better absorbed than from vegetable foods. Dietary factors which influence absorption are several: phytates, oxalates, tannins, and milk all inhibit while vitamin C enhances absorption. Iron is toxic in excess.

7. Sodium and chloride. Meta-analyses of epidemiological and experimental work confirm the view that a general reduction in intake would reduce the incidence of essential hypertension. Ways of reducing salt intake are given on page 134.

8. Potassium, present within cells, is supplied by vegetables and fruits. A high potassium intake may reduce the risk of hypertension. An excess is harmful only in those with impaired renal function, such as the elderly. High potassium salt substitutes should be used at table only and not in cooking to avoid excess.

9. Magnesium is in many foods. There is little evidence of deficiency except in alcoholics. It is not toxic.

10. Zinc is present in a number of enzymes and therefore has many functions, including growth, taste acuity, and wound healing. Elderly people and small eaters are at risk of mild deficiency. A number of conditions increase urinary loss.

11. Copper is also part of many enzymes, including those which quench free radicals. Deficiency occurs only in special situations

like infants fed milk too long, chronic malabsorption syndrome, kidney dialysis.

12. Selenium is also part of enzymes, including free radical quenchers. Deficiency is unknown in the UK.

13. Iodine forms part of the thyroid hormone molecule. Deficiency is rare in the UK. Iodized salt is available for those not eating animal foods.

14. Fluorine, though not essential to life, is protective against tooth decay. Excess causes fluorosis, with mottling of teeth. Found in tea, seafood, toothpaste.

15. Molybdenum, manganese and chromium are also essential.

8 Dietary energy

This chapter describes the need for dietary energy, its units of measurement, requirements and factors determining them and appetite control. Obesity, its definition, measurement and treatment, illustrated with some case studies, are discussed along with its metabolic effects. Starvation, anorexia nervosa and bulimia are covered briefly. Advice on food choice, with the energy values of some common foods, is given.

The need for dietary energy

The living organism uses energy to live. We need energy:

- to produce *heat* to maintain the body temperature at a higher level than the environment;
- for the *synthesis of large molecules* from smaller ones (for the normal replacement of muscle fibres, hormones, enzymes and for tissue growth) and sometimes for their transport in the body, and
- for the *contraction of muscle fibres*, for breathing, the beating of the heart and for all movement.

The efficiency of the use of food energy for the last two purposes is about 25%, the other 75% appearing as heat (Garrow and James, 1993).

Energy expenditure is often divided into two components: resting or basal metabolic rate and total metabolic rate.

Basal metabolic rate (BMR; see Box 8.1) is the rate of energy expenditure under standardized conditions of complete rest (Table 8.1). When the precise conditions specified for BMR are not met it is referred to as **resting metabolic rate**.

Note: equations for estimating the basal metabolic rate for older children, adolescents, adults and the elderly are given in the COMA Report 41, *Dietary Reference Values for Food Energy and Nutrients for the UK*, page 202 (Department of Health, 1991)

BMR may be expressed as energy expenditure per kg body weight or as the total for the individual. BMR correlates well with the *lean* body

Basal Metabolic Rate (BMR) is measured with the subject lying down at complete physical and mental rest, at least 12 hours after the last meal and comfortably warm. An over-active thyroid causes a marked increase in BMR and vice versa.

Table 8.1 Average normal values for resting energy requirement

Weight (kg)	Resting energy requirement	
	kcal (MJ)/day	kcal (MJ)/kg/day
Infant, 1 year old 10	500 (2.1)	50 (0.21)
Child, 8 years old 25	1000 (4.2)	40 (0.17)
Adult woman 55	1300 (5.4)	25 (0.1)
Adult man 65	1600 (6.7)	25 (0.1)

(From *Manual of Nutrition*, (1995). Crown copyright is reproduced with the permission of the Controller of HMSO).

mass which, being more metabolically active than adipose tissue, is the main contributor to energy expenditure at rest. BMR falls with increasing age, and this is one of the reasons why most people need less food energy as they get older. Total BMR is obviously also determined by body size.

Metabolic rate

This is the total expenditure of energy, expressed per unit time (per day or per hour) and sometimes also per unit body weight. It is the sum of energy expended as BMR, plus physical activity, thermogenesis (caused by diet or in response to cold) and the production of any new tissue.

FACTORS INFLUENCING METABOLIC RATE

Physical activity

Including walking, running, and so on, this will increase the metabolic rate above the resting level and may be a major factor in determining energy requirements. In fact in our society, where most people are sedentary, activity contributes only about 15% of total energy expenditure.

The energy costs of various activities have been measured and average values are available. Energy expenditure obviously depends on size since of course it requires more work to move a 20-stone (125 kg) body upstairs than one of only 5 stone (30 kg).

BOX 8.2

ENERGY EXPENDITURE OF VARIOUS ACTIVITIES OF MODERATE
DURATION GROUPED ACCORDING TO PHYSICAL ACTIVITY
RATIO (PAR)

PAR 1.0–1.4

- Lying at rest, sitting at rest, standing at rest

PAR 1.5–1.8

- Sitting and knitting, driving, playing piano
- Standing and doing washing up, ironing, general office and laboratory work

PAR 1.9–2.4

- Standing and doing household cleaning, washing small clothes, cooking, hairdressing, snooker, bowling

PAR 2.5–3.3

- Standing and dressing, showering, hoovering, making beds
- Walking at 3–4 km/hour, playing cricket
- Some industrial tasks like painting and decorating, electrical work

PAR 3.4–4.4

- Standing and mopping floor, gardening, cleaning windows, table tennis
- Walking at 4–6 km/hour and golf
- Motor vehicle repairs, carpentry, joinery, bricklaying

PAR 4.5–5.9

- Standing and polishing furniture, chopping wood, heavy gardening, volley-ball
- Walking at 6–7 km/hour
- Dancing, moderate swimming, gentle cycling, slow jogging
- Labouring, hoeing, road construction, felling trees

PAR 6.0–7.9

- Walking uphill with load or cross-country, climbing stairs
- Average jogging, cycling
- Football, more energetic swimming, tennis, skiing

Modified from COMA 41 (Department of Health, 1991). Details of methods for estimating requirements of energy are to be found in the Coma Report 41.

The method now used to estimate the cost of activity is the **physical activity ratio** or **PAR** which is the *multiple of an individual's BMR for the particular activity*. For walking on the level at an average pace, the PAR is 4 which means that the energy cost of walking will be four times the BMR of an individual (Box 8.2).

Although the brain has a high consumption of oxygen, this does not seem to alter with intellectual activity.

Age

Various factors determine the changes in energy expenditure with age. These are growth, body weight, activity and BMR. Growth increases energy requirements and so does the increase in size during childhood. Levels of activity vary with age and the BMR gradually falls. Generally energy requirements peak in adolescence, when high growth rate and high activity levels coincide.

Gender

Men have, on average, a higher BMR per kg body weight than women, probably due to a higher proportion of lean tissue. They are also usually heavier. These two factors increase their *total* metabolic rate. Activity levels may or may not be higher.

Body weight

Clearly the heavier the body the more energy will be required to maintain it and to move it about, as every athlete knows. But it is also true that heavy people often move less and more slowly than lighter ones.

Growth, pregnancy and lactation

During these stages new tissue is being produced and so increased supplies of energy and of some nutrients are required. Appetite increases during growth spurts, as it sometimes does in pregnancy. Part of the energy cost of lactation is met by the utilization of fat stores.

Dietary thermogenesis

When a fasting person eats, the production of heat rises. **Postprandial thermogenesis (PPT)**, refers to the increase which begins within 10 minutes of eating and may continue for several hours and **dietary thermogenesis** refers to the general increase in BMR which occurs with overfeeding.

Normally PPT accounts for an increase in energy expenditure (and therefore heat production) of 5–10% over basal rate. In practical terms, the value of food in preventing hypothermia in the elderly in winter is confirmed.

Exposure to cold

Cold weather stimulates the appetite and it certainly causes changes in food choice. Exposure to cold means that heat production must be increased to maintain body temperature. It is very difficult to measure this increase because of the problem of designing an experiment in which *all* the conditions except ambient temperature are kept the same. For this reason quantitative estimates of the increase in metabolism are not available. However, the effect of extreme cold and great activity increased the energy intake of Sir Ranulph Fiennes and Dr Michael Stroud *fourfold* in their Arctic expedition.

Brown adipose tissue (BAT) is a specialized type of fat which has a high heat-producing capacity, around ten times that of skeletal muscle. It plays an important role in the maintenance of body temperature in the new-born. It has been shown to persist in adulthood in the male at least. Noradrenaline greatly increases its activity after a meal and during exposure to cold. It has been suggested that obese humans have less active BAT than lean ones, therefore have a reduced postprandial thermogenesis and so store more of the food they eat as fat. To support this view, it is found that genetically obese strains of mice and some other species lack BAT. However, its role in the development of human obesity is not supported by subsequent research (Lindberg, 1970).

State of health

Illness affects both the level of activity and the appetite. Injuries such as burns and lacerations greatly increase energy requirements, which further increase dramatically if sepsis is added to injury (Windsor, 1988). An intravenous drip, containing glucose, will be able to provide a patient with 400 kcal (1.7 MJ)/day, when they probably need at least 2000 kcal (8.4 MJ). A recent study of a large sample of patients found that 40% lost weight in hospital (see Chapter 18).

Individual variations in metabolism

The food energy required by any one person will be that amount which balances his or her expenditure.

A striking fact is the very wide variation in the food intake (and therefore the energy requirement) between *apparently similar* individuals. This was first shown clearly by McCance and Widdowson, who, in the

1930s, measured the food intake of 63 men, all of whom were healthy and sufficiently well off to eat well. Physical activity might, obviously, have varied between them. However, their energy consumption (and therefore their energy expenditure) varied widely from 1772 kcal (7.5 MJ)/day to 4955 kcal (20.8 MJ)/day. So the largest eater consumed almost three times as much as the smallest (Widdowson, 1936). These findings have been confirmed many times since. Morgan, in 1982, classified subjects as large or small eaters. The large eaters ate 15 MJ/day and were, on average, leaner than the small eaters who consumed only 7 MJ/day. Why? Presumably the requirement for food energy is normally distributed, as mentioned in Chapter 1. Everyone has observed these differences for themselves. It is extremely important that health visitors and other advisers realize how great the variation may be. Inexperienced mothers do not realize that, even if their child appears to eat 'nothing', if he or she is growing normally and is active and well, then a small appetite simply reflects a low energy requirement.

COMPONENTS OF ENERGY EXPENDITURE

Basal metabolism
Energy cost of growth, repair, pregnancy and lactation
Physical activity
Thermogenesis — dietary
              cold

Units of energy measurement

Dietary energy is measured in kilocalories (kcal) or in kilojoules or megajoules where:

1 kilojoule (kJ) = 1000 joules (J)
1 megajoule (MJ) = 1000 kJ = 239 kcal
1 kcal = 4.184 kJ

Although the joule is the SI unit and so should be the unit of choice, the calorie is so firmly embedded in popular use that both units will be given.

DIETARY REFERENCE VALUES (DRVs) FOR ENERGY

Only the Estimated Average Requirements (EARs; Department of Health, 1991) have been calculated for energy (see Box 8.3; Table 8.2).

EARs have been set on the basis of current estimates of energy expenditure (Box 8.4), which has been falling throughout this century as we become more sedentary.

BOX 8.3

WHY THE EAR ONLY?

In prescribing therapeutic diets, the RNI for *nutrients* is used because this means that an individual's needs will almost certainly be met and anyway an intake moderately in excess of requirements will have no adverse effects. This is *not* true for energy, where an excessive intake would be stored as fat. So the RNI for energy really has no use.

The EAR is suitable for planning food supplies for a large group; the big eaters will be balanced by those with small requirements.

Table 8.2 Estimated Average Requirements (EARs) for energy, MJ/day; (kcal/day). (From COMA 41, Department of Health, 1991) Crown copyright is reproduced with the permission of the Controller of HMSO.

Age	Males	Females
0–3 months	2.28 (545)	2.16 (515)
4–6 months	2.89 (690)	2.69 (645)
7–9 months	3.44 (825)	3.20 (765)
10–12 months	3.85 (920)	3.61 (865)
1–3 years	5.15 (1230)	4.86 (1165)
4–6 years	7.16 (1715)	6.46 (1545)
7–10 years	8.24 (1970)	7.28 (1740)
11–14 years	9.27 (2220)	7.92 (1845)
15–18 years	11.51 (2755)	8.83 (2110)
19–50 years	10.60 (2550)	8.10 (1940)
51–59 years	10.60 (2550)	8.00 (1900)
60–64 years	9.93 (2380)	7.99 (1900)
65–74 years	9.71 (2330)	7.96 (1900)
75+ years	8.77 (2100)	7.61 (1810)
Pregnancy		+0.80* (200)
Lactation		
1 month		+1.90 (450)
2 months		+2.20 (530)
3 months		+2.40 (570)
4–6 months (Group 1)		+2.00 (480)
4–6 months (Group 2)		+2.00 (570)
> 6 months (Group 1†)		+1.00 (240)
> 6 months (Group 2‡)		+2.30 (550)

* Last trimester only.
† Group 1, lactating mothers: where breast milk is total or main part of diet.
‡ Group 2, lactating mothers: where breast milk is supplemented.

BOX 8.4

METHODS OF MEASURING ENERGY EXPENDITURE

Energy expenditure can be measured in the following ways:

- by direct calorimetry, when all the heat produced by an individual is measured
- by measuring oxygen consumption, for which there are various techniques
- by the use of doubly labelled water, the most recently developed method, which does not curtail normal activity and food intake, but which is technically difficult.

Is the energy intake adequate?

The simplest way to check the adequacy of a healthy individual's diet for energy is to observe their weight over a few weeks. Is it steady? If so, they are in energy balance, even though their actual weight may not be ideal. If it is falling, then there is an energy deficit; if rising, then there is an excess of dietary energy, providing of course that the individual has stopped growing and is not pregnant.

Appetite and hunger

The amount of food eaten is regulated by the sensations of hunger, appetite and satiety. These sensations are the body's response to signals from a variety of receptors, in the mouth, stomach and elsewhere (see also Chapter 9).

Generally over a period of several days (although not necessarily day-by-day) the amount of food eaten matches energy output and the body is in energy balance. After a period when too little food has been eaten, due to scarcity or illness, appetite will be increased until the weight lost has been replaced. In our society there are several factors which make it very easy for the normal regulating mechanism to be overcome, leading to obesity.

Obesity

A healthy body contains some fat mainly in fat cells or adipose tissue. Sex and other genetic factors determine its distribution. Typical values for body fat content for men and women in their twenties are 14% and 25% respectively.

The amount and distribution of fat is a characteristic of the individual's particular **somatotype**. The three main types are shown in Figure 8.1, though few of us are a 'pure' type.

Obesity is defined as an excessive accumulation of adipose tissue. But what is excessive? The distribution of the amount of body fat through the population is continuous (that is, everyone has some degree of this

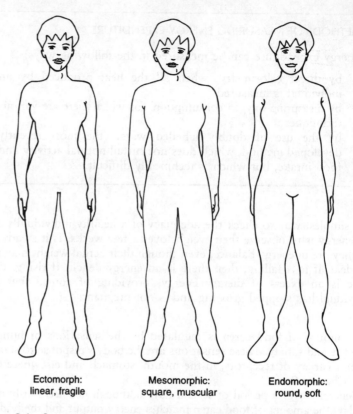

| Ectomorph: | Mesomorphic: | Endomorphic: |
| linear, fragile | square, muscular | round, soft |

Figure 8.1 Somatotypes; genetically determined body characteristics, although few of us are a 'pure' type.

characteristic, unlike measles, which you have or have not, a discontinuous distribution) and, as for other biological variables, the dividing line between normal and abnormal is artificial. Extreme obesity is visually obvious, but the dividing line between plumpness and obesity is not.

Desirable or optimal body weight has been defined from the data of Life Assurance Companies as the weight at which there is the lowest risk of death. Such data reveals a *range* of desirable weights at each height. For example, for a woman of 5'6" (1.7 m), it is between 54 kg (8.5 stone) and 66 kg (10.5 stone).

MEASUREMENT OF BODY FAT AND DIAGNOSING OBESITY

There are various ways of measuring body fat. These include underwater weighing, nuclear resonance scanning and X-ray scans. None of these is feasible in ordinary medical practice. For this the methods commonly used are:

- visual inspection
- weight-for-height tables
- skin-fold callipers
- Body Mass Index.

Garrow (1988) has defined three grades of obesity, I, II and III, of increasing severity.

WEIGHT-FOR-HEIGHT TABLES

A typical weight-for-height table is shown in Figure 8.2.

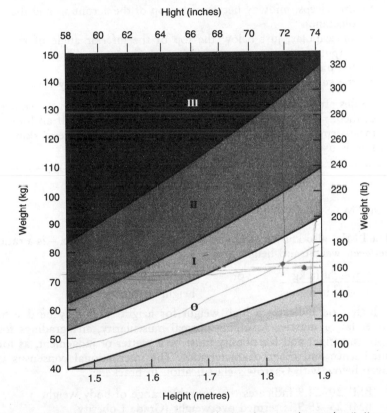

Figure 8.2 Desirable range of weight for height, showing the grades (I, II and III) of obesity. Desirable range of weight for height – optimal. (Redrawn from Garrow, J.S. and James, W.P.T. (eds) (1993) *Human Nutrition and Dietetics*, 9th edn, Churchill Livingstone, London.)

SKIN-FOLD CALLIPERS

Much of the body fat is deposited beneath the skin so the thickness of this layer can be used as an estimate of obesity (Figure 8.3). Harpenden or Holtain callipers are used to measure skin-fold thickness at four sites (Box 8.5).

BOX 8.5

QUANTIFYING OBESITY

Sites for measurement of skin-fold thickness using Harpenden callipers include:

- the triceps, midway between the top of the acromion and the olecranon
- subscapular, just below the top of the inferior angle of the scapula
- the biceps, mid-point
- the suprailiac, over the iliac crest in the mid-axillary line.

Tables are available which give the relationship between the sum of these measurements and the percentage of body fat. If all four measurements are not possible, measurement of the triceps' skin-fold is useful.

BODY MASS INDEX (BMI)

The BMI – also known as Quetelet's index, or obesity index – is a ratio between weight and height and is expressed as

$$\frac{\text{weight in kg}}{\text{height}^2 \text{ in metres}} \qquad \text{or} \qquad \frac{\text{weight in lb} \times 703}{\text{height}^2 \text{ in inches}}$$

A high ratio indicates a high weight for height. This may be due to either fat or muscle. Assuming normal muscularity, any gradings for optimal weight and for obesity must be a matter of judgement, as for intelligence and other characteristics. The international consensus is given below with Garrow's classification in brackets:

- BMI 20–24.9 indicates the desirable range of body weight
- BMI 25–29.9 is termed overweight (Grade I obesity)
- BMI 30–40 is obese (Grade II obesity)
- BMI > 40 is termed very obese (Grade III obesity) (see Figure 8.4).

These ratios are not applicable to children.

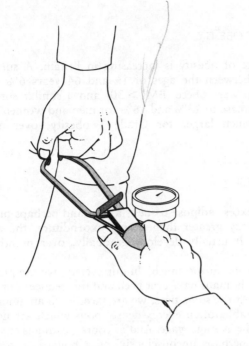

Figure 8.3   Using Harpenden callipers. The fold of skin and subcutaneous fat is raised and the thickness measured with the callipers.

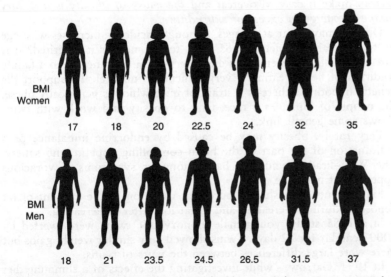

BMI Women: 17, 18, 20, 22.5, 24, 32, 35

BMI Men: 18, 21, 23.5, 24.5, 26.5, 31.5, 37

Figure 8.4   Silhouettes showing a range of Body Mass Indices. (From material of the Canadian Dietetic Association.)

INCIDENCE OF OBESITY

The prevalence of obesity is increasing in Britain. A survey in 1987 showed that between the ages of 16 and 64 years 6% of men and 8% of women were obese (BMI > 30) and a similar survey in 1993 showed an increase to 13% and 16% for men and women respectively. Figures are much larger for Grade 1 obesity, over 50% of the population.

CAUSE OF OBESITY

The cause of excess adipose tissue is a past and perhaps present intake of dietary energy greater than energy expenditure, the excess being stored as fat. It usually develops gradually, over months and even years.

What makes us eat too much? In our society, we are probably more sedentary than humans have ever been and this reduces our food energy requirements. At the same time, we are faced with an abundant supply of highly palatable, often energy-dense foods which are not expensive in relation to the average wage. And of course, eating is enjoyable; food may be seen, perhaps unconsciously, as a reward, a comfort or an escape from boredom. The trend from set meal times to snacking or 'grazing' has also made frequent eating socially acceptable. All these factors make it easy to overeat and *the cause of obesity is a dietary intake of energy in excess of expenditure*.

Obesity may occur at all ages, although incidence increases with age up to 50 years for men and 65 years for women. Is it inherited? It *is* often familial. Whether this is due to genetic inheritance or to a family tradition of hearty eating is very difficult to unravel. To support the genetic hypothesis there is a strain of mice which is genetically obese, the people of Pima, as a race, tend to obesity and work with twins shows some genetic link.

Very rarely, obesity may be caused by endocrine imbalance or a malfunction of the part of the brain controlling appetite and satiety. The Willi–Prader syndrome has, among its symptoms, a voracious appetite but it is rare.

Experiments have shown individual variation in the amount of fat deposited during overeating and in fat loss after undereating.

In a 1985 study, young male monozygotic twins were overfed by 4000 kcal/day for 22 days. Twins showed very similar weight gains but there were large differences between the pairs of twins.

In 1991, Garrow – while investigating the effects of a slimming diet of 800 kcal/day over three weeks, in more than 100 people – found that weight loss varied from 1.5 kg to a maximum of 11 kg, following a normal distribution. This fact, like the variation in energy requirement, must be remembered when helping people to slim.

Some people store fat more readily than others and slimming diet will vary in its effectiveness between persons.

THE EFFECT OF OBESITY ON HEALTH

Obese people are more liable than those of optimal weight to a number of diseases, such as heart disease, hypertension, stroke, non-insulin dependent diabetes and some cancers which are sensitive to sex hormones (Garrow, 1991a).

If BMI exceeds 30, then mortality from these causes increases. In moderate obesity (BMI 25–30) although increase mortality is much less, the risk of disability, for example from musculoskeletal and cardiovascular diseases, is greater than for normal-weight people.

The distribution of fat varies, and some research suggest that the waist-to-hip circumference ratio is significant, and that if high (the 'apple shape'), there is a greater likelihood of the metabolic complications of obesity (see Figures 8.5 and 8.6).

The major metabolic change in obesity (shown in experimental obesity in normal young men and in experimental animals) is a decreased sensitivity to insulin, which is reversible on weight loss. This

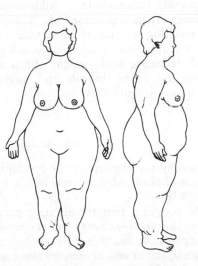

Figure 8.5   The peripheral distribution of adipose tissue, with a waist/hip ratio of 0.66. (Provided by the Medical Illustration Department, Withington Hospital, Manchester.)

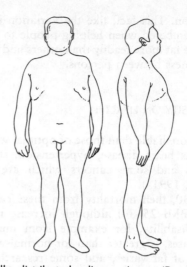

Figure 8.6 Centrally distributed adipose tissue. (Provided by the Medical Illustration Department, Withington Hospital, Manchester.)

change causes others. Decreased glucose tolerance is paralleled by increased susceptibility to arterial disease, and it is also strongly correlated with hypertension. Obesity is also associated with high levels of low density lipoprotein (a risk factor for coronary artery disease) and high serum triglyceride concentrations. Additionally, adipose tissue contains the enzyme system aromatase, which converts androgens to oestrogens; the resulting hormonal imbalance may contribute to infertility. Gallstones, abnormal liver function and gallbladder cancers are also increased. Increased body weight affects the weight-bearing joints, making exercise more difficult and increasing the risk of musculoskeletal diseases (Figure 8.7).

TREATING OBESITY

The target proposed by the Department of Health is that by the year 2000 the proportion of obese adults should be 7% or less (Secretary of State for Health, 1991).

Garrow (1991b) proposes that for effective prevention *the public must be informed about the range of weight-for-height that is associated with appreciable health risks* in order to warn those who should be taking some action and *to reassure those who should not* (see page 155). Secondly, he suggests that there must be *affordable slimming groups open to the public for sound advice about dieting.* (**Note:** Harrow Health District has been running such a scheme for

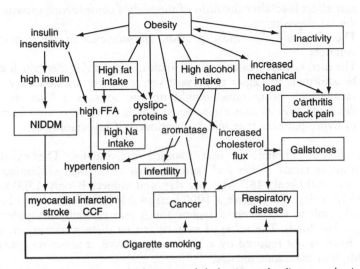

Figure 8.7 The effects of obesity and behaviours leading to obesity on important causes of death and illness. Important diseases are shown in black boxes; some alterable life-style factors which predispose to these diseases are in white boxes. NIDDM, non-insulin-dependent diabetes mellitus. (Redrawn from Garrow, J.S. and James, W.P.T. (eds) (1993) *Human Nutrition and Dietetics*, 9th edn, Churchill Livingstone, London.)

some years; Bush *et al.*, 1988.) Finally, there should be a *policy in primary schools to identify children starting school who are above the 90th centile of weight-for-height and to provide facilities to reduce their weight gain as they grow* in height.

For obesity, prevention is certainly better than cure. A huge number of people (many unnecessarily) are trying to lose weight at any one time and successful and lasting weight loss is notoriously difficult to achieve. It is a behavioural problem.

Any slimming regime must fulfil the following *nutritional criteria*:

1. An *energy imbalance* must be achieved, so that energy expenditure exceeds intake, either by reducing dietary intake or increasing exercise or both.
2. *Adipose tissue* rather than lean tissue must be lost. This is achieved by *slow* loss of weight (for example 0.5–1 kg/week) which may be required over many months. Crash diets (that is, semi-starvation) have been shown to cause the loss of lean tissue as well as fat. Muscle is better maintained if exercise is part of the regime. If rapid loss of lean and adipose tissue occurs, followed by weight gain, the

nett effect is to alter the ratio of the body's constituents, increasing the fat deposits.

3. The slimming diet must provide *all nutrients* in the required amounts.

4. The dietary modifications must result in a *palatable* diet which can be afforded. Strategies to prevent severe hunger are necessary.

5. Ideally, the programme should not be seen as a 'diet' to be discarded after its aims are achieved, but as a *long-term modification* to living patterns that will be continued, if less rigorously.

A slimming regime is best planned individually. The existing situation, in terms of diet and exercise, must be established. Subject A may eat 4000 kcal (16.7 MJ) per day and subject B only 1500 kcal (6.2 MJ) a day. To suggest a 1000 kcal (4.2 MJ) daily intake to both would result in too severe a regime for A and probably insignificant weight loss for B. The value of exercise is that dietary restrictions are less, BMR is not reduced by a low energy intake, it improves general health, and maintains muscle.

Some general *practical points* are:

1. Wherever possible an increase in exercise is beneficial, for example a daily 20-minute walk, not using the lift at work, swimming, and so on.

2. Recommend a diet which promotes satiety by including food which requires chewing and so prolongs the duration of eating, for example, fruits, salads and beans.

3. Use sensible pre-prepared snacks (carrot, celery, pepper sticks, sugar-free jelly, suitable fruits).

4. A meal pattern which avoids long periods without food is advisable, otherwise ravenous hunger causes will-power to evaporate. It has been shown, too, that fat deposition is less when food is eaten in small, frequent meals rather than in one or two large ones.

5. Meals should not be unrealistically small, as there is then a tendency to fill up with less nutritious and more calorie-dense foods.

6. Use a small plate, remove food after taking a helping, so that 'seconds' are not available: small tips like these may be helpful.

7. Many people find late evening a danger time. A hobby (embroidery?) which needs both hands, so that eating is impossible, may be helpful.

8. Do not be over-ambitious. A recent study showed that among groups given varying dietary prescriptions, the group given the smallest reduction in energy intake (about 500 kcal (2.1 MJ)/day, with a mean energy prescription of 1700 kcal (7.1 MJ)/day) showed the greatest weight loss, presumably due to better compliance.

COMMERCIAL SLIMMING AIDS AND PROGRAMMES

Weight Watchers

This well-known organization supplies a great deal of sensible, structured information about diet and exercise. It has the added incentive of specific advice, regular weight checks and it costs money, so that slimmers want to see some result. It provides useful menus and recipes, though there is a lot of material to read through so it is not for the faint-hearted.

Rosemary Conley's Hip and Thigh diet and Inch Loss Plan

This contains nothing which is really new and follows the traditional pattern of recommending exercise and a low energy diet. It is, however, presented in an attractive way. The suggested diet is very low in fat and would cause, in most people, a fairly rapid weight loss.

The Cambridge Diet

This is advertised as 'a revolutionary approach to safe and effective weight loss'. This product is available in two forms: a powder providing 110 kcal (460 kJ) per serving, which represents one meal. Three servings supply 330 kcal (1.4 MJ) and the US RDA for vitamins, minerals and trace elements. There is also a meal replacement bar, providing 160 kcal. Clients are advised to drink an additional 4 pints (2.2 litres) of liquid a day and to keep to the diet for a maximum of 4 weeks, then to take an extra meal for 1 week and then return to the strict diet. This is a very low energy intake. Weight will be shed quickly, probably with loss of lean tissue (Department of Health, 1987).

WHEN SHOULD A PATIENT BE REFERRED TO A DIETICIAN?

All patients in the upper end of Grade 2 and those of Grade 3 obesity should be referred.

SOME CASE STUDIES

John

John, aged 57, not seriously overweight but with a gradually increasing tummy. John achieved a 10 lb (4.5 kg) weight loss over 18 months with no dieting at all. After taking early retirement from a desk-bound job, he began to walk an average of 6 miles daily. This was apparently enough to produce a small energy deficit and his tummy disappeared. The effect on his weight was slight but he became fitter, lost fat and gained muscle.

Sally

Sally, aged 17, again not seriously overweight, was nevertheless a bit plumper than she liked. Working for A-levels, she was very sedentary, doing her school work and then watching television. She joined an athletics club, trained around 5 hours a week and trimmed down nicely. The exercise also lifted her mood, having a noticeably cheering effect and it helped rather than hindered her A-level preparation.

Margaret

Aged 22, Margaret had been severely overweight since her early teens. At 20, she weighed 20 stones (127 kg). Over 2 years she halved her weight. This required a lot of self-discipline and she had to plan her food each day, aiming at 1000 kcal (4.2 MJ). Breakfast was fruit (apple, orange, and so on), for lunch a selection of fruit and salads, perhaps with soup on a cold day and she had a carefully balanced meal at night – lean meat or fish, a lot of vegetables (obviously avoiding chips) and fruit, low-fat yoghurt or sugar-free jelly for pudding. She found these jellies very useful and sometimes used them as a drink. She also took some form of exercise daily. Obviously Christmas and other celebrations interfered with her steady weight loss, but this she accepted, being aware of the hazards of obsessional slimming. She kept a supply of carrot and celery sticks handy for nibbles and sometimes went to bed early to avoid eating more. Margaret easily gains weight and it seems, unless she takes up a very energetic life-style, will have to continue to be careful.

Edward

Edward, aged 22, became plump around the age of 8. A rather inactive little boy, he had lifts to and from school and was fond of watching television and of eating. Though not severely obese, he was overweight. His mother did nothing about it, hoping that the adolescent growth spurt would solve the problem. In fact he solved the problem himself around 16. He bought some body-building weights, did daily exercises and cut out between-meal snacks and sugar in tea. After 6 months, he was attractively leaner and fitter. He still ate substantial meals, though fewer chips, but indulged in the occasional chocolate bar and the more frequent Guinness. The great benefit of this sequence of events was that a lot of probably useless nagging was avoided. Had the problem been more serious, and if there had been bullying or teasing at school, then an earlier intervention would have been required.

Pauline

Pauline, aged 40, was a fat child. Part of this was due to an indulgent father, who would treat her to cream cakes. Again, little was achieved in the childhood years, probably because family harmony was at stake. A chance remark by a relative that 'Pauline would look really lovely if she lost some weight' triggered her first really motivated attempt to slim at 22. Losing weight she has remained slim, with some fluctuations, since.

Richard

Parental divorce and a child minder who gave him chips every day caused Richard, now 11, to put on weight, so that he began to be teased at school. He lost this weight over the long summer holidays, by a planned combination of exercise, no chips and more salads. Richard himself was unaware of the plan. This is often sensible for children: who wants to worry about dieting at 11?

Joyce

Joyce, aged 70, likes food and has always had a tendency to put on weight easily. She now has arthritis and moves little and slowly. Thus, all her energy deficit has to come from calorie reduction. Only by severely reducing fat-rich foods can she do this and still have meals bulky enough to satisfy her. This means always choosing low fat foods, like fruit for snacks, lots of vegetables with main meals, perhaps a clear soup instead of a pudding or gelatine-type desserts rather than creamy ones. With these alternatives, an adequate supply of vitamins and minerals would be provided along with non-starch polysaccharides to prevent constipation. This situation, where exercise is severely limited, is very difficult and diet has constantly to be watched.

Sir Ranulph Fiennes and Dr Michael Stroud

Walking in the Arctic and pulling heavy sledges, both these men lost weight in spite of eating 5200 kcal (22 MJ)/day. This must be the proof that exercise alone can cause loss of body weight. For an Arctic husky race, the Iditarod, an average food supply of 6000 kcal (25 MJ)/day is recommended.

MORE EXTREME TREATMENTS FOR OBESITY

These have been used under medical supervision, with varying degrees of success.

1. Waistcord: a non-stretch cord is fitted and sealed around the waist, so that it becomes tight and uncomfortable after eating a large amount, thus giving an additional signal of satiety.
2. Jaw-wiring, so that liquid food only can be taken, through a straw.
3. Oesophageal banding has been used in Scandinavia, so that the particle size of swallowed food is restricted and eating slowed.
4. Surgical procedures of gastric partition, gastric balloon, gastric bypass all reduce the storage capacity of the stomach, so reducing the amount that can be eaten at one time. Jejunoileal bypass and biliopancreatic bypass both reduce the absorption of nutrients.
5. Lipectomy, where fat cells are removed by suction, is used for reducing fat stores.
6. Pharmacological agents, such as appetite-suppressants, enzyme inhibitors and thermogenic drugs have been used. Prolonged treatment with ephedrine has shown to have some success, presumably by activating brown adipose tissue.

COMMON MYTHS

'It's my bones'
No. Bones, being a dry material, are relatively light in weight. Build is a different matter and a broad mesomorph will inevitably weigh more than a slight ectomorph of similar height.

'It's my glands'
Very unlikely, although obesity is common in hypothyroidism, hypogonadism, hypopituitarism and Cushing's syndrome. It is a common experience that female sex hormones influence appetite (as in the often-increased appetite of pregnancy and in the last half of the menstrual cycle) but this does not usually cause obesity.

'It's in the family'
True, obesity certainly is familial (see page 158).

'I eat nothing but I get fat'
Although obesity is always the result of too much food, some people, especially if sedentary, do require very little (around 900 kcal, for example) to maintain their body weight and therefore very easily

exceed this. The solution is to find some acceptable way of regularly increasing their energy expenditure.

DANGERS OF SLIMMING

There is a growing lobby *against* slimming diets. There are very many people who are constantly preoccupied with what they eat and their weight, often quite unnecessarily. Obsessional slimming can lead on to anorexia nervosa. A balanced view, with a realistic idea of the optimal range of body weight and an active enough life-style to permit a healthy appetite, is ideal (Anonymous, 1994).

For details, refer to Holland *et al*. (1991).   **Food choice**

Energy values:

- Water   zero
- Protein   4 kcal (17 kJ)/g
- Fat   9 kcal (37 kJ)/g
- Carbohydrates   3.75 kcal (16 kJ)/g

General rules:

- The drier the food, the more calories
- The more fat, the more calories
- Water gives bulk without energy
- Non-starch polysaccharides are often thought not to be metabolized, but they are broken down to some extent and may therefore contribute to a minor degree to energy intake.

MILK

Choose semi-skimmed or skimmed, compensating for loss of vitamins A and D with oily fish. For example:

- Whole milk (1 glass):   130 kcal (544 kJ)
- Semi-skimmed milk (1 glass):   85 kcal (355 kJ)
- Skimmed milk (1 glass):   64 kcal (274 kJ)

YELLOW FAT SPREADS

Avoid wherever possible or spread thinly. Use butter when soft, or margarine. Fat-reduced spreads better but may be more expensive.

- Butter, 10 g: 74 kcal (304 kJ)
- Margarine, 10 g: 73 kcal (300 kJ)
- Low-fat spread, 10 g: 36 kcal (150 kJ)

MEAT

Choose lean cuts or remove fat. Discard excess fat from mince after initial cooking.

FISH

Oily fish, although more calorific than white, should be eaten once a week for its fat-soluble vitamins. Add flavour to white fish with herbs. Frying in batter more than doubles the calorie content.

- Typical oily fish, 100 g: 250 kcal (1045 kJ)
- Grilled cod, 100 g: 108 kcal (454 kJ)
- Cod fried in batter, 100 g: 235 kcal (982 kJ)

Note: oily fish includes sardines, herring, salmon, pilchard and mackerel.

CHEESE

Edam is lower in fat than most hard cheeses. Cottage cheese is substantially lower in energy, but also in many nutrients.

- Cheddar cheese, 50 g: 203 kcal (841 kJ)
- Edam cheese, 50 g: 160 kcal (682 kJ)
- Cottage cheese, 50 g: 48 kcal (201 kJ)
- Cream cheese, 50 g: 230 kcal (978 kJ)

CREAM AND CREAM SUBSTITUTES

- Cream, single, 50 g: 97 kcal (403 kJ)
- Double, 50 g: 223 kcal (920 kJ)
- Fromage frais (plain), 50 g: 56 kcal (234 kJ)
- Evaporated milk, 50 g: 74 kcal (310 kJ)
- Custard, 50 g: 59 kcal (248 kJ)
- Yoghurt (low fat, natural) 550 g: 32 kcal (138 kJ)

BREAD AND BREAD SUBSTITUTES

There is virtually no difference in energy value between the different types of bread, white, wholemeal and so on. Many people believe that Ryvita, cream crackers and similar products are useful foods for slimmers. They are actually more energy dense than bread, having less moisture.

- 1 slice white bread, 27 g: 66 kcal (276 kJ)
- 1 slice wholemeal bread, 27 g: 61 kcal (255 kJ)
- 1 Ryvita, rye crispbread, etc.:   100 kcal (418 kJ)
- 1 cream cracker: 33 kcal (138 kJ)
- 1 pitta bread, 27 g: 69 kcal (288 kJ)
- 1 roll: 86 kcal (359 kJ)

BISCUITS

There is a large variation in energy value, dependent on the fat content. Values for one biscuit:

- Bourbon cream: 63 kcal (263 kJ)
- Garibaldi: 33 kcal (138 kJ)
- Iced shorties: 39 kcal (163 kJ)
- Wafer: 47 kcal (196 kJ)
- Jam rings: 62 kcal (259 kJ)

CAKES

There are two things to consider, the fat content and the size of the slice. Scones are not highly calorific, but with butter and jam, may become so. Values are given for an average slice or an individual bun.

- Dundee cake: 95 kcal (397 kJ)
- Chocolate gateau: 128 kcal (535 kJ)
- Fruit bun: 85 kcal (355 kJ)
- Yule log: 127 kcal (530 kJ)
- Swiss roll: 110 kcal (460 kJ)

PUDDINGS

Values are for average helpings.

- Ice-cream: 100 kcal (418 kJ)
- Jelly: 19 kcal (79 kJ)
- Cheesecake: 240 kcal (1003 kJ)
- Apple pie: 370 kcal (1546 kJ)

VEGETABLES

- Green, leafy vegetables: 15–20 kcal (63–84 kJ)/100 g
- Root vegetables (not potatoes): 14–44 kcal (58–184 kJ)/100 g
  depends on sugar content.
- Boiled potatoes, 100 g: 76 kcal (322 kJ)
- Fried chips, 100 g: 234 kcal (983 kJ)
- Oven chips, 100 g: 162 kcal (687 kJ)
- Roast potatoes, 100 g: 150 kcal (632 kJ)

FRUIT

- Oranges, apples, melon, etc., 100 g: 23–46 kcal (96–192 kJ)
- Bananas, 100 g: 76 kcal (326 kJ)

Grapes, depending on sweetness, fall between these values.

SNACKS

Snacking is so much part of our life-style that the choice of snacks is important. Some energy values are given below.

- 1 carrot, 100 g: 28 kcal (117 kJ)
- 1 stick celery, 100 g: 8 kcal (33 kJ)
- 1 apple, 120 g: 65 kcal (271 kJ)
- 1 banana, 70 g: 63 kcal (263 kJ)
- 1 orange, 120 g: 50 kcal (209 kJ)
- 1 tbsp sultanas: 71 kcal (297 kJ)
- 1 packet crisps: 150 kcal (627 kJ)
- 1 Mars bar: 128 kcal (535 kJ)
- 1 Cornetto: approx. 200 kcal (836 kJ)
- Polo peppermints, 1 tube: 110 kcal (460 kJ)
- 1 chocolate: approx. 50 kcal (209 kJ)

DRINKS

Coffee and teas: calories only from added milk and sugar.
Milk: see earlier list.

- Orange squash, 25 g diluted to 1 glass: 24 kcal (100 kJ)
- Orange juice, 1 glass: 140 kcal (585 kJ)
- Coca-Cola, 1 can: 140 kcal (585 kJ)

- Diet Coke, 1 can: less than 1 kcal
- Beer, ½ pint: 96 kcal (400 kJ)
- Wine, 1 glass: 96 kcal (400 kJ)

Starvation

The world has much experience of famine. A classic experiment by Keys in Minnesota in 1944 elucidated the effects of severe energy deficit on fit young men.

These can be summarized as follows: there is loss of tissue. Decreased secretion of insulin leads to loss of fat deposits and muscle mass is reduced, especially from the gastrointestinal tract. The heart also wastes and the weight of the liver falls markedly. There is no evidence of change of weight of the brain, nor of mental ability, although there are psychological changes, an obsession (not unnaturally) with food, apathy and self-centredness. Basal metabolic rate is reduced (due in part to reduced cell mass) and total energy expenditure is minimized by behavioural changes, such as curtailing all unnecessary movements. The skin sometimes shows pigmentation and people feel cold. Famine oedema may occur due to a fall in plasma protein concentration (Keys et al., 1950; Cahill, 1976).

Starvation is rare in the western world. But some commercial diets are near starvation level and the psychiatric disorder of anorexia nervosa causes some to starve themselves.

Thinness

A BMI below 20 is related to increased mortality. Some people are very thin and cannot easily put on weight. For those who have lost weight due to illness a reversal of the advice for slimming is required, that is, choose calorie-dense foods, add nourishing drinks to meals (milk, for example) and so on. Keys, in the Minnesota experiment, found that at the end, when the subjects regained lost weight, they first gained fat and only regained their former muscularity after 9–12 months.

For thinness in children and old people, see Chapters 11 and 13.

Anorexia nervosa

The term anorexia means, simply, loss of appetite. Anorexia nervosa is a psychiatric condition in which the patient, despite often extreme emaciation, denies that he or she is thin, never admits to hunger and seldom to fatigue. Bruch (1974) claims that it is the disturbance of perceived body image which is unique and central to the condition.

Anorexia nervosa occurs most frequently but not exclusively in intelligent girls from affluent families. Anyone with experience of adolescents will know that many become temporarily obsessed about their weight: the emphasis on slimness in our society fosters this and it is wise to turn a blind eye to such *temporary* phases. Where slimness is vital and therefore emphasized, as for ballet dancers and gymnasts, the incidence of anorexia nervosa is increased, though usually triggered by some underlying problem. The condition becomes serious, requiring treatment, when a female subject's weight falls below that compatible with menstruation, on average 46 kg. Although dietary supervision and advice is necessary, the problem is essentially one for a psychiatrist.

Some good results have been reported using zinc supplements; anorexia is a symptom of zinc deficiency and a long period of slimming may greatly reduce zinc status. On the other hand, the increased appetite which results may exacerbate the psychiatric condition (Bruch, 1974; Scott, 1988).

Bulimia   Bulimia, a condition where gorging is followed by vomiting, is also indicative of psychiatric disturbance.

Key points   1.   Food supplies chemical energy for movement, synthesis of new compounds, and heat. The rate of energy expenditure is measured as Basal Metabolic Rate (at complete rest) or as metabolic rate, the energy production at any one time.

2.   The Estimated Average Requirement is the only Dietary Reference Value. There are very big differences in the energy requirements of individuals, depending on age, weight, gender, activity, state of health, environmental temperature and on individual metabolic characteristics.

3.   The sensations of appetite, hunger and satiety regulate energy intake and normally intake balances energy expenditure, indicated by a steady body weight.

4.   Obesity is defined as an excess of adipose tissue, but this begs the question of what is excess. Diagnosis is by visual inspection, use of weight-for-height charts, Harpenden callipers to measure skin-fold thickness, or the Body Mass Index.

5.   The incidence of obesity is rising in the UK; the cause of obesity is a period of excessive energy intake.

6.   Obesity affects health by increasing the risk of coronary heart disease, hypertension, stroke, non-insulin-dependent diabetes and some cancers which are sensitive to sex hormones.

7.   Treating obesity is not easy; it is a behavioural problem. Any slimming diet must supply adequate nutrients but a deficit of dietary energy must be achieved, either by increasing exercise or decreasing calorie intake, or both. Weight loss should be slow, to avoid loss of lean tissue.

8. Various practical strategies, varying from food choice to joining a slimming club, will help. Exercise is extremely valuable.
9. Starvation causes changes in body composition (loss of adipose tissue, muscle from gut, heart, reduction in liver weight, but not in brain) and psychological changes. In recovery fat is regained first and normal muscularity after several months.
10. Anorexia means loss of appetite. Anorexia nervosa is a psychiatric illness in which hunger is denied and body weight falls dramatically. Bulimia is a condition where binge-eating is followed by vomiting.

Part Two
Dietary planning

A healthy diet 9

In this chapter the typical British diet and meal patterns will be examined, along with ways of interpreting nutrient goals in a healthy diet which are flexible enough to give a variety of solutions.

A healthy/balanced/ prudent diet

All these terms are used to describe a good diet. We know that, for health, we need nutrients in adequate amounts; that some, like the fat-soluble vitamins, are toxic in excess and that others, like some fats or a general excess of energy, may cause ill-health in the long term: that individuals vary very much in what they need: and that appetite usually ensures adequate energy supplies but not optimum nutrient selection.

The particular advice given in any place at any one time varies, simply because it aims at correcting the *particular* deficits or excesses of the average diet in the light of current knowledge. Today, in the UK we are advised to reduce fat, sugar, salt, alcohol and energy and increase the amount of non-starch polysaccharides (NSP, dietary fibre) and starch, eating more fruit and vegetables. This advice, with some variation as to the precise amounts, is given by the WHO and various expert committees in the USA, the UK and a number of other industrialized countries.

In the developing world the advice would be different; it might well be to eat *more* fat, for example.

OVERVIEW

What we eat today

Of course the range of diets eaten is enormous, but *average* intakes and the trends in our diet in the UK are calculated from the National Food Survey (MAFF; annual reports), which is carried out annually on more than 7000 private households throughout Great Britain. It measures all food brought into the households for a week. Because of the increasing amount of food and drink eaten outside the home, information on this food has recently been collected for some households. Additional information comes from occasional surveys, like the Survey of British Adults (Gregory *et al.*, 1990), and from firms such as Taylor Nelson AGB, a market research company.

MEAL PATTERNS

The typical meal pattern today is a light breakfast or none, a series of snacks during the day and a main meal in the evening.

Taylor Nelson found that most of us, if we eat breakfast, have a light meal with bread in some form and tea or coffee (with consumption of cereals, dried fruits, cheese and yoghurt increasing), then a snack lunch and a main meal in the evening, often later than 6.30 pm. Afternoon tea, which was once – like the cooked breakfast – a British institution, is now the preserve of the under 5s and over 65s (Burnett, 1989). Breakfast is a non-event for many people. Taylor Nelson found that on a sample day no breakfast was served in 2.6 million households, with children between 11–16 and men aged 17–24 most likely to go without (Burnett, 1989).

These changes show how we have moved from formal meals to snacks, with consumers putting an increasing stress on *convenience*, showing greater demands for *variety* and a *growing interest in health*.

FOODS AND NUTRIENTS

In terms of foods and nutrients, the changes year by year are not dramatic, although clear trends can be seen. A comparison between the beginning of the century and today would show striking differences, especially in the poorest groups. The extreme poverty of those earlier days is illustrated by two memories. A baker, calling at a house, allowed the youngest child to lick her fingers and press them into the crumbs at the bottom of his basket; the child remembered this as a great treat. In another case, a young girl lost her job as a domestic servant. Her mother's cry of horror was 'What about my dripping?' for the girl had brought home a basin full every second week. People on a low income still find it difficult to eat well, but the scale of the problem today is quite different.

We now spend on average only 12% of our total expenditure on food. The average expenditure in 1993 was £15.02 per person per week, including drinks and sweets, and 2.91 meals per person per week were eaten outside the home.

The changes of the last 10 years or so are as follows.

- *Bread*: the domestic consumption of bread, which had been falling continuously between 1950 and 1980, has steadied. Wholemeal bread has increased greatly in popularity, while consumption of white bread is still declining.

- *Sugar, biscuits and confectionery*: there is little change here except in the fall in packet sugar and rising chocolate consumption. The consumption of confectionery in the UK is one of the highest in the world, at over 200 g per person per week.
- *Fat*: average visible fat consumption is around 300–350 g per person per week. It has been falling slightly, with butter declining and soft margarine increasing. The average percentage energy from fat remained remarkably steady for years, between 42.8 and 42%, but fell to 39.7% in 1993 along with a decrease in total consumption.
- *Milk*: milk consumption started to decline in the late 1970s and has continued to do so. Liquid whole milk has fallen by more than 20% since 1991. Low-fat milks show a steady increase and their total consumption is now greater than for whole milk. More flavoured milk drinks are being consumed. Yogurt consumption has grown steadily.
- *Cheese*: consumption continues to fall.
- *Meat and meat products*: there have been recent small falls in this area; the average consumption is between 140–160 g per person per day. We are eating more poultry and less beef and lamb. Sausages have suffered from adverse publicity, while consumption of frozen products, paté, salami and others has increased.
- *Fruits and vegetables*: the UK consumption is one of the lowest in the developed world at a total in 1993 of 109.1 ounces (3052 g) per person per week (MAFF, 1991).

NUTRIENT AND ENERGY INTAKE

What does this mean in terms of nutrients and energy intakes? Our average energy intake has fallen. The energy content of the diet fell steadily from 1970 to 1990 and then stabilized. In 1993 it averaged 1830 kcal (7656 kJ) per person per day, soft and alcoholic drinks adding another 100 kcal (418 kJ) to this. In spite of this obesity is increasing, as we become less active (see Box 9.1).

Using a new and accurate technique (the doubly labelled water technique) changes in energy expenditure of British women between the 1960s and 1980s has been calculated (Figure 9.1).

Research in Cambridge has shown that a typical woman spends only 550 kcal (2301 kJ) a day on all her activities above that required for sleeping all day. This shows how easy it is to exceed energy requirement. Perhaps it is necessary to do so to obtain all the other necessary nutrients?

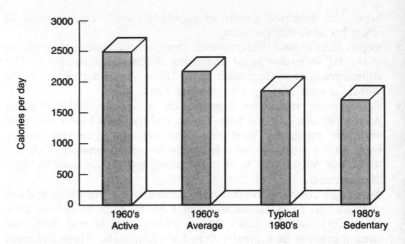

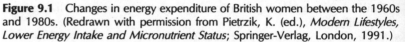

Figure 9.1 Changes in energy expenditure of British women between the 1960s and 1980s. (Redrawn with permission from Pietrzik, K. (ed.), *Modern Lifestyles, Lower Energy Intake and Micronutrient Status*; Springer-Verlag, London, 1991.)

The National Food Survey gives no evidence of undernourishment, although in 1993 the average intake of NSPs was found to be 11.9 g/day, a good deal below the suggested intake for adults of 18 g/day. But there were changes between 1992 and 1993 in the right direction; intakes of both total fat and saturated fats fell, and so did added (non-milk extrinsic) sugar consumption.

The effect of the fall in energy consumption on micronutrient intake is difficult to assess. The National Food Survey showed intakes of iron, zinc, magnesium and potassium below the RNI in most categories of household, but we must remember that the RNI is a generous standard. Intakes of magnesium and potassium rose between 1992 and 1993, those of iron, calcium and sodium fell. Intake of all the vitamins which were calculated were well above the RNIs.

BOX 9.1

> RNI: the Reference Nutrient Intake, which represents the estimated amount of a nutrient which would be enough or more than enough for 97% of a population.

It has been noted in earlier chapters on micronutrients that there is little evidence of overt deficiency in the UK, and we know that there is adaptation to low intakes. However vulnerable groups who are at risk of intakes which are less than ideal have been identified. These include those with very low energy intakes, smokers, those with high alcohol consumption and must also include people on very low incomes, especially the very young and the elderly.

Early nutrition may affect later health and there is no doubt that a lifelong good diet, beginning *in utero*, is a major factor in maintaining health and minimizing disease.

DIET OF SUB-GROUPS

Of course diet in the UK is not uniform. There are regional differences as well as differences according to income, household size and ethnic origin. The figures given below are taken from the National Food Survey, 1993.

Regional differences

There are considerable regional variations in the amounts of different *foods* eaten, but less difference in *nutrient* intakes, since the dietary variations are often between similar foods, for example beef instead of lamb. Intakes of food energy, and therefore of most nutrients, were higher in England than in Wales or Scotland.

Consumption of dairy foods was greatest in the South-West. Intakes of fish, sugar and preserves were low in Scotland. Vegetable consumption was highest in the South-West and West Midlands [269.4 and 273.4 ounces (7540 and 7665 g) per person per week] and lowest [243.3 ounces (6810 g) per person per week] in the North. Carcass meat was lowest in Scotland and highest in the South-West. Expenditure on food is highest in the South-East/East Anglia at £16.31 per person per week (1993) compared with the lowest total of £13.36 in the East Midlands.

There are other local differences in diet, some of them specific to quite a small area: the popularity of home-made leek soup in a small area east of Manchester or leek pudding in Newcastle are two examples.

Differences between income groups

The results of the National Food Survey are analysed according to income group. The data for the lowest income group is valuable since it is quantitative and the intakes of nutrients have been calculated, unlike most other surveys of those on low incomes.

In 1993 the average expenditure on household food increased with the income of the head of the household, from £11.51 per week in income group D to £15.62 in income group A. The highest expenditure was £17.64 in group E1. In group D more vegetables and much less fruit was eaten. Cereals, including bread, rose as income fell.

There was, however, no clear relationship between intake of most vitamins and minerals and income except for vitamin C, which is highest for group A. *Per capita* expenditure on meat and vegetables was highest in a household with two adults.

Interestingly, higher-income households had the highest proportion of energy from saturated fatty acids and the highest intake of non-milk extrinsic sugars. The lower-income households had the lowest percentage energy from fat.

Differences in household composition

Household composition has a major effect on diet. Expenditure per head decreased as household size increased in all types of household. This does not necessarily mean a poorer diet or less food, since a larger household can benefit from better value for money by buying large sizes of items and, if children are part of the household, they will usually have lower food requirements than adults.

However, household composition has a greater effect on nutrient intake than income. Households with children had lower intakes of all nutrients per person than households of adults and the difference increased with the number of children.

Variations in diet with age

The National Food Survey analyses the results according to the age of the diary keeper, that is the person who did most of the shopping and cooking. The average expenditure per person per week was lowest when the diary keeper was under 25 years of age and it increased with age up to the age of retirement. This is not surprising, since food is often not a major priority for the young, who may also eat out more and who may simply have less money than older people.

Life-style

Life-style is described by the World Health Organization (1988) as 'a cluster of closely interrelated behaviour patterns that depend on social and economic condition, education, age and many other factors' (Pietrzik, 1991). It is difficult to analyse these various differences into components which can be measured and related to diet.

As noted above and in Chapter 6, smoking and heavy alcohol consumption are two aspects of life-style which have important adverse effects on diet and nutrient requirement. Vegetarianism is another, where the effect is usually beneficial.

Most of the major characteristics of life-style will be examined in the chapters which follow.

What we are advised to eat

The goals advised by expert bodies (Table 9.1) have already been mentioned. These guidelines are proposed *for populations* and, in the field of public health, provide goals against which the diet of the nation can be assessed. Their precision does not represent exact knowledge. It is the best judgement of experts and, in the words of one report, 'should not be over-interpreted'.

The guidelines are for *healthy adults* and should not be rigidly applied to children under five years old, pregnant and breast-feeding

Table 9.1 (a) Population nutrient goals

	Limits for population average intakes	
	Lower	*Upper*
Total energy	See*	
Total fat (% total energy)	15	30†
Saturated fatty acids (% total energy)	0	10
Polyunsaturated fatty acids (% total energy)	3	7
Dietary cholesterol (mg/day)	0	300
Total carbohydrate (% total energy)	55	75
Complex carbohydrate‡ (% total energy)	50	70
Dietary fibre§ (g/day):		
As non-starch polysaccharides	16	24
As total dietary fibre	27	40
Free sugars** (% total energy)	0	10
Protein (% total energy)	10	15
Salt (g/day)	–††	6

* Energy intake needs to be sufficient to allow for normal childhood growth, for the needs of pregnancy and lactation, and for work and desirable physical activities, and to maintain appropriate body reserves of energy in children and adults. Adult populations on average should have a body mass index (BMI) of 20–22 (BMI = weight in kg/(height in m)^2).

† An interim goal for nations with high fat intakes, further benefits would be expected by reducing fat intake towards 15% of total energy.

‡ A daily minimum intake of 400 g of vegetables and fruits, including at least 30 g of pulses, nuts, and seeds, should contribute to this component.

§ Dietary fibre includes the non-starch polysaccharides (NSP), the goals for which are based on NSP obtained from mixed food sources. Since the definition and measurement of dietary fibre remain uncertain, the goals for total dietary fibre have been estimated from the NSP values.

** These sugars include monosaccharides, disaccharides, and other short-chain sugars produced by refining carbohydrates.

†† Not defined.

(b) Intermediate and ultimate nutrient goals for Europe

	Intermediate goals		Ultimate goals
	General population	Cardiovascular high-risk group	
Energy (%)* derived from:			
Complex carbohydrates†	>40	>45	45–55
Protein	12–13	12–13	12–13
Sugar	10	10	10
Total fat	35	30	20–30
Saturated fat	15	10	10
P:S ratio‡	≤0.5	≤1.0	≤1.0
Dietary fibre (g/day)§	30	>30	>30
Salt (g/day)	7–8	5	5
Cholesterol (mg/4.18 MJ)	–	<100	<100
Water fluoride (mg/1)	0.7–1.2	0.7–1.2	0.7–1.2

* All the values given refer to alcohol-free total energy intakes.
† The complex carbohydrate figures are implications of the other recommendations.
‡ This is the ratio of polyunsaturated to saturated fatty acids.
§ Dietary fibre values are based on analytical methods that measure non-starch polysaccharide and the enzyme-resistant starch produced by food processing or cooking methods.
Alcohol intake should be limited. Iodine prophylaxis should be applied when necessary and nutrient density should be increased. A BMI of 20–25 is both an intermediate and an ultimate goal, although this value is not necessarily appropriate for the developing world, in which the average BMI may be 18.
Data from Garrow, J. and James, P. (1993) *Human Nutrition and Dietetics*, Churchill Livingstone, London.

women, frail, elderly people, and those who are ill or on a therapeutic diet. All these groups have special nutritional needs.

If these goals were achieved by the adult population, significant falls in the incidence of coronary heart disease (CHD), hypertension, some cancers and obesity are predicted.

Rigid goals for the diets of *individuals* should be applied cautiously and advice depends on many factors. The risk of, say, a raised blood cholesterol to a particular individual may not be severe, if their genetic predisposition to CHD is low and no other risk factors may exist. The individual may therefore feel that is not worth while to severely limit the fat content of their diet. But for the government, providing expensive health care, it is advisable that the population as a whole shifts its blood cholesterol levels downwards. This would reduce the risk of CHD both for the few with very high cholesterol and for the multitude with much lower cholesterol and *apparently* lower risk, who, because of their numbers, represent most of the patients in hospital.

The dietary goals represent a dietary change for most people. This change must, if it is to be followed, be interpreted as a pleasant and palatable diet.

WHAT MAKES PEOPLE EAT AS THEY DO?

What made you decide to have a curry from the take-away last night? Fed up? Too tired to cook? You needed a treat and a take-away was cheaper than going out to eat? All these and other factors operate, namely:

- culture;
- personal preference;
- available resources; shops, time, money, cooking facilities and skills;
- psychology;
- social pressures;
- nutritional knowledge;
- health.

The relative importance of these factors varies. For someone on the poverty line money is an ever-present restraint; for others it might not matter at all.

Cultural background

An individual's cultural background is still, even in this multicultural society, one of the strongest influences on food choice. It includes religious rules (as in Judaism and Islam) and national, local and family traditions. Culture determines the foods which are suitable for breakfast as well as those necessary for a celebratory meal. It pervades the whole of the diet and, to an extent which depends on the individual, it determines its framework.

Available resources

The *availability of food* varies widely. In a large city, there may be a choice of several supermarkets and open-air markets as well as smaller shops. In the country, the choice is likely to be between the village shop (if there is one) and a journey to a supermarket. The possession or not of a car makes a great difference to the accessibility of food retailers.

The *money available* is often, after cultural influence, the limiting factor in food choice. Also important are *cooking facilities* and *cooking skills* and the *time* available to use them.

Individual likes and dislikes

Everyone has likes and dislikes. The flavour, texture and appearance of food are important. Taste acuity (or sensitiveness) varies, decreasing with age and in smokers. Food preferences often change with age; for example, most children seem to dislike the texture of lettuce, cabbage and Brussels sprouts but this usually lessens as they grow up.

Moral and political convictions may lead to vegetarianism or to the avoidance of foods produced in particular countries.

In many households the food provider has to tread a very careful path between individual likes and dislikes.

Psychological influences

Food, often used as a reward or a comfort in childhood, may remain a comfort in depression, loneliness or boredom in adult life. Sweet foods are particularly used like this. Some foods are liked because they are associated with home; others are avoided because their consumption coincided with illness or vomiting, or the person was made to eat them as a child.

Anorexia nervosa and bulimia are conditions where psychological influences override all others to an extent which is pathological.

Social pressures

These range from children who *must* have crisps in their lunch box or on the way home from school, to the business executive who is obliged to eat rich meals when entertaining clients.

Nutritional knowledge

There is a great deal of information and misinformation about food and nutrition today. The extent to which it influences diet varies. For some people nutritional considerations may be very important. They may be advised by their doctor to alter their diet to reduce the risk of CHD, for diabetes and so on.

The stage of life has an influence. Adolescents and new mothers are particularly likely to seek information and to follow it.

For others, nutrition may not be considered at all and there is some backlash against the plethora of advice and against the social pressures for slimness.

It is not easy to give accurate nutritional advice. For example, whole milk is recommended for children aged under two. At grandma's, only semi-skimmed is available. This *does not matter*; semi-skimmed milk is not harmful, it simply is not the best choice for everyday use at this age, because it has less energy and fat-soluble vitamins than whole milk.

Misinformation may be followed and result in absurd food fads. One example is a preparation of enzymes which is claimed to cause food to be used more efficiently. This is nonsense; the absorption of fats, carbohydrates and proteins is well over 90%, but such products are often persuasively marketed.

Health

When health is good, so, usually, is appetite. But illness may affect diet in many ways. There may simply be a loss of appetite, or discomfort on eating (as in gastric or duodenal ulcers) or concern about triggering an attack of migraine. All of these affect food intake and may do so for months and even years.

Appetite

Obviously appetite determines how much, and to some extent, what is eaten. Experiments in rats have shown that areas in the hypothalamus are involved in eating behaviour, receiving and processing signals from various receptors. This area of the brain then sends impulses to the cerebral cortex, resulting in feelings of either appetite or satiety.

Concentrations of blood glucose, the hormones insulin, glucagon, and adrenaline, the amount of liver glycogen and body weight are among the factors which have been shown, in laboratory experiments, to influence feeding behaviour.

Exactly what makes a person stop eating? This must be from a range of signals from mouth and stomach. There is also evidence that we unconsciously learn the energy value of food by experience and adjust our subsequent intake accordingly. New foods, of which we have no experience, cannot be judged like this and so it seems that a series of new foods in the diet could upset energy balance.

Variety stimulates appetite. This has been shown conclusively and is part of everyone's experience. Today, both novelty and variety in foods are common, perhaps causing us to eat more than we need.

There *is* long-term control of intake, though again the mechanisms by which this occurs are unclear. Underfed and underweight children eat twice the average energy intake until their body weight-for-height is normal, when their appetite suddenly falls. Similarly, adults fed very dilute foods will, over a few days, increase their intake to get enough energy.

Obesity is common in rich, industrialized countries. Lack of activity, a wide variety of foods and a high fat intake contribute to this. Grazing (or a series of snacks) may also be a factor, not only by adding new tastes and variety, but because, although a carbohydrate snack 30–60 minutes before a meal reduces food intake (the basis of that old warning, 'don't eat that now dear, you'll spoil your dinner'), a snack 2 hours before a meal does not and so can contribute to an increased energy intake.

Planning a good diet   The problem in dietary planning is to interpret nutrient advice in terms of foods, recipes, meal plans which are practical, palatable and possible. Planning cannot and need not be exact. There is considerable latitude in dietary needs. But a knowledge of the main nutritional characteristics of foods is valuable.

Many foods are excellent but *none is essential* for a good diet. The present tendency to classify foods as 'healthy' and 'unhealthy', although it has a rational basis, can be unhelpful. Sugar is *not* a 'healthy' food but it has great value in some diets and makes a lot of foods palatable. Similarly, fruit and vegetables are 'healthy' but would provide a low-calorie, bulky and unbalanced diet if eaten alone. People with obsessive tendencies about food can rigidly avoid 'unhealthy' foods and so eat an unsuitable diet.

There are various ways of planning diets, which will be discussed here in outline. More specific and practical advice will be given in the following chapters.

VARIETY AND MODERATION

This is the simplest message for a healthy diet. Add to it a good level of activity, and avoidance of excessive alcohol and of smoking and many risks to health are avoided.

Variety means that meals should not always centre round biscuits, chips and burgers, but should include a variety of protein sources, as well as plenty of fruit and vegetables. It means chips, say, are not eaten *every day* but *once a week*, with boiled or jacket potatoes, rice, pasta, bread on the other days. The greater the variety of foods, the less likelihood there is of deficiency or excess. Of course the variety has to be 'real' and not just a variation in flavour, as in cheese and onion crisps versus salt and vinegar.

An excess of any food, even one which is 'healthy' can be bad. An example is the effect on children of very large amounts of fruit juices and squash (page 228).

FOOD GROUPS

Food can be divided into four main groups (see Tesco's booklet, *Healthy Eating*) based roughly on the nutrients they provide. The advice which is usually given on this basis is as follows:

- bread and cereals group: four servings daily
- fruit and vegetables group: four servings daily
- milk products group: three servings daily
- meat, poultry, fish and alternatives group: two servings daily.

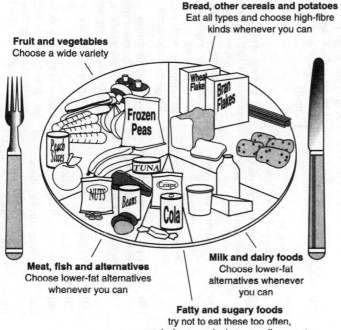

Fruit and vegetables
Choose a wide variety

Bread, other cereals and potatoes
Eat all types and choose high-fibre
kinds whenever you can

Meat, fish and alternatives
Choose lower-fat alternatives
whenever you can

Milk and dairy foods
Choose lower-fat
alternatives whenever
you can

Fatty and sugary foods
try not to eat these too often,
and when you do, have small amounts

Figure 9.2 The balance of good health. (Redrawn with permission from *The National Food Guide*, Health Education Authority, 1994.)

Foods like biscuits, cakes, sweets and chocolate should be added in moderation. Fats and oils should be used sparingly.

Another way of giving the same information is the *food pyramid*. Based on these groups, bread and cereals form the base of the pyramid, eaten in greatest quantity, then fruit and vegetables, then meat and alternatives, and finally the smallest amount from dairy produce. The same message is often illustrated on a plate (Figure 9.2).

MEAL-BY-MEAL PLANNING

Most people think meal-by-meal, or snack-by-snack, rather than for a whole day. What shall we have tonight? What can I eat now?

For main meals a tried and tested method is to choose the protein food (for example, meat, fish, cheese, lentils), to add vegetables (usually one, but two or more would be better), and finally the starchy filler

Table 9.2 Illustrative example of changes to National Food Survey results if COMA'S recommendations were met. The figures represent national averages, not recommendations for individuals. Food and drinks provided and eaten away from home would be additional to the amounts shown below. (From Report on Health and Social Subjects no. 46. *Nutritional Aspects of Cardiovascular Disease*, HMSO, London, 1994b.)

Food group	Average household food consumption 1992 (National Food Survey)		Illustrative example of average household food consumption meeting COMA recommendations		Comment
	g/person/ week*	Rough equivalent in terms of portions	g/person/ week*	Rough equivalent in terms of portions	
Milk	1960 (ml)	1 glass whole milk plus 1 glass semi-skimmed milk each day	2140 (ml)	½ glass whole milk and 1¼ glasses semi-skimmed milk each day	Continues trend to low-fat milk. Cheese consumption is currently steady
Other milk and cream	260 (ml)	1 tablespoon cream each day	130 (ml)	½ tablespoon each day	
Cheese	115	filling for 2–3 sandwiches each week	60	filling for 1–2 sandwiches each week	
Carcass beef and lamb	210	2 portions each week	210	2 portions *lean* meat each week (trimmed of visible fat)	For carcass meat the amount is left unchanged but a switch to leaner meat assumed; for meat products the example shows reduced consumption with no change in fat content
Pork and poultry	300	3 portions each week	300	3 portions each week	
Other meat and meat products	440	7 portions each week	220	3½ portions each week (assumes 30% reduction in sodium content)	
Fish and fish products	140	1 portion white fish or fish products plus ½ portion oily fish	190	1 portion white fish or fish products plus 1 portion oily fish	In effect this means doubling the number of people eating sardines, salmon, etc. in any week
Eggs	60	1 egg each week	60	1 egg each week	Assumes no change
Butter	40	spread for 3 slices bread each day	20	spread for 1½ slices bread each day	
Margarine	80		40	spread for 2½ slices bread each day	
Low and reduced fat spreads	50	spread for 1 slice bread each day	120		Continues switch to low-fat spreads and move from butter/margarine/lard to vegetable oils for cooking
Vegetable oils	50	4½ tablespoons each week	100	9 tablespoons each week	
Other fats	25	1½ tablespoons each week	10	¼ tablespoon each week	

Potatoes	900	1 small portion potatoes (2 egg-sized potatoes) each day	1260	1 medium portion potatoes (3 egg-sized potatoes) each day	Assumes 50% increase in main categories: present trends are for fruit to increase (mainly juice) but potatoes and bread falling
Potato products	170	each week either: 2 potato croquettes or 1 medium portion chips	80	each week either: 1 potato croquette or small portion chips	
Vegetables and products	1130	2–3 portions each day	1690	4 portions each day (assumes 30% reduction in sodium content of processed vegetables)	
Fruit and products	930	1½ pieces fruit each day	1290	2 pieces fruit each day	
Bread	750	3 slices each day (of which 1½ slices wholemeal)	1130	4½ slices each day of which 1 slice wholemeal (assumes 30% reduction in sodium content)	
Buns, cakes and biscuits	290	3–4 biscuits each day	145	1–2 biscuits each day	Assumes 50% reduction, with no change from current composition
Breakfast cereals	130	1 bowl each day	130	1 bowl each day	Assumes no change
Other cereals	285	1 serving pasta or rice each day	285	1 serving pasta or rice each day	
Sugar and preserves	200	6 teaspoons sugar each day (or good spread for 2 slices bread)	190	5 teaspoons sugar each day or (or thin spread for 2 slices bread)	Continues trends on sugar/preserves and move to low-calorie soft drinks. Assumes small reduction in consumption of confectionery
Soft drinks (containing sugar)	720 (ml)	2 cans each week	360 (ml)	1 can each week plus any amount sugar-free drinks	
Chocolate confectionery	35	1 small bar each week	30	¼ small bar each week	Consumption of soft drinks and confectionery is probably heavily under-stated because much is bought for consumption away from home
Sugar confectionery	15	3 boiled sweets each week	15	3 boiled sweets each week	
All other foods	440	2 tablespoons pickle or dressing each day	440	2 tablespoons pickle or dressing each day	Assumes no change

* Unless otherwise stated

(potatoes, rice, pasta) according to energy needs. To this 'meat and three veg', a pudding or sweet is often added. This can add useful nutrients to a meal, but soup or a salad (as in the American tradition) as a starter are alternatives which add vegetables to the diet instead, possibly, fat or sugar (Department of Health, 1994a).

There are a huge number of leaflets and recipe books with very good ideas, but a lot of people don't have the time to sit and plan their diet carefully, or are constrained by their family's likes and dislikes or their reluctance to try new foods or by poverty. But often the best way to eat a good diet is to plan for the week ahead.

ADJUSTMENT OF THE AVERAGE DIET

To show how dietary goals can be achieved, the results of the National Food Survey of 1992 have been analysed and the suggested changes made to it (Department of Health, 1994a) (see Table 9.2). This gives one example of good food choice, but it is only one. There are innumerable ways of interpreting the dietary goals.

ORGANIZATION OF MEALS

The common pattern of very little breakfast, a light lunch and then a main evening meal, with the evening often spent 'grazing' is not ideal. It can result in feeling hungry for most of the day. It has been shown that a good breakfast improves work performance in the morning.

Children need food fairly regularly throughout the day and the family meals should, if possible, be arranged to suit them. For example, most children come in from school very hungry and often fill up on cakes and biscuits. It is better if their evening meal is eaten early or after-school snacks are foods like sandwiches or toast (with peanut butter, Marmite, jam) or breakfast cereals with milk.

For retired people at home it is often convenient to have the main meal in the middle of the day. Of course, adults form habits which suit them and meal patterns to which they have adapted.

Finally, food is one of the great pleasures of life and should be enjoyed. It seems to me silly to prevent children or adults enjoying traditional party food occasionally because it is not 'healthy'. It is the *totality* of the diet which is important and, for children, too firm a hand at home often means increased skills in circumventing it.

Achieving change   Primary health care practitioners are in a key position to give advice about diet. Advice from practice nurses is often very well received. Health visitors, hospital nurses, and doctors all have a part to play and it has been shown that brief interventions of advice, information and counselling may be effective in helping people to change their behaviour (Douglas, 1976; Baron *et al.*, 1990). The skills required for advising on diet are the same as those used in other situations, those of sympathetic questioning, active listening, and of giving clear, appropriate advice in a non-judgemental manner.

EDUCATION THEORY

There is a theoretical basis for the process of helping people change. The sequence proposed by Prochaska and DiClemente (1986) has a sound research base and has been shown to be valid in different countries and with different behaviours. It can be summarized as the process of thinking about change, preparing to change, making changes and maintaining them (Figure 9.3). Relapsing, irritatingly, is a normal part of the process.

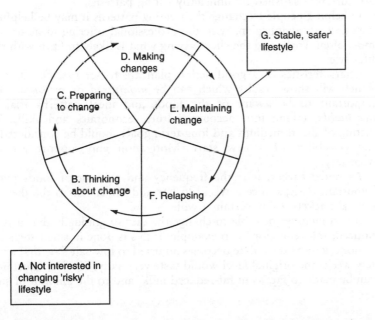

Figure 9.3 The process of change. [Redrawn from Health Education Authority Trainer's Manual; Health Education Authority, Hamilton House, Mabledon Place, London WC1 9TX; adapted from Prochaska, J.O. and DiClemente, C.C. (1986) Towards a comprehensive mode of change, in *Treating Addictive Behaviours: Process of Change* (eds W.R. Miller and W. Heather), Plenum, New York.]

Raising the issue

There are often opportunities for the health professional to ask about risk factors in a client's life-style. The defensive reaction of 'mind your own business', the fear of being judged or of being pushed into action before they are ready for it may be obstacles. If a person is not interested in changing, then there is no point in offering advice.

Thinking about change

Typically people balance the pros and cons of the situation. Information about health risks is necessary. It is important that enough time is given for the client to talk about their situation.

Making changes

Human beings use the easiest, most convenient and effective ways of meeting their needs. In changing behaviour will-power is rarely enough and it is necessary to find alternative ways of meeting the needs which are currently satisfied by unhealthy eating patterns.

In helping people to change their eating patterns it may be helpful to negotiate an action plan, with the professional offering ideas of what most often works and the client saying what is likely to fit in with their life-style.

Characteristics of a good action plan are to set *specific objectives* which will show results which can be *monitored or measured*. It is important to be aware of the foods and meal patterns that are *acceptable*, taking into account culture, economics and skills. The setting of short, medium and long-term goals should be considered, or the possibility of a new start. Motivation and support are also necessary.

As noted earlier, it is the frequency and amount of foods that is important. Crisps once a week do not add much salt to the diet, but several packets a day certainly will.

It is sometimes possible to change the diet so gradually that it is not noticed; salt reduction is an example. If this is done in small steps, it is unnoticeable as the palate becomes adjusted to low salt flavours; after a few weeks the original level would taste very salty. Similar adjustments can be made to fat, as in fat-reduced milk, and to the amount of sugar used.

Maintaining change

Group support, as in Weight Watchers, can be useful. Rewards for 'good behaviour' and strategies for avoiding or dealing with 'temptation' should be considered (Douglas, 1976).

Relapses

Relapses are not inevitable but they are common. The client should identify situations where relapses are likely to occur, so that avoiding action can be taken and should realize that the occasional relapse does not mean total failure.

EDUCATION RESOURCES

Food and nutrition are being taught in primary schools and the British Nutrition Foundation has produced a pack for this, *Food – A Fact of Life*.

In secondary schools, nutrition is taught in home economics and in biology. The British Nutrition Foundation and MAFF are producing resource material for this age range as part of their *Food – A Fact of Life* programme. Changes of emphasis in home economics and the introduction of technology have reduced the time for teaching cooking skills. There is a 'Get Cooking Campaign' which aims to rectify this.

There are many leaflets with information and/or recipes for the general public and the popularity of television programmes testifies to the attraction of cookery demonstrations.

The Health Education Authority has been training people to help people change with reference to smoking, alcohol consumption, eating and physical activity.

Key points

1. The dietary advice for a population aims to rectify the common excesses and deficiencies of the target population as identified with the present state of knowledge. Dietary goals for the developed world and for the developing countries will therefore be different.
2. Dietary goals for the UK are to eat enough to avoid obesity, to reduce intake of fat, especially saturated fats, and sugar, to increase intakes of starch and NSP and to avoid excessive alcohol consumption. These goals are for healthy adults and not for under five-year-olds, pregnant and lactating women, the frail elderly, the sick and those on therapeutic diets.
3. The average UK diet is adequate for all nutrients, except for NSP. The % energy from fat is higher (at 39% energy from fat) than is advised.
4. The typical meal pattern is a light breakfast or none at all, a snack lunch and a main evening meal, often later than 6.30 pm.
5. Factors which determine choice of food are culture, personal preferences and appetite, available resources, psychological factors, social pressures and nutritional knowledge.

6.   There are several ways of planning a diet: the simplest is variety and moderation. Food groups may be used or meal-by-meal planning. Ways to adjust the average national diet to meet the dietary goals are given.
7.   The health professional can have a key role in helping people to improve their diets. Prochaska and DiClemente (1986) have proposed a scheme for achieving change.

Pregnancy and lactation 10

This chapter deals with the requirements and common dietary problems for the preconceptual period and for pregnancy and lactation, discussing issues such as the role of folate in prevention of neural tube defects.

A woman's diet is very important both preconceptually and during pregnancy. Pregnancy is also a time when many women become very anxious about their weight gain and their diet in general, and often seek advice. The worry that a special diet is required is unnecessary as an ordinary balanced diet will normally fulfil all requirements.

Preconceptual nutrition for women

Since pregnancy increases metabolic demands, the nutritional status of the mother at conception is important. In the first weeks, which are crucial for the normal development of the fetus, a woman is unaware that she is pregnant and therefore ideally anyone likely to become pregnant should be eating a good diet and so be ready for the physiological demands of pregnancy. This is particularly important for folate, since a deficiency increases the risk of neural tube defects and the harm is done before a woman realizes she is pregnant (Thomas, 1994).

BODY WEIGHT

Body weight at the start of pregnancy influences outcome. Ideally the prospective mother should be within the optimal weight range (see page 155). There are hard data relating low pre-pregnancy weight to low birth weight, the major effect of *severe maternal underweight* being fetal growth retardation. Women who are *severely overweight* before pregnancy have an increased risk of complications such as hypertension. For these women some loss of weight *before* pregnancy is desirable, although it is difficult to decide how much, either from a physiological standpoint or practically, and any calorie reduced diet must be adequate in micronutrients.

Women who are recovering after anorexia nervosa may become pregnant as their fertility recovers and need special care.

NUTRIENT STORES

Some of the demands of pregnancy are met from body stores and it is therefore beneficial for these to be high, especially for folate and zinc, both essential for normal cell division.

VITAMIN SUPPLEMENTS

These are advisable for women who are, or who have been, on a slimming diet. However, megadoses of vitamins A and D can cause fetal malformations and high doses should be discontinued before conception.

ALCOHOL

Because of the fetal alcohol syndrome (see page 207) alcohol should be avoided at this time.

ORAL CONTRACEPTION

Oral contraceptives may affect micronutrient status and so it is advised that a different method of contraception is used for 3–4 months before trying to conceive.

Preconceptual nutrition for men   There is little evidence for specific needs in humans and therefore the only advice that can be given is the consumption of a good diet, and a reduction of an excessive alcohol intake. Severe obesity or underweight should be treated if possible.

Recent reports claim that there has been a fall in the average sperm count in the past 50 years and suggest that environmental oestrogens might be responsible. Both claims are extremely difficult to prove and the topic is covered concisely and readably by Vines (1995).

Pregnancy   Nutrient requirements are increased during pregnancy. This increase is met by a combination of altered metabolism, by the use of the body stores and by diet.

Pregnancy is a strongly anabolic state; there is increased retention in the body of nutrients to form new tissue. The changes are complex. Thomsom (1973) gave the following description of a pregnant woman; 'she gains weight extremely rapidly. She may be sluggish and often complains of digestive upsets. Body temperature is slightly raised and pulse, respiration and basal metabolic rate are also increased. Haematological changes suggest anaemia. The erythrocyte sedimentation rate is characteristic of chronic infection and the reduced level of serum albumin, often accompanied by oedema, suggests severe malnutrition' (Pietrzik, 1981). A higher incidence of abnormal nutritional status measurements suggests multiple micronutrient deficiency. Nevertheless, nearly always a perfectly healthy baby is born from a healthy mother.

The fetus is totally dependent on the mother and for some nutrients, like iron, acts as a true parasite, while for others, such as folate, the infant suffers more than the mother from a deficiency.

NUTRIENT REQUIREMENTS DURING PREGNANCY

These are even more difficult to estimate than for other population groups. Values given in the COMA report 41 are listed in Table 10.1.

The striking thing about the information in Table 10.1 is the small size of the nutrient increases. They represent the judgement of the Coma Committee on the scientific evidence available and the report notes that *these recommendations depend on adequate nutrient stores.* Where such stores are unlikely, a multi-vitamin supplement is recommended.

The difficulties in deciding on requirements can be illustrated from the estimates of vitamin B6 requirements in pregnancy. Depending on the chosen criterion for need, they range from 1.4 mg/day to 15–20 mg/day. Examples of the criteria used are the total amount of the vitamin transferred to the fetus (giving an estimate of 1.4 mg/day), optimum Apgar score at 1 minute after birth (7.5 mg/day) and maximum cord plasma levels of pyridoxal phosphate (7.5 mg/day). Does this uncertainty matter in practical terms? In this case, since B6 is widely distributed in foods, it is largely academic and it must always be remembered that the DRVs are estimations for populations rather than precise requirements for individuals.

Weight gain and appetite

The average weight gain for the whole of pregnancy is 10–12.5 kg (22–28 lb). A woman who is very thin at the beginning of pregnancy will obviously be likely, and will need, to gain more. During the first

Table 10.1 Dietary Reference Values for the pregnant woman. (From COMA Report no. 41, Department of Health, 1991) Crown copyright is reproduced with the permission of the Controller of HMSO.

Nutrient	Female (aged 19–50 years)	Pregnancy	Lactation
Energy (EAR)	1940 kcal, 8.10 MJ	+200 kcal, 0.80 MJ*	+450 kcal (1.9 MJ)– 570 kcal (2.4 MJ)
Protein (RNI)	45 g/day	+6 g/day	+11–8 g/day
Thiamin	0.8 mg/day	+0.1 mg/day*	+0.2 mg/day
Riboflavin	1.1 mg/day	+0.3 mg/day	+0.5 mg/day
Niacin	12 mg/day	No increment	+2 mg/day
Vitamin B6	1.2 mg/day	No increment	No increment
Vitamin B12	1.5 μg/day	No increment	+0.5 μg/day
Folate	200 μg/day	+100 μg/day	+60 μg/day
Vitamin C	40 mg/day	+10 mg/day	+30 mg/day
Vitamin D	0	10 μg/day	10 μg/day
Calcium	700 mg/day	No increment	+550 mg/day
Magnesium	270 mg/day	No increment	+50 mg/day
Iron	14.8 mg/day	No increment unless stores low	No increment
Zinc	7.0 mg/day	No increment	0–4 months, +6mg/day; 4+ months, +2.5mg/day
Copper	1.2 mg/day	No increment	+0.3–5 mg/day
Selenium	60 μg/day	No increment	+15 μg/day

Note: where a range of values is given for lactation, this refers to the different stages of lactation.
* Last trimester only.

trimester weight is usually gained slowly or even lost due to nausea and/or vomiting. Thereafter, weight gain is fairly steady, falling off at the end of pregnancy. Adipose tissue is gained most rapidly in mid-pregnancy and is deposited in the abdominal, subscapular and upper thigh areas (Table 10.2).

Table 10.2 Components of weight increase during pregnancy (maternal and foetal tissues) (From Thomas, B., 1994.)

Component	Increase (%)
Water	62
Fat	30
Protein	8

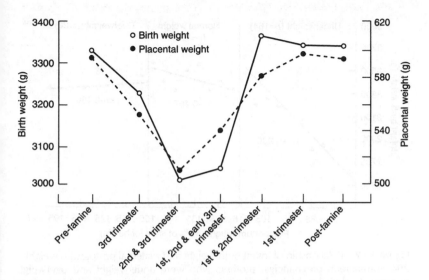

Figure 10.1 Effects of severe under-nutrition on birth weight and placental weight: this graph shows the dramatic effects of severe under-nutrition, especially when it occurs during the second and third trimester of pregnancy. (Redrawn with permission from Winnick, M., *Nutrition, Pregnancy and Early Infancy* (1989), Williams & Wilkins, Baltimore, London.

Both pre-pregnancy weight and the weight gain in pregnancy influence the health of the child, as shown in Figures 10.1 and 10.2.

From this it is clear that an underweight woman who gains little weight during pregnancy has a baby at far greater risk of perinatal death than normal, while an overweight woman has a similar increased risk, whatever her weight gain in pregnancy.

The additional energy requirements for a pregnant woman living in the UK are estimated to be quite small and several dietary surveys of pregnant women have shown little increase in food intake except at the end of pregnancy. However, dietary surveys often underestimate consumption and there is much anecdotal evidence of increased appetite during pregnancy, as well as records of marked increase in food intake in pregnant experimental animals.

Energy requirements will vary greatly according to activity. A woman pregnant for the first time may take care to rest while a woman who already has two small children will inevitably be very active. Appetite is, as always, a good guide to requirement. Weight gain is monitored throughout pregnancy and so a sudden increase, which may be due to water retention, will be noted. Pregnant women are often worried about their weight and ask 'how much should I eat?' It is

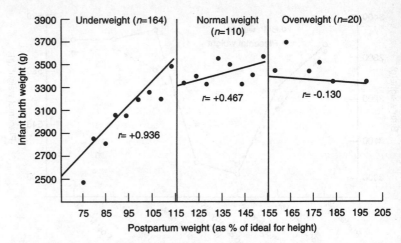

Figure 10.2   Relationship of infant birth weight and maternal postpartum weight in 294 normal-term pregnancies: mothers who were underweight and overweight (measured after the birth) had smaller babies than normal-weight women. (Redrawn with permission from Worthington-Roberts, B. and Rodwell-Williams, S., *Nutrition in Pregnancy and Lactation*, 5th edn.; Mosby, London, 1994.)

important that advice is tailored for the individual; as we have already said, a normally slim woman who loses weight readily will be able to, and should, gain more weight than a plumper person.

There is some fascinating work being done comparing the energy costs of pregnancy of women in developing and developed countries and showing huge differences, women in developing countries having lower energy intakes. This is not relevant to women in the UK but does emphasize the enormous variations in nutritional needs.

Protein

There is increased need but this is not normally a problem in the UK where protein intakes are nearly always higher then the RNI. Nitrogen balance is positive in pregnancy. In the first half, extra protein is deposited in the maternal muscle tissue, and this is reused in the second half of pregnancy to supply amino acids to the fetus.

Fats

Long-chain n-3 fatty acids are needed for development of the fetal nervous system and fetal requirements are high in the last trimester.

These acids are found in oily fish, liver and egg yolk and in soya bean and rapeseed oils.

Vitamins

Vitamin A

A deficiency during pregnancy has been linked with low birth weight and premature birth while excessive consumption may cause fetal defects. Therefore pregnant women are advised not to take fish-liver oil tablets or vitamin A supplements, nor to eat liver, which may, due to current animal feeding practices, be very high in the vitamin. On the other hand, oily fish weekly is a good idea.

Vitamin D

A deficiency may cause maternal osteomalacia and in the new-born, reduced birth weight, low blood calcium (hypocalcaemia) and tetany. Dietary vitamin D (from margarine, evaporated milk, oily fish) is therefore important, as well as exposure to sunlight.

Vitamin K

This is important as maternal deficiency causes haemorrhagic disease of the new-born, which can be fatal. All babies in the UK are given vitamin K by injection or orally at birth.

Thiamin (B1)

There is increased need for thiamine which is water-soluble and destroyed by heat (as in the cooking of vegetables and the toasting of bread). Breakfast cereals and Marmite or wheatgerm may be useful sources.

Folate

There is a substantially increased need for folate. Deficiency during pregnancy causes megaloblastic (large-celled) anaemia in the mother and is linked with a range of problems, including increased rates of spontaneous abortion, premature delivery, low birth weight and foetal malformation. Most importantly, neural tube defects (spina bifida, anencephaly) are due, in the vast majority of cases, to a metabolic block in folate metabolism. This block can be overcome by the intake of high levels of folate preconceptually. In a recent study of more than 20 000 pregnant women the incidence of neural tube defects were reduced by

75% when 4 mg folate was given as a supplement early in pregnancy (Scott *et al.*, 1994). However, this amount is very large and the results could be due to a pharmacological effect.

The Department of Health recommends that all young women should have 0.4 mg folic acid daily to ensure adequate stores for pregnancy. Women who have had a child with neural tube defects should take 4 mg daily before and during a subsequent pregnancy.

Such intakes would be provided by the following average helpings:

- Marmite and Bovril (1 tsp):   50 μg
- Broccoli: 50 μg
- Cabbage, spring, boiled: 15 μg
- Cauliflower, cooked: 40 μg
- Orange, one, fresh: 42 μg
- Peanuts, 1 ounce (28 g):   28 μg
- Egg, one, size 2:   23 μg
- Wholemeal bread, two slices: 28 μg
- Beetroot: 50 μg
- **Total:**   **415 μg (0.4 mg approx.)**

Other rich sources are:

- Liver, lamb, 90 g: 216 μg (but not advised during pregnancy, as levels may be higher than this)
- Spinach, cooked: 228 μg
- All-Bran, 45 g: 240 μg

As you see, folate is present mainly in fruit and vegetables and so it is easy for intake to be low. It is also easily lost in cooking and people who eat a lot of take-away or restaurant foods may eat vegetables in which very little of the vitamin remains.

Vitamin B12

Deficiency of B12 is a separate and independent risk factor for neural tube defects (Scott *et al.*, 1994). Care is needed for vegans and Rastafarians since this vitamin is found only in animal foods. Some vegetarian foods are fortified with the vitamin (for example, some soya milks, some yeast extracts). (Details are obtainable from the Vegan Society, 7, Battle Road, St Leonards-on-Sea, East Sussex, TN37 7AA.)

Ascorbic acid (vitamin C)

There is increased need for vitamin C in the last trimester. This is easily supplied by fruit or fruit juices or vegetables. Those not able to afford much fruit must take care to cook vegetables so that vitamin C is retained and when buying fruit to choose those richest in the vitamin, citrus fruits rather than apples, for example.

Minerals

There is adaptation to increased need by increased absorption of calcium, iron and zinc from the gut during pregnancy.

Calcium

There is increased requirement, particularly in the last few weeks of pregnancy. During this period, maternal calcium stores decline. Achieving the increased calcium intake is easy if milk and cheese are eaten. White bread and canned oily fish like sardines and pilchards, where the soft bones are eaten, are also good sources. Vegans appear to get adequate supplies from vegetable foods.

Iron

There is increased need and iron deficiency in pregnant women is not uncommon. The fetus is a true parasite for iron and obtains its requirements at the expense of the mother. Groups most at risk of iron deficiency are those on low incomes, teenagers and multiparous women. Where maternal haemoglobin levels fall below 10 mg/dl (1.55 mmol/l), there is evidence of increased occurrence of prematurity, low birth weight and perinatal mortality.

In contrast a recent large study showed that the highest mean birth weight occurred in women whose haemoglobin during pregnancy fell to between 8.5 and 9.5 mg/dl (1.3 and 1.5 mmol/l) (Sterr et al., 1995). This study supports the view that routine iron supplements are rarely necessary for health of the fetus.

The present decline in eating red meat, a good source of well-absorbed iron, particularly by the young, is of concern although it is quite possible to gain enough iron from a good meat-free diet. Iron supplements are no longer routinely given, but haemoglobin levels are monitored and so reveal any need for supplementary iron.

MEAL PATTERNS

Fasting is not desirable for pregnant women and therefore regular meals are sensible. Today's common meal pattern of eating very little all day until the evening meal is not the best and a modification to increase the amount eaten at breakfast and midday would be sensible.

FOOD POISONING

Salmonellosis

The principal symptoms of salmonellosis are diarrhoea, abdominal pain, fever, nausea, vomiting. The carrier state can last for three months and sometimes there are complications. Salmonella is most commonly found in raw chicken and raw eggs. Both should be well-cooked (eggs hard-boiled) to kill the organisms. Good kitchen hygiene should be observed, especially avoiding using a chopping board for cooked meat or other foods which will not be cooked, after cutting raw chicken on it.

Listeriosis

Listeriosis, caused by infection of the bacterium *Listeria monocytogenes*, is a rare illness, though with a high mortality rate. In pregnant women it usually causes a mild influenza-like illness. Infection of the fetus can lead to abortion, stillbirth or delivery of an acutely ill infant.

Listeria may be in soft cheeses (Brie, Camembert, Stilton, Danish Blue) and these should be avoided in pregnancy. Undue anxiety is unnecessary, however, since very few cases in the UK have been attributed to food.

Toxoplasmosis

This infection is caused by a parasite which may be found in raw meat and unpasteurized (green top) milk and cats' faeces. It causes a mild flu-like illness in the adult but may cause abortion, blindness and mental retardation in the fetus.

NAUSEA AND VOMITING

Particularly common in the first 14 weeks of pregnancy (and indicating a lower risk of miscarriage than average), nausea and vomiting usually occur in the morning but may continue all day. Small, frequent meals (up to eight for those with severe nausea) are advised, avoiding fatty foods. Sometimes eating a dry biscuit or dry toast before getting out of bed in the morning is helpful. Where the vomiting is excessive (hyperemesis), medical help should be sought. Dehydration and fasting must be avoided.

CONSTIPATION

Gastrointestinal motility and tone decrease during pregnancy and this may cause constipation. Increasing intake of NSP through whole cereals and fruit and vegetables will help. If wholemeal bread is disliked, there are some white breads with additional NSP. Nuts may also be useful. Adequate liquid intake is essential.

HEARTBURN

This is caused by the reflux of acid from the stomach which burns the oesophageal lining. Sitting up or using several pillows for sleeping, small frequent meals and drinking milk (not fruit juice) to neutralize the gastric juice may be helpful.

ALTERATIONS IN TASTE

These are not uncommon. Pregnant woman often 'go off' tea or coffee or alcohol, or notice a persistent metallic taste.

PICA

This is a craving for particular, often bizarre, substances, which may be foods or things like soil or coal. It is thought that this reflects a lack of iron in the diet. Its frequency has fallen greatly in recent years.

ALCOHOL

Excessive intake in early pregnancy may cause the fetal alcohol syndrome, characterized by mental and physical retardation, and facial changes, a high forehead, prominent cheekbones and wide epicanthal folds. It does not appear to be dose-related and so the most prudent course is to avoid alcohol preconceptually and in early pregnancy, after which the occasional drink is harmless. A *safe* amount is very difficult to determine but current advice is to drink a maximum of four units per week which is two pints of beer, or four small glasses of wine. Women who have drunk socially during the early days should be reassured that the possibility of damage to the fetus is remote. (With the multiplicity of advice and warnings given today, it is possible to produce great anxiety in the pregnant woman.) (Bourne, 1989; Winick, 1989; Garrow and James, 1993).

It has been shown that the levels of vitamins and minerals in the body return to normal about six weeks after the birth, but levels of serum

After pregnancy

folate, ferritin (iron storage), and plasma PLP (pyridoxal phosphate), zinc and selenium remain low. Women with pregnancies in quick succession may therefore be at risk of developing inadequate nutritional status of these nutrients and may need supplements.

Lactation   The production of milk inevitably, like growth, requires a supply of nutrients. Some, such as energy, will be partly met from the maternal stores. The estimated increases, from COMA Report 41 are given in Table 10.1.

The requirements of the lactating woman are similar to those of pregnancy. She will need to drink plenty, feeling thirstier than usual, and this is a good way of including extra nutrients, by taking a variety of drinks, like milk, Marmite and fruit juices. Dietary vitamin D is required and this may be needed from a supplement. There is no estimated extra need for iron, since there is no iron loss from menstruation. Once again, appetite should be a good guide to food requirements.

Some undesirable substances do pass into the milk and so should be avoided. These are alcohol, caffeine, nicotine (from smoking), senna and alkaloids (from green potatoes). Many drugs also pass into the milk.

Key points
1. The nutritional status of a woman at the time of conception is important; good nutrient stores are beneficial, especially for folate, a deficiency of which is linked to neural tube defects. Body weight at the start of pregnancy influences outcome.
2. There is little evidence about the importance of preconceptual nutrition for men.
3. Pregnancy is a strongly anabolic state, with increased retention of nutrients. The Dietary Reference Values do not estimate large increases in requirements but assume adequate nutrient stores. The most important points are that a good diet is eaten, that long-chain n-3 fatty acids (oily fish, liver, egg yolk), folate, iron, calcium are taken in adequate amounts. Vitamin B12 supply needs care for vegans. Excessive intake of alcohol should be avoided.
4. Pregnant women may have various minor problems, like constipation, heartburn and so on, and these are discussed.
5. Pregnant women should be careful to avoid salmonellosis (undercooked poultry and eggs), listeriosis (soft cheeses) and toxoplasmosis (raw meat, unpasteurized, green-top, milk).

Feeding children 11

This chapter gives an outline of the processes of growth and covers the feeding of infants and children up to adulthood. References are given for a range of literature from academic reviews and papers to the advisory leaflets for the general public. As always the organization of the material posed questions. Thus some topics, like faddiness, are dealt with under pre-school children but, of course, are not confined to that age group. Dental health is covered in Chapter 3 and obesity in Chapter 8.

Growth

Growth is the process by which the original, single, fertilized cell increases to many millions of cells, differentiated into various types to form the organs of the human body. The rate of growth and the final size of a person are influenced by genetic make-up and by environmental factors. Growth is a regular, orderly process, controlled by the coordinated action of several hormones. The raw materials are the nutrients supplied by the diet. The hormones involved are the growth hormone, which acts through somatomedin (a substance produced in the liver and kidney), the thyroid hormone, androgens and insulin.

Growth is a word which is often used without much thought as to its precise meaning and it is usually taken to mean an increase in height. To assess growth, height-for-age or, much less commonly, the height velocity curve (the rate of increase in height over time) can be used.

The most *commonly used* measurement, though, is weight, particularly for young children. Weight is much easier to measure than height and often a fall in weight is the first indication that growth is slowing and that something is wrong.

Another index which is used is *head circumference*, measured in all new-born babies. It is relatively independent of diet and therefore may be used as an indication of the baby's expected size.

Standards for growth are obtained by measuring the growth of a healthy population. This data is then used to produce centile (also called percentile) charts, showing the typical height-for-age or weight-for-age for boys or girls. The 50th centile line gives the growth rate for those children who lie exactly in the middle of the population, the 90th, for those who are in the biggest tenth of the population and so on. There are many height and weight tables. New UK standards were produced in 1990; they are called the 1990 nine centile United Kingdom charts and are published by the Child Growth Foundation. The US National Center for Health Statistics (NCHS) standards are also available and are given in Thomas (1994). They are based on US data of the late 1960s and early 1970s.

The centile lines on standard weight charts do not define a 'normal' pattern of growth. The crossing of centile lines is more common than most people think.

These charts are commonly used by health professionals to monitor the growth of children up to about nine years old. After this the adolescent growth spurt, which may occur at widely different ages, confuses the issue. The growth spurt is flattened out in the centile charts by the averaging of many such spurts. As for all biological characteristics, the range of normality is wide. It is the convention that those falling outside the 3rd and the 97th centile should be investigated for possible pathology. Accurate measurements are essential.

The view of Tanner's (1989) is that height velocity is the best general monitor of health that we have and nutrition is one of the major factors influencing the rate of growth. Nutrition reflects family income, maternal skills and behaviour, all of which influence the diet. The happiness of the child is also significant, since psychosocial stress slows growth. This was shown clearly in McCance and Widdowson's work in German orphanages after the Second World War. Here, children who had been short of food for a long time were given extra food. Eating exactly the same rations, children in the care of a sympathetic matron grew faster than those supervised by a severe woman who made mealtimes a time of conflict.

Growth velocity is a very sensitive indicator of the child's *total environment*.

There are two periods of increased growth rate (growth velocity) for height. These are just after birth and during adolescence. On average boys complete their growth by 17.5 years (± two years) and girls two years earlier.

Infant feeding   BREAST FEEDING

Every authority recommends breast feeding for the first 4–6 months for healthy, full-term babies. It has huge advantages, which cannot be overemphasized, for both mother and child (Edsall Summaries, 1984; Winick, 1989; Walker, 1990). Women who are HIV-positive are advised not to breast feed because of the possibility of the virus being present in the milk. Women in developing countries where there is little alternative to breast feeding may be advised differently.

Present-day practice

Breast feeding declined in the earlier part of this century, picking up again in the early 1970s. By 1985, over 50% of babies were exclusively breast fed at least for the first week or two. The proportion was higher for first babies and in socioeconomic groups A and B (Mills and Tyler, 1992).

Advantages of breast feeding for the mother

Breast feeding is, for most people, *pleasurable*, once it is established and the early discomforts of engorged breasts are over. The obvious enjoyment of the baby, the chance to sit down during a busy day, even the fact that there is a free hand to hold a book or a displaced toddler, all add to its satisfaction, although some women do find it distasteful. Breast feeding is also easy, there is no preparation or washing up, and it is *cheaper* than bottle feeding, even allowing for extra food for the mother. Immediately after birth it causes *uterine contractions* (which may, in second and subsequent babies be painful), and so aids the return of the uterus to normal size. Breast feeding delays the return of menstruation and, if frequent and continuous, has a *contraceptive effect*, although this should not be relied upon. This effect is beneficial, though, where contraception is unavailable or not acceptable. Finally, most breast-feeding mothers find that they *lose the extra fat* laid down during pregnancy. Some worry that the shape or size of their breasts will alter. The degree to which this occurs varies and is minimized if a good supporting bra is worn.

Disadvantages for the mother

The mother is *tied* to the baby and cannot hand over for someone else to feed, except by expressing milk in advance. *Fatigue* may become a problem, through disturbed nights. There may be some *discomfort* from sore or cracked nipples.

Inverted nipples may be a problem and can be corrected by the wearing of specially designed plastic shields which fit inside a bra. These should be worn continuously for the last six weeks of pregnancy and between feeds if necessary.

Mastitis and breast abscesses may occur but they are infrequent.

Table 11.1   Composition per 100 ml (3½ oz) of colostrum, human and cows' milks. (From Edsall Summaries for Health Professionals, 1984)

Nutrients	Units	Colostrum 1–5 days	Transitional human milk (6–10 days)	Mature human milk*	Mature cows' milk
Energy	kcal	58	65	67	66
	kJ	240	265	275	270
Protein	g	2.7	1.6	1.2	3.3
Fat	g	2.9	3.6	3.8	3.7
Carbohydrate	g	5.3	6.6	7.0	4.8
Sodium	mg	48	29	15	58
Potassium	mg	74	64	55	138
Calcium	mg	31	34	33	125
Phosphorus	mg	14	17	15	96
Iron	mg	0.09	0.04	0.08	0.10
Copper	μg	50	50	40	30
Vitamin A	μg retinol eq.	108	94	58	40
Vitamin C	mg	4.4	5.4	4.3	1.6
Vitamin D (fat soluble)	μg	–	–	0.01†	0.06

* Figures taken from the Department of Health and Social Security Report on Health and Social Subjects 12 (1977).
† 0.8μg vitamin D sulphate also present.
eq. equivalent

Advantages of breast feeding for the baby

Nutritionally, breast milk is an ideal food. *Colostrum* is the name given to the milk produced during the first few days after birth, to be followed by *mature* milk. The composition of the two varies (Table 11.1).

Lactose accounts for 40% of the energy of human milk and the galactose component (see page 39) is necessary for the development of brain tissue. The *fat* is well absorbed and contains the *essential fatty acids*, important in the development of the nervous system. Fat supplies between 40–50% of the energy of milk. Interestingly human milk has a high, though variable, level of *cholesterol*. The *protein* in human milk differs from cows' milk and forms a soft, easily digested curd in the stomach. The concentration of protein is relatively low, but the quality is high so that it is fully used for body building. This means that the excretion of urea from surplus amino acids is minimal. The risk of dehydration is therefore reduced (the infant kidney cannot concentrate urine as efficiently as the mature kidney and so excretion of a substance like urea requires excretion of water along with it) and so is nappy rash, because it is the urea which is converted to ammonia by bacteria on the bottom and this ammonia burns the skin. Breast milk has a high concentration of glutamine which has a beefy taste; perhaps this influences later food preferences? It has a *low sodium content* and, overall, a lower mineral concentration than cows' milk which, again, is beneficial for kidney function.

All other nutrients are provided and there is no risk of too concentrated a feed. The absorption of iron from breast milk is extraordinarily high, around 20–50%. Obesity is less common in breast-fed babies than in formula-fed ones. Finally, brain development and function may benefit from breast feeding (Lucas *et al.*, 1992).

Protection from infections

Breast milk is sterile, although the baby ingests normal skin flora (Staphylococci) from the skin around the nipple. If the mother has an infection, there is no need to stop feeding. Bacterial infections will normally be treated promptly with an antibiotic and viral infections will not normally be transmitted to the baby.

Thus, the most common infection of babies, gastroenteritis, is both less common and less severe in breast-fed babies compared with bottle-fed babies. The more difficult the living conditions and the more hard-pressed or uninterested the mother, the more valuable this protection.

Breast milk protects against other bacterial and viral infections because it contains the protective agents. These are macrophages, lymphocytes, the bifidus factor (which inhibits growth of *Lactobacillus bifidus*) and antibodies.

Protection against allergy

Although some allergens are excreted in breast milk, it is much less likely to provoke an allergic response than other milks.

Disadvantages for the baby

An inadequate milk supply may occur, particularly if the mother is overworked and tense. Some mothers 'follow the book' so conscientiously that they will not give supplementary feeds even if the baby is clearly unhappy and hungry. Milk supply is increased by frequent suckling and if supplementary feeds are given, they should be given after the breast feed.

Contraindications to breast feeding

Illness of either the mother or baby, low birth weight and physical problems like cleft palate are situations where breast feeding may not be possible.

Note that there are *no dietary reference values* for breast-fed babies.

Practical points

A series of booklets produced by SMA Nutrition may be helpful in this area.

Starting to feed

Breast feeding is an art which has to be learned. If the baby is put to the breast immediately after birth, it suckles readily and usually all is well. Some delay in putting the baby to feed, due perhaps to a Caesarean section, means that this early reflex is less strong and a new mother usually will require help in getting the baby to latch onto the nipple. A pillow over a sore tummy is useful.

Frequency of feeding

The supply of breast milk is determined by demand and is stimulated by frequent suckling. The more a baby takes, the more will be produced. In the first few days feeding 2–3-hourly for a few minutes at each breast is good practice. Complementary feeding should not be given at this stage.

Once breast feeding is established, the advice today is to allow the baby to empty one breast and offer the other, beginning with alternate sides. Normally a baby will get all they need in the first 10 minutes of feeding.

Lactation will normally become fully established within 3–6 weeks. During this period fairly frequent feeding (ideally every 3–4 hours) is advisable to maintain milk production. Once established the frequency is less critical.

Expressing milk

It is quite easy to express milk, either manually or with a breast pump, into a sterile container, which can then be frozen and given later from a bottle by a minder, while the mother is out or to allow her to miss a night feed. It is useful to try this fairly early on. Once the baby is fully used to the nipple they *may* be reluctant to take the bottle, which requires a different sucking technique. Perseverance and trying different shaped teats should solve this problem if it occurs.

COMPOSITION OF HUMAN MILK AND FORMULAE

The composition of human milk and commonly available formulae is shown in Table 11.2. Note that similar figures for casein dominant and for soya based infant formulae are given by Thomas (1994).

Table 11.2 Composition of human milk and whey-dominant infant formulae. All values are per 100 ml reconstituted feed. (Reproduced with permission from Thomas ed, *Manual of Dietetic Practice*, published by Blackwell Science Ltd, Oxford, 1994)

Constituent		Mature breast milk	DHSS Guidelines (1980)	Cow & Gate Premium	Wyeth SMA Gold	Farleys Oster-Milk	Milupa Aptamil
Major nutrients							
Protein	g	1.2–1.4	1.2–2.0	1.4	1.5	1.45	1.5
Casein: whey ratio		40:60	As for human milk	40:60	40:60	40:60	40:60
Fat	g	3.7–4.8	2.3–5.0	3.6	3.6	3.8	3.6
Essential fatty acid ratio Linoleic:α-Linolenic (ω6):(ω3)		5:1	5–15:1	5:1	14:1	Trace of α-linolenic acid	9:1
Carbohydrate	g	7.1–7.8	4.8–10.0	7.1	7.2	7.0	7.3
Minerals							
Calcium	mg	32–36	30–120	54	42	39	59
Phosphorus	mg	14–15	15–60	27	28	27	35
Calcium: phosphorus ratio		2.3:1	1.2:1–2.2:1	2:1	1.5:1	1.4:1	1.7:1
Sodium	mg	11–20	15–35	18	15	17	18
Potassium	mg	57–62	50–100	65	56	57	85
Chloride	mg	35–55	40–80	40	40	45	38
Magnesium	mg	2.6–3.0	2.8–12	5	4.5	5.2	6.5
Iron	μg	62–93	70–700	500	600	650	700
Zinc	μg	260–330	200–600*	400	450	340	400
Iodine	μg	2–12	ns	7	6.0	4.5	4
Manganese	μg	0.7–1.5	ns	7	15	3.4	4.2
Copper	μg	37–43	10–60*	40	47	42	46
Potential Renal Solute							
Load	mosmol/l	86	79–143	92	92	93.5	100
Vitamins							
A Retinol	μg	40–76	40–150	80	60	100	61
D₃ Cholecalciferol	μg	na	0.7–1.3	1.1	1.0	1.0	1.0
E dl-α-Tocopherol	mg	0.29–0.39	0.3–ns	0.8	0.64	0.48	0.7
K₁ Phytomenadione	μg	na	1.5–ns	5	5.5	2.7	4.0
B₁ Thiamin	μg	13–21	13–ns	40	67	42	40
B₂ Riboflavin	μg	31	30–ns	100	100	55	51
B₆ Pyridoxine	μg	5.1–7.2	5–ns	40	42	35	30
B₁₂ Cyanocobalamin	μg	0.01	0.01–ns	0.2	0.13	0.14	0.16
Nicotinic acid	μg	210–270	230–ns	800	500	1200	400
Pantothenic acid	μg	220–330	200–ns	300	210	230	400
Biotin	μg	0.52–1.13	0.5–ns	1.5	1.5	1.0	1.1
Folic acid	μg	3.1–6.2	3–ns	10	5.0	3.4	10
C Ascorbic acid	mg	3.1–4.5	3–ns	8	5.5	6.9	6
Choline	mg	na	ns	7	4.7	4.8	nd
Energy							
	kJ	270–315	270–315	277	274	284	281
	kcal	65–75	65–75	66	65	68	67

na, not available; nd, not declared; ns, not specified; *, tentative guideline

BOTTLE FEEDING

Dietary reference values have been set for bottle-fed babies. The fact that the efficiency of absorption may be less than for breast milk has been taken into account in their determination. The DRVs for some nutrients may be higher than those obtained from some brands of infant formulae but these formulae are within the ranges permitted in the UK (Department of Health and Social Security, 1980).

Infant formulae, of which there are many, are produced to resemble human milk as far as possible (see Table 11.2). The protein is usually from milk and skimmed milk, or it may be demineralized whey. A few use soya protein (Wysoy, Wyeth and Formula S, Cow and Gate). The fat content is nearly always a mixture of milk (cows') fat and vegetable oils.

Advantages of bottle feeding for the mother

It is a solution for the woman who finds breast feeding distasteful, while some mothers are reassured to be able to see the amount of milk the baby is getting. It is useful for some working mothers (although it is possible to work and breast feed, with careful management) and for women whose nutritional status is poor and not up to the demands of lactation.

Disadvantages for the mother

Formula feeding creates extra work in the preparation and sterilizing of the bottles, which must be properly done to avoid gastroenteritis. It is much more expensive than breast feeding, even taking into account the cost of the extra food required for lactation.

Advantages of bottle feeding for the infant

Satisfactory formula feeding is obviously better than inadequate breast feeding and since babies are sensitive to the mood of their carers, a happy bottle-feeding mother is better than a tense and anxious breast feeder. Innumerable healthy children testify to its nutritional adequacy.

Disadvantages for the infant

The protection against infections and allergens, conferred by breast milk, is absent. The physical closeness between mother and infant *may*, or *may not* be less than for the breast-fed child. Bottle-fed infants tend to swallow more air than breast-fed and so need to be winded more often. Constipation is more common and this may be helped by giving cooled boiled water between feeds.

It is important that, whichever method is used, once the decision has been taken, the mother does not feel guilty.

Practical points

Preparation of formulae

The instructions given on the packets should be closely followed and instruction into what is a level measure must be clear to avoid an over-concentrated feed. The importance of not adding an extra bit 'for luck' must be emphasized.

The choice of milk

This decision is often made on quite irrational grounds or outdated advice. All milks on the market follow the Department of Health and Social Security guidelines and so personal preference, cost, availability and ease of use are the factors to be considered.

Soya infant formulae should not be the first choice unless there is a *specific* reason for excluding cows' milk formulae from the diet. Non-milk sugars are used in soya-based formulae and therefore, to protect dental health, cup feeding should replace bottle feeding after one year and drinks of soya milk between meals and at bedtime are not recommended (SMA Nutrition, Iron a Nutritional Guide; see also Chapter 3). Special milks for low birth weight infants are available.

Choice of teat

Teats vary in shape and trial and error will determine which suits an individual baby. Some have an automatic vacuum release so that there is a continuous flow of milk from the bottle.

Position of the baby

The baby should be held comfortably and the bottle tilted so that the teat is always full of milk, to prevent the baby swallowing air.

Amount of feed

Guidelines, based on *average* requirements, are given but individual babies vary widely and current advice is to feed on demand.

Adding cereal to the bottle

This used to be a common practice, particularly for the last feed, to encourage the baby to sleep through the night. It is not recommended. It may give too high a solute load for the infant kidney and does not help in the development of feeding skills.

Heating milk

Bottles should not be heated in microwave ovens because uneven heating may occur, with some of the milk getting too hot.

THE LOW BIRTH WEIGHT BABY

Breast milk produced after a premature birth differs from mature milk and the premature baby is best fed with its mother's milk. Details of feeding low birth weight infants are given by Thomas (1994), Edsall Summaries (1984) and Walker (1990).

Weaning   Milk is a dilute food, low in iron and in vitamin C. As a baby grows and requires more energy and nutrients, more concentrated foods are necessary. Therefore the baby is weaned (Department of Health and Social Security, 1980; Edsall Summaries, 1984; Winick, 1989; Lucas *et al.*, 1992; Mills and Tyler, 1992; Department of Health, 1994; Thomas, 1994). This means that other foods are introduced, at first as a smooth purée with a gradual progression to the full range of foods and textures. Weaning causes a lot of anxiety among mothers, about the timing, what to give and how much. Some mothers, faced with an array of 'special' foods feel that it is not possible to give a baby ordinary food at all. While the baby foods are convenient and well-formulated, home-prepared food is cheaper and just as good.

THE AIMS OF WEANING

Weaning is the intermediate stage between a diet of milk and a 'normal' diet. It aims gradually to increase the nutrient density of the diet, to introduce a full range of food textures, and to establish a sensible dietary pattern. It causes new mothers a great deal of anxiety while for second and subsequent babies it often happens naturally without any stress.

GUIDELINES FOR WEANING

- The *age* at which weaning should begin varies with individual babies but will normally be between *4–6 months*. The guide will be the baby's appetite. If he or she is obviously getting hungrier so that the intervals between feeds are decreasing rather than increasing, then weaning should be considered. Physiologically the important factors are nutrient requirements and the maturity of the alimentary canal. When it was the custom to introduce foods very early, they often were excreted more or less unchanged. By four months the gut epithelium has 'closed' to foreign protein molecules which could cause an allergic reaction and the kidneys are better able to excrete a sodium load. Some of the current prohibitions, such as not introducing the foods most likely to be allergenic in susceptible babies, are blanket recommendations to protect the minority. These foods could probably be given earlier – with no ill effects – to most babies, but the safety first approach is recommended.
- Weaning is a *gradual* process and if the introduction of foods other than milk is at first unsuccessful, then it should be left for a few days before trying again. Immediate responses are often misleading – the baby who at first wrinkles its nose may soon accept the food placidly.
- The first weaning foods are not nutritionally important, since very small amounts are taken and milk is still the main food. The aim however is to attain a *nutritionally balanced pattern*, which combines starchy foods (cereals, bread and potatoes and pasta) for increased energy, fruit and vegetables for micronutrients and protein foods (meat, fish, cheese and pulses) for body building. All three are required.
- Babies should never be forced to take food they do not want. This could be the beginning of constant battles over food. No infant or child will starve itself voluntarily when there is food available and a relaxed approach (always remember that no adult is still refusing solid food) is essential.
- None of the advice given need be followed to the letter. Babies vary enormously in their requirements and in their development and intelligent observation of their needs is vital. Mother, usually, knows best.

STAGES OF WEANING

Weaning is usually divided into three stages (For details see Department of Health and Social Security, 1980; Tanner, 1989; Winick, 1989; Walker, 1990; Lucas *et al.*, 1992). The first, when smooth puréed foods are introduced, the second when purées are replaced with an increasing range of minced and chopped foods is given, and the third when the baby begins to eat more or less the same food, though chopped, as the family.

The role of milk in the first year

Milk remains an important food, valuable for protein, calcium and other nutrients throughout the first year. After breast milk has stopped, formula milk can be given until one year (some are iron-enriched, which is useful). After that cows' milk can be given. Obviously these are guide-lines only, although young mothers get so much advice, that they often like to have a definite recommendation.

'Follow-on' milks are available. They are expensive, some are very high in sugars but they are usefully iron-enriched. Some health visitors have found that babies who are used to them do not accept cows' milk well, presumably because it is much less sweet.

The introduction of cows' milk is postponed until one year because it is high in sodium, low in iron and vitamin C and possibly an allergen. Skimmed and semi-skimmed milks are not suitable for infants who need *more*, not less, concentrated foods, but there is no harm in using them for prepared foods. Evaporated milk is simply concentrated cows' milk and condensed milk has sugar added. Neither is suitable for babies.

It is recommended that about 1 pint (568 ml) of milk is given daily, in drinks or with foods (like cereals, potato) and in dishes like rice pudding, custard, cheese sauce.

Goats' and *sheep's milk* should not be given to infants and if used after one year, they must be boiled before use because they are not pasteurized by law (Armstrong et al., 1990). Goats' milk is low in folic acid.

Other drinks

Water can always be given. It should be boiled for the first six months and then tap water is acceptable. Bottled waters are not necessary. Most are suitable, however, but some may be too high in minerals. Fruit juices are a useful source of vitamin C. Those formulated specially for infants may be high in sugar and therefore cariogenic, so they should be given at meal times only. If ordinary fruit juice is given, it should be diluted.

Tea and coffee are not necessary or desirable. The stimulant effects of caffeine on the nervous system are undesirable and the tannin in tea reduces the absorption of iron.

Stage one weaning

This is the first introduction of solids, usually around 3–4 months.

Suitable foods

Baby rice puréed with breast milk, infant formula or boiled water. Puréed fruit or vegetables. Bananas are useful. Foods should be made quite sloppy at first so that they can be 'sucked' from the spoon and should start with 1–2 spoonfuls gradually increasing in amount and in firmness. Salt should not be added (partly because it is not necessary and because the infant kidney is not able to excrete a high solute load) and most literature includes sugar too. This is sensible, but it is worth remembering that baby is used to a milk which is sweet and it is sensible to include enough sugar to make fruit palatable.

Foods to avoid

The foods which most commonly cause allergic reactions should be avoided as a precaution. These are foods containing gluten (bread and flour, oats, rye, barley products), as well as cows' milk and eggs, nuts and citrus fruits. These foods can be added gradually to the diet after six months, one at a time, in case of an allergic reaction. It should be noted that the majority of children will have no such allergies.

Foods high in NSP (fibre) like Weetabix and All-Bran are unwise. Very fatty foods and anything containing chillies should also be avoided. Cabbage and broccoli are included by some authorities in this list.

Saving time in preparation

Such small amounts are needed at first that inevitably some is wasted, so it is useful to use powdered foods at this time. Note that they do not keep for very long (see use-by date). Once puréed foods are accepted it is a good idea for them to be cooked in bulk, enough for a week say, and frozen in ice-cube trays. Then one or two can be popped out for each meal, defrosted and heated thoroughly before use. In preparing the food, good hygiene must be practised: after cooking, the food should be cooled quickly and immediately frozen in containers which have been rinsed in very hot or boiling water. Where good practice is unlikely, these time-savers are not sensible. Some health visitors advise mothers to get a store of puréed food made well ahead of weaning so that they are prepared. To purée, a food blender or a Mouli can be used. A hand-held blender is very useful for small quantities as it can be used in a cup.

When to give solids

A time should be chosen which is convenient to both mother and child, when the baby is happy, and there is time to be unhurried. The new food should be given either before the milk feed or half-way through if the baby is very hungry. Gradually increase the amount to about one tablespoon at 2–3 meals a day.

A typical plan would be:

- breakfast: cereal and milk
- midday: protein and vegetables, like potato mashed with milk and carrots, home-made chicken soup (no stock-cube because of its salt content) which has been put through a food processor, or a strained ready-prepared dinner
- teatime: banana mashed with milk or puréed apricots, plums or pears or puréed vegetable.

How to feed

A sterilized, shallow, plastic baby spoon should be used and the dish should be sterilized also. At first an eggcup or the top of the feeding bottle will be big enough.

Stage two weaning

During this stage the balance between milk and solids is gradually altered in the favour of solid foods, which are offered in a firmer state and in more variety. It occurs normally around 5–6 months.

Suitable foods

More foods can be given, such as eggs (cooked until the yolk is firm to avoid danger of *Salmonella* poisoning), fish (no bones, canned sardines and tuna are good, but not in brine because of salt content), lentils and baked beans. A home-made stew can be mashed and given, adding the salt and pepper after the baby's portion has been removed. It is sensible now to use more of the family food for the baby, although ready-prepared foods are useful when visiting and travelling.

Foods to avoid

Wheat-based foods, fatty or fried foods, nuts and spicy foods, bran and bran-based cereals.

Time-saving preparation

A bowl of grated cheese kept in the refrigerator is useful for a quick meal. Canned fish such as sardines, tuna or pilchards are handy. Adjusting family main meals so that they are suitable for the baby, for example bolognaise sauce, with seasoning added after removing the baby's portion, casseroles and stews, soups. Rice pudding, custard, milk jelly are all useful.

Vitamins

Vitamin drops are recommended from *6 months* to *2 years*. They are available from the child health clinic or from chemists. One of the reasons for this is to prevent vitamin D deficiency. Few foods are rich in vitamin D (exceptions are egg yolk, oily fish, cheese) and exposure to sunlight is often low and associated with skin damage. Asian babies are at the greatest risk of vitamin D deficiency (see page 96).

Breast milk may be low in vitamin D and otherwise well-nourished infants, who may or may not have the typical deformities of rickets, may be hypocalcaemic. Two cases were recently described where infants presented with stridor and intermittent sudden airway obstruction due to laryngospasm. Both had severe hypocalcaemia due to nutritional deficiency of vitamin D (Train *et al.*, 1995).

Stage three weaning

Around 9 months, the food is now mashed or finely chopped or minced with the 'bits' gradually getting larger as the baby chews better. The range of foods can also be increased.

Additional foods

Bread, pitta bread and chapatti. Bread can be toasted (or not) and given as a finger-food or mashed with milk and grated cheese. Other finger-foods, including pieces of fruit, vegetables (celery, carrot, cucumber), and pieces of cheese can be given. Citrus fruits can be included and spreads such as smooth peanut butter, or Marmite. In fact now the baby can eat nearly all the usual family foods with the exceptions of highly spiced and very fatty foods. Most babies love sweet foods and this taste should not be over-indulged.

Practical points

A plastic sheet or newspaper under the baby's high chair to catch the dropped food is useful if the room is carpeted. Allowing the baby to feed him/herself when he/she wants to means that they will enjoy eating and learn the necessary skills quickly.

The aim is to adopt a sensible pattern, based on the family meals, which means that constant decisions (what shall I give him/her now?) are avoided.

However, 'normal family meals' vary greatly. Where these consist of convenience foods and ready-made meals they may not be suitable for young babies, being perhaps too high in salt, or fat or too highly spiced. Family meals which *are* suitable are things like stews and casseroles, pasta dishes, a mix of rice, tuna and sweet-corn, shepherd's pie, macaroni cheese, fish in white sauce. A diet which is healthy for a sedentary middle-aged man is not necessarily ideal for a baby in that high fibre and low fat foods do not meet the needs of an active, fast-growing infant with a small stomach.

Snack foods like crisps are not a good food for babies.

Ill children

Even when suffering from a minor infection, children nearly always lose their appetite. Drinks are essential to prevent dehydration and appetite will return on recovery.

Rusks

Even low sugar rusks, are a sweet food.

Gravy

This may be added to mashed potato and vegetables, but it is not a protein food and is likely to be a salty liquid. It is better to give the baby milk and perhaps some grated cheese if the meat part of the meal is not suitable.

Iron-deficiency anaemia

This is common after six months because by this time the stores of iron, present at birth, are exhausted. A study in Bradford found that nearly 25% of the children in the sample were anaemic (Erhardt, 1986). Children from deprived backgrounds and of Asian and Afro-Caribbean origin were found to be particularly at risk. Too heavy a dependence on milk and vegetarian diets may be reasons for iron deficiency.

At the Montpelier Health Centre in Bristol all children are offered screening for iron-deficiency anaemia when they attend for the measles, mumps and rubella immunization at 13–14 months. Those who are found to be iron deficient can then be given dietary advice. A programme of dietary education reduced the prevalence of iron deficiency from its original 25% to 8%. Iron-rich foods are meat, oily fish, liver, pulses, rusks, cocoa (see page 128) and a useful booklet (SMA Nutrition) gives very valuable tables of the iron content of food.

Advice on weaning

A commercial formula manufacturer, on interviewing mothers to determine their needs, found that mothers not only wanted information early, but also wanted advice on:

- what types of food to give;
- quantities of food to give;
- when to give them;
- menu/meal plans;
- use of tinned foods;
- food allergies;
- vegetarian foods;
- suitable milks to follow on after breast or formula;
- safety;
- vitamin supplements;
- practical and handy tips;
- food hygiene;
- diet and illness;
- dental hygiene.

For details about food intolerance, which includes allergies, see Chapter 19.

IMPORTANCE OF EARLY GROWTH ON HEALTH IN ADULT LIFE

There is recent evidence which suggests that the nutrition of the infant and of its mother are important in determining the later risk of coronary heart disease. Examination of the detailed records of people, born between 1910 and 1930 in Hertfordshire and Preston, has shown that poor prenatal and postnatal growth (as shown by birth weight and weight at one year) are strong *predictors* of risk of death from coronary heart disease and that the systolic blood pressure in adult life is *related* to both placental weight and to birth weight. Thus, adult systolic blood pressure fell on average by 11 mmHg, as birth weight increased from 5.5 lb (2.5 kg) or less to over 7.5 lb (3.4 kg). These relationships were independent of raised body mass index and alcohol consumption, both of which increase blood pressure (Barker *et al.*, 1989, 1990; Barker, 1995).

Relationship does not necessarily mean cause and this work is still in its infancy. If it is confirmed then the health of girls and young women will be an important issue in preventive medicine.

Children

Children are *not* mini-adults, but the scientific basis for estimating their nutrient intakes is meagre. There is data on requirements for energy, protein, vitamin D and calcium, but very little for the other nutrients. We also have relatively little information about what children actually eat. Many questions cannot be answered; for example, what is the effect on adult health and longevity of a high fat intake in childhood?

It is important to encourage a healthy eating pattern because there is general agreement that the food habits developed in childhood often continue into adulthood. Many children are quite adventurous about food and this should be encouraged.

The pre-school children

The pre-school child needs a balanced and fairly nutrient-dense diet which they enjoy eating, which sounds simple enough, yet problems with food loom large in many households. This is sometimes caused by the parents' loss of control over how much the child eats as he/she asserts his/her own will.

A large survey of children aged 1–4 years in 1995 showed that there has been an increase in average height since the last survey of 1967–1968. Average intakes of thiamin, riboflavin, niacin, vitamins B6 and B12 and folate were satisfactory. But iron deficiency was found in almost one-quarter of those aged 1–2 years. Leafy green vegetables were eaten by only 39% of the sample (National Diet and Nutrition Survey, 1995).

APPETITE

Appetite often declines after the first birthday as the rate of growth slows. The ravenous hunger of the first year is replaced by a fussier approach to food. This causes problems as there is nothing more irritating for a parent than the disdainful refusal of carefully prepared food. But no child ever starved voluntarily and there is no point in coaxing, forcing or bribing a child to eat (Illingworth, 1986). Attractive nutritious meals should be offered, if possible, at table with the rest of the household, and the child should eat as much as he or she wants with *unobtrusive* supervision. If almost nothing is eaten, there is no need to worry. *But,* this deficit should not be made good with offers of biscuits, sweets, and so on. Instead, the child should be allowed to wait until the next meal. If necessary and possible, this could be given earlier than usual. The amount of food required by individual children varies as much as it does between adults. The important issue is whether the child is healthy, happy and growing normally and not whether it eats as much as its parents expect. It is also true that children, unlike adults, have no *habit* of eating. Their appetites may vary greatly from day-to-day or week-to-week and this variation may be due to differences in activity. A healthy child will eat as much as it wants and needs.

MEAL PATTERNS

Small children have small stomachs and so they need more frequent meals or snacks than adults. An early breakfast may mean that a mid-morning snack is necessary. The important thing is that such snacks are nutritious, for example a banana, a piece of toast, a piece of apple, a cheese biscuit. Ideally they should be sugar-free and sugary foods given only at the three main meal times (see Chapter 3).

On the other hand, some children will eat a big breakfast, are not very hungry at midday and eat a large tea. This is fine.

NUTRITION REQUIREMENTS

The requirements for nutrients in relation to energy are relatively high in children and therefore the young need a nutrient-dense diet; that is to say, they cannot eat a lot of sugary foods, low in nutrients, and still eat enough 'good' food to satisfy their nutrient requirements. This applies particularly to children with small appetites. Therefore the food offered, based on ordinary family food, must be well-chosen and *what the child will eat*. Bread, cheese, milk, potatoes, meats, fruit and vegetables should be the basis of the meals. The *healthy eating guidelines for adults* are not intended for active, fast-growing children. Of course nutritious foods are required but a very low-fat and high-fibre diet is not suitable, because it does not provide enough calories.

The type of fats eaten are probably important (the evidence on this score is scanty), so unsaturated fats rather than saturated ones should predominate. A high sugar intake is undesirable both from the point of view of nutrients supplied and dental health (Chapter 3). Similarly, there is no need for a high salt intake and this should be avoided.

DRINKS

By giving a variety of drinks the nutritional balance of the diet can be improved. Milky drinks (adding drinking chocolate will increase iron content), fruit juices and Marmite (which is sugar-free and so useful between meals) as well as water can be given. Diet drinks are sometimes given since they are sugar-free and so do not cause tooth decay but they have no value in a child's diet.

Frequent amounts of high-energy drinks, like squash and fruit juice, have been shown to lead, in some children, to poor appetite, irritability, diarrhoea and poor weight gain. The collective symptoms have been called 'the squash-drinking syndrome' and were found in a group of children who received more than 30% of their daily energy intake from drinks other than milk. Very few of the children drank water and the researchers note 'Children are targeted consumers being unwittingly conditioned not to drink plain water' (Hourihane et al., 1995).

LIKES AND DISLIKES

Children's taste sensations are more acute than those of many adults and they are very aware of food texture, so that when they dislike a food, this distaste tends to be strong. Few young children seem to like lettuce for example. Some are much fussier than others. What to do? A consistent approach is vital. It is no good being strict one day and lenient the next. My own view is that it is best not to insist on the child eating what he or she does not like; this way a lot of friction is avoided and tastes generally widen as the years go by. Children usually eat better when their behaviour is not the centre of attention, which is why many mothers find that when guests or friends are present, eating problems temporarily disappear. The importance of a relaxed atmosphere was shown by McCance and Widdowson's famous work in orphanages in Germany after the Second World War (page 210).

FADS

It is also true that children often become 'hooked' on a particular food, or like some bizarre combinations. These phases pass and really do not matter. My youngest children had a phase of liking tomato sauce sandwiches made with white sliced bread, no butter or margarine, just tomato sauce. Or 'the red dish' becomes the only receptacle from which food will be eaten. These things are important to children and can easily be indulged.

CHOICE

As children grow it is possible to offer some choice. This should not be too wide. For example, 'how would you like your egg?' offers enough choice for a 3 or 4-year-old. My son's answer was always 'hard-boiled, hot, in the shell'.

ILLNESSES

Illness will always cause a loss of appetite. Drinks *must* be given. Growth will cease but will begin again as soon as the illness is over and appetite restored.

SWEETS AND TREATS

These are an enjoyable part of normal life but they are a cause of tooth decay. Sweets should either be given at the end of a meal (when there is a good flow of saliva, reducing chance of dental decay) or, say, once a week, on Saturday morning, after swimming or whatever. As long as sweets and crisps do not become a *major* part of the diet, all is well. Of course it is sensible to keep a young child in ignorance of them for as long as possible since habits are quickly formed, and yet this is surprisingly hard to do. It seems so mean not to give them just a taste of chocolate.

Salt-free crisps should be given for preference. Fizzy soft drinks should be counted as sweets and offered in the same way.

DENTAL HEALTH

See Chapter 3.

EXERCISE

Pre-school children are very active. The value of exercise and the opportunity to run about in the fresh air should not be underestimated. It will increase the appetite of 'picky' eaters and strengthen muscles. Swimming always seems to make children hungry.

Heinz Company Limited and SMA produce suggested menus which are a useful source of ideas for mothers.

Most children in the UK are adequately nourished and there is little frank nutrient deficiency, but more evidence of excess in the form of overweight. The concerns about children's diets lie in the groups at risk of sub-optimal intakes, and the possible effects of high intakes of

The school-age child

Table 11.3 Estimated Average Requirements (EARs) for energy kcal/day (MJ/day) (From COMA 41, Department of Health, 1991)

Age (years)	EAR value in kcal/day (MJ/day)	
	Males	Females
4–6	1715 (7.16)	1545 (6.46)
7–10	1970 (8.24)	1740 (7.28)
11–14	2220 (9.27)	1845 (7.92)
15–18	2755 (11.51)	2110 (8.83)

Table 11.4 Reference Nutrient Intakes for protein (g/day) (From COMA 41, Department of Health, 1991)

Age (years)	Males	Females
4–6	19.7	19.7
7–10	28.3	28.3
11–14	42.1	41.2
15–18	55.2	45.0

Crown copyright is reproduced with the permission of the Controller of HMSO.

fat and salt on future health. Although more non-milk-extrinsic sugars are eaten than recommended, the amount of dental decay has fallen.

Details of vitamin and mineral requirements are given on pages 87 and 116 respectively. The limitations of these estimates has already been mentioned.

Tables 11.3 and 11.4 show that, not surprisingly, average energy requirements rise with age, with boys needing more than girls. The RNIs for protein rise sharply and the requirements for vitamins and minerals to a lesser degree. These increases reflect the increasing size of the child and the usually increased level of activity.

What school-age children eat

There is not very much data on the eating patterns of children and young people. In the past 15 years some 10 studies have been carried out and only three of these have samples of more than 1000 (Department of Health and Social Security, 1989). These surveys show that energy intake are generally adequate. It is estimated that 10% of children are overweight. The Body Mass Index (BMI) tends to increase from the age of four and the earlier this increase, the greater the likelihood that the child will be overweight in adolescence and adulthood. Activity levels were found to be low (Armstrong et al., 1990).

Other points of concern are the generally low intakes of vitamin E and folate and in adolescents, low intakes of iron and calcium. One in nine children do not eat breakfast, with this proportion rising in teenage girls. A significant proportion eat crisps, snacks and biscuits instead of an evening meal. This confirms the importance of the school dinner for a large number of children and of nutrition education to enable a sensible choice to be made.

PROBLEMS IN PROVIDING GOOD NUTRITION FOR SCHOOL-AGE CHILDREN

Control of diet

The child now spends more time away from home, at school, with friends and so on and increasingly chooses his or her own food. So, a common pattern is a rushed breakfast or none at all, a school dinner offering free choice on a cafeteria basis, and the parent providing the evening meal only, and having little idea of what the child has eaten during the day. Provision of nutritious snacks for when they come home from school and a good evening meal are important.

Ideas for after-school snacks

Cheese scones, apple cake, carrot cake, banana and milk, carrot and other vegetable sticks. Sandwiches, toast, or breakfast cereals and milk.

Nutritious main meals

See page 365. For older children it may be useful to give a soup and then a main course, rather than a pudding.

Breakfasts

See pages 353–6.

School dinner versus packed lunch

The decision should be made considering all the factors which operate for a particular child. Are the school dinners 'set' or cafeteria-based? If the latter, what sort of choices are being made? Does he or she eat much of the school dinner or leave a lot on the plate? Do all his/her friends have packed lunch? A packed lunch can be just as good as 'a proper cooked meal' but it must be well chosen. Ideas for packed lunches are given on page 402.

Vitamin supplements

Vitamin supplements should not be necessary after two years of age if the child is eating a good diet. They may be useful, though, after an illness or for a child whose appetite has suffered through anxiety.

The thin child

Some children are naturally thin. If they are healthy, there is no need to worry. To increase food intake, some foods can be enriched (for example, mashed potato can be enriched with milk, dried milk, cheese), appetite stimulated by offering a variety of food (when sandwiches are offered with one type of filling only or with a variety, more of the latter will be eaten). The amount of exercise should be considered, since this increases appetite. A sweet course at the end of a meal is often a way of increasing the amount eaten.

The obese child

See Chapter 8.

The future

A Mori poll survey found that of a group of children aged between 7–15 years, only 38% could cook a jacket potato and only 54% a cake. There is a 'Get Cooking' project initiated by the National Food Alliance and the BBC *Good Food Magazine* which will perhaps replace the skills formerly taught at school in home economics.

The adolescent

The nutrient and energy requirements of the adolescent are high, for most people the highest they will ever require. This is due to the combined effects of the adolescent growth spurt and a high level of activity. The growth spurt occurs at different times in different individuals; for the DRVs the period of 15–18 years is used. The energy needs of the male adolescent are particularly high and it is usually need and not greed that makes them eat so much. Bread and potatoes are excellent fillers. A sandwich toaster is useful.

Girls have increased iron requirements because of menstrual losses. Iron deficiency is a risk in this age group and iron-deficiency anaemia is not uncommon, especially in those who become pregnant.

NUTRITIONAL PROBLEMS OF TODAY'S ADOLESCENT

The loss of the traditional meal pattern and the increase in snacking and in take-away meals mean that sensible individual choice is vital (Woodward, 1985a,b; Bull, 1985).

Slimming diets

Many adolescents, especially girls, periodically try to lose weight. This is not necessarily a bad thing if the weight loss is *necessary* and is carried out sensibly, but often the slimmer is not overweight and a very restricted diet is taken, or meals are simply missed out. This behaviour often reflects the unhealthy cult of thinness in our society and anorexia nervosa is a risk, especially in the high-achieving perfectionist (see Chapter 8). Sometimes nutrition education, by overemphasis on a division between 'healthy' and 'unhealthy' foods, can add to such problems, with adolescents eating only what they see as 'healthy' foods and avoiding starches, sugars and fats.

Vegetarianism

A well-chosen vegetarian diet is a perfectly healthy one. It is easier to provide all nutrients from a lacto-ovo vegetarian diet than it is from the more restricted vegan diet. The vegan must get protein, iron and vitamin B12, which are normally obtained largely from animal foods, from vegetable sources. One report found that vegan children have lower energy, fat and calcium intakes and higher fibre, iron and antioxidant vitamins than non-vegan children (Sanders, 1986). For more detail about vegetarianism, see Chapter 15.

Commonly held myths

- *That chocolate and fatty foods cause acne vulgaris*; there is no evidence to support this. Acne is related to hormonal changes rather than diet. But fairly high intakes of vitamin C may help (personal experience) and can do no harm. *Very* high intakes are not necessary or wise since they may, when stopped, cause rebound vitamin C deficiency.
- *That 'natural' foods like honey, brown sugar, organically grown produce are better, nutritionally, than ordinary versions*; this is wrong. There are differences in taste but no nutritional advantage.

Key points

1. *Growth* is an ordered process, controlled by hormones and influenced by genetic inheritance. It is modified by environmental factors, including nutrition and the psychosocial situation.
2. *Infant feeding*: breast feeding is recommended for its nutritional superiority, emotional bonding, convenience, and protection against infection and allergic reactions. There are no DRVs for breast-fed infants.

3. *Bottle feeding*: formulae based on modified cows' milk or soya protein are available and DRVs have been set.

4. *Weaning*: there are four stages of weaning from a diet of milk to one of varied foods and textures. A gradual process, with individual variation in timing, the aim is to achieve a good dietary pattern.

5. *Pre-school children*: appetite varies greatly between children and in one child from day-to-day. Appetites seem small and food fads may occur. Cheerful provision of a good mixture of acceptable foods and enough exercise to stimulate appetite are required and the child's appetite is then the best guide.

6. *School-age children*: the change in focus from home to school means that parental control is reduced. After-school snacks and evening meals must be nutrient-dense to achieve a good diet.

7. *Adolescence* is the time of the highest nutritional requirements. Iron intake for girls must be adequate. Sensible dietary adaptation is necessary for vegetarians. Excessive slimming should be avoided.

Diet in adult life 12

This chapter reviews the dietary guidelines for adults, and looks at the role of diet in common pathologies which may occur prematurely in middle age. Nutritional aspects only are discussed and so, for example, the effect of the contraceptive pill on blood clotting is not mentioned although it may be more important than its nutritional effect on folate status.

Dietary guidelines

The dietary guidelines for adults, both from the World Health Organization (WHO) and those of several expert committees, summarized by James, 1988, have been given on pages 183–4. There are also the recommendations of the Coma Report 46 (Department of Health, 1994) on the nutritional aspects of cardiovascular disease, which are very similar to those mentioned above and which also give recommendations for average intakes of specific foods. The Nutrition Task Force (page 6) had the responsibility for producing a plan of action to achieve the specific dietary and nutritional targets in the White Paper, taking into account these guidelines.

By the middle years some acquired habits may have an adverse effect on nutritional status, for example, a lack of exercise and a rich diet, or a high alcohol intake. But the quality of the diet in maintaining health is important.

Cancers and cardiovascular disease are together the major causes of both total and premature death in the UK. For cardiovascular disease, the mortality of the 40–60-year age group in the UK is one of the highest in the world. In both, diet is a significant factor.

Alcohol

A high intake of alcohol affects nutrition in several ways. It influences food intake, the digestion and absorption of nutrients and their transport, storage and excretion. Fat digestion may be impaired because of effects on pancreatic secretion, reduced bile salt secretion and/or changes in the intestinal mucosa. The availability of the fat soluble vitamins may therefore also be reduced.

Thiamin status may be reduced, leading in severe cases to the Wernicke–Korsakoff syndrome (see page 100). This is alleviated by thiamin supplementation. Other nutrients where status may be adversely affected are B6, folate, iron, calcium, magnesium and zinc (Pietrzik, 1991).

So, excessive alcohol consumption has a marked effect in reducing nutrient status. High alcohol intake is also a risk factor for CHD and a cause of hypertension, causing increased risk of stroke. Alcohol is second to smoking as a proven cause of cancer.

What is a safe level of intake? Alcohol consumption is associated with increased morbidity and mortality, increasing the likelihood of hypertension and stroke, liver cirrhosis and deaths from accidents. The relationship between alcohol consumption and age of death gives a U-shaped curve, however, with moderate alcohol consumers at the lowest point, indicating that a moderate intake may be beneficial (Marmot et al., 1981).

In addition, an association between national average wine consumption and national CHD mortality has been shown, wine-drinking communities having a lower CHD mortality than similar non-wine-drinking populations. This may be due to the presence of flavonoids, which are anti-oxidants, in red wine. Males drinking up to 30 units of alcohol a week are less likely to die from CHD than non-drinkers, but this is offset, even at fairly low levels of consumption, by increased morbidity and mortality from all causes.

The current recommendations are that 21 units of alcohol weekly for women and 28 units weekly for men are safe (Department of Health, 1995). (See pages 339–40 for alcohol content of different drinks.)

There is, however, more than one view about the safe level of alcohol consumption, some arguing that it is currently set too low, although no one would argue against moderation.

Oral contraceptive pill Folate status is reduced in women who, after long-term oral contraceptive medication, have repeated pregnancies (see page 105).

Obesity This has been dealt with in Chapter 8, where the causes, treatment and effects of obesity on health are discussed. Factors which may cause a positive energy balance for the middle-aged are lack of time for exercise, frequent business lunches, a very fatty diet, or a high alcohol intake. Increased earning power may make eating out a more frequent occurrence. Obesity often develops very slowly over years.

Diet and cancers Cancers are a major cause of death and morbidity. Environmental factors play a causative role in a number of cancers. This is indicated by the facts that incidence varies considerably between different countries and that rates in migrants alter to match those of the host population within one or two generations (Garrow and James, 1993). Diet is one of these environmental factors although the evidence is, in most cases, incomplete.

Experimental studies in animals, however, have shown clearly that diet can influence the incidence of cancer by a number of mechanisms, for example by affecting the metabolism of carcinogens and the body's reaction to them, as well as being a source of carcinogens.

Epidemiological studies support the hypothesis that diet is probably a major factor in the development of cancers of the large bowel and stomach and that it may possibly be so for cancers of the breast and prostate. Table 12.1 summarizes the position (Austoker, 1994).

A more detailed analysis from WHO, describing possible associations between diet and cancer is shown in Table 12.2.

Table 12.1   Current hypotheses relating diet and cancer. (Reproduced with permission from Austoker, J., (1994), British Medical Journal 308.)

Possible protective factors	Possible risk factors
Fruit	Meat
Vegetables	Total fat
Non-starch polysaccharides	Saturated or animal fat
Anti-oxidant nutrients:beta-carotene, vitamins C and E	Preserved foods
Fish oils	Alcohol
Plant-derived oestrogenic compounds	Salt

Table 12.2   Associations between cancer and diet. (From Austoker, J., 1994)

Site of cancer	Increased fat intake	Increased body weight	Increased fibre intake	Increased fruits and vegetable intake
Lung	Possibly increased			Decreased
Breast		Increased*		
Prostate	Possibly increased			
Endometrium		Increased		
Cervix				Decreased
Bladder				Decreased
Oral cavity				Decreased
Oesophagus				Decreased
Stomach				Decreased
Colon/rectum	Increased		Decreased	Decreased

* Postmenopausal women only.

This evidence endorses the current dietary recommendations and it is important, for the UK, to find acceptable ways of increasing our fruit and vegetable intakes.

- *Colon cancer*: the incidence of colon cancer is related to dietary fat intake and to meat consumption in between-country epidemiological studies. A large study in women in 1990 showed an increased risk with high intakes of saturated and monounsaturated fats, and with high meat intake. A high intake of NSP (non-starch polysaccharides) has been shown to be protective. Most studies of colorectal cancer have found a protective effect from vegetables, perhaps from fruit but not from cereals (Austoker, 1994).
- *Breast cancer*: incidence of breast cancer is increasing. Epidemiological studies between countries show a consistent relation between dietary fat and breast cancer incidence *but*, as in some other relationships, this is not demonstrated *within countries*, perhaps because the range of fat intakes is too narrow to show an effect. There is increased risk of breast cancer in post-menopausal women who are obese.
- *Prostatic cancer*: prostatic cancer shows a similar association as breast cancer with fat intake between countries and also, between *counties* in the USA.
- *Stomach cancer*: the rate of stomach cancer is declining in the UK. Diets rich in fruit and vegetables (and in garlic) are protective. Diet in early life may be important since changes in incidence in migrants occur later than for other cancers (Garrow and James, 1993).

PROTECTIVE EFFECTS

The protective effect of *fruit and vegetables* appears to be strong for cancers of the respiratory and digestive tracts, but absent for hormone-related cancers (breast, prostate). Smokers who eat a lot of vegetables and thus increase their plasma beta-carotene level may reduce their risk of developing lung cancer by 60%. Heavy drinkers who also have a low fruit and vegetable intake have the highest risk of oral, pharyngeal and oesophageal cancers.

There is no conclusive evidence that vitamin supplements protect against cancer, nor that food additives are a risk.

Smoked, cured or pickled foods are not eaten normally in sufficiently large amounts in this country to warrant concern. Mouldy foods should be avoided, which is not normally difficult.

The term cardiovascular disease covers many specific pathologies. Coronary (or ischaemic) heart disease and stroke are the two where dietary considerations are important. An excellent account of the nutritional aspects of cardiovascular disease is given in COMA number 46 (Department of Health, 1994).

Cardiovascular disease

DIETARY FACTORS

To quote COMA 46, diet is 'a major and modifiable cause of cardiovascular disease and is therefore central to prevention', although of course it is only *one* aspect.

The recommendations of this report, which are targets for *populations* and therefore proposed *average* intakes, are based on the available evidence of the relationships between diet and CHD and stroke (Department of Health, 1994).
They are that:

- people should maintain a desirable body weight (BMI between 20 and 25; see page 156);
- the average contribution of saturated fatty acids to dietary energy be reduced to no more than about 10%;
- there should be no further increase in average intakes of n-6 polyunsaturated fatty acids (PUFA);
- average consumption of long-chain n-3 PUFA be doubled;
- *trans* fatty acids should provide no more than about 2% of dietary energy;
- the average contribution of total fat to dietary energy be about 35%;
- average daily intake of cholesterol should not rise;
- average intake of sodium should be reduced by about one-third;
- average intake of potassium should increase to about 3.5 g/day.

Food recommendations are that:

- two portions of fish are eaten (one oily) per week;
- reduced fat spreads and dairy products are used instead of full-fat products;
- there is an increase of at least 50% in the consumption of vegetables, fruit, potatoes and bread.

These recommendations should bring about a beneficial change in blood lipids, a reduction in incidence of essential hypertension and in obesity.

CORONARY (ISCHAEMIC) HEART DISEASE

What is it?

Coronary heart disease (CHD) occurs when the coronary arteries are occluded to a greater or lesser extent by cholesterol-containing atheromatous plaques (Box 12.1).

BOX 12.1

> ATHEROSCLEROSIS
>
> In this condition the arterial lining is thickened by the accumulation of lipid and by the migration of smooth muscle fibres from deep layers of the wall, which proliferate. Atherosclerosis begins with fatty streaks which may develop into atherosclerotic lesions or atheroma.

These plaques cause a reduction in the blood flow to heart muscle and symptoms of ischaemia of the cardiac muscle (inadequate supply of blood) may occur during exercise. This is called angina pectoris and the symptoms are breathlessness and pain or discomfort in the chest, sometimes radiating down the left arm and to the neck and brought on by exercise or stress.

Atherosclerosis is a condition which develops gradually, perhaps over decades and this is one of the reasons why investigation into its cause(s) is so difficult.

Blood clotting (thrombosis) may occur at the site of the atheroma. A thrombus (clot) may cause total occlusion of the artery and so a 'heart attack'. This is a sudden or acute event. It is possible that it has the same or different cause(s) from the development of atheroma and this obviously complicates research.

Epidemiological evidence of cause

In most industrialized countries CHD is the most common cause of death, although rates vary considerably (Figure 12.1).

In the UK, *premature* death from CHD is high (Figure 12.2). Rates are higher in men than in women (and this is the reason why so many trials have been done on men, since a smaller sample is needed) (Figure 12.3).

CHD is, today, more common in lower-income groups than in higher ones (Figure 12.4). This is in contrast with the 1930s, when CHD was nearly four times as common in social class 1 as in classes IV and V. By 1950, this class differential was reduced by half and since then has reversed.

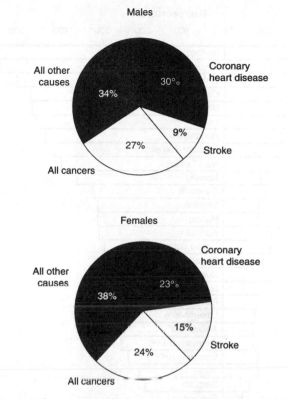

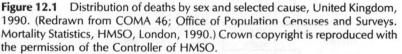

Figure 12.1 Distribution of deaths by sex and selected cause, United Kingdom, 1990. (Redrawn from COMA 46; Office of Population Censuses and Surveys. Mortality Statistics, HMSO, London, 1990.) Crown copyright is reproduced with the permission of the Controller of HMSO.

In the 50 years up to 1960, the incidence of CHD in the UK rose. Although there were changes in diagnosis, there is no doubt that this rise was a real one. Since about 1978, incidence has been falling for both sexes and all ages (Figures 12.5 and 12.6).

In view of the link between CHD and dietary fat, the trends in fatty acid consumption are shown in Figure 12.7.

What is the cause of CHD?

The truth is that we do not know. A very large number of risk factors have been identified, that is, factors which increase the likelihood of the individual suffering from CHD. This leads to the conclusion that the cause is multifactorial rather than a single agent.

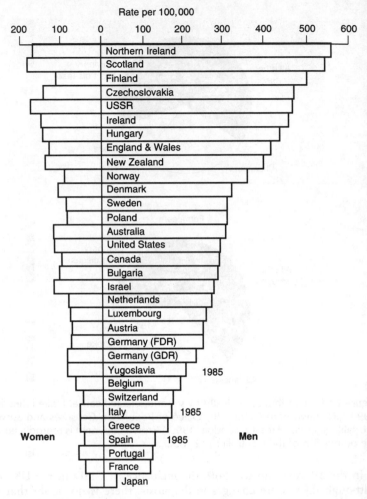

Figure 12.2 Coronary heart disease rates in 32 countries for men and women aged 40–60. Values are age-standardized rates per 100 000 for 1986 (unless otherwise stated). This figure shows the variation between countries and between males and females. (Redrawn from Eastwood, M., Edwards, C. and Parry, D., *Human Nutrition, a Continuing Debate,* Chapman & Hall, London, 1992.) ·

The risk factors can be classified into several types:

- inherent biological characteristics, like age, sex and family history of CHD

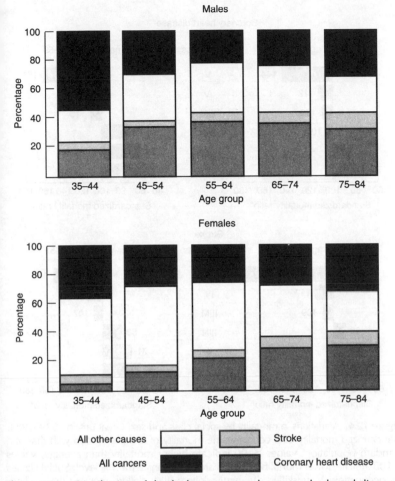

Figure 12.3 Distribution of deaths by age group by sex and selected disease, United Kingdom, 1990. (Redrawn from COMA 46; Office of Population Censuses and Surveys. Mortality Statistics, HMSO, London, 1990.) Crown copyright is reproduced with the permission of the Controller of HMSO.

- modifiable physiological characteristics, such as raised plasma cholesterol and raised blood pressure, which have been repeatedly shown to be major risk factors. Obesity and diabetes also fall into this group, as do weight at birth and at one year
- behaviours, such as cigarette smoking, high alcohol consumption, and a diet high in saturated fat, low in fruit and vegetables
- social characteristics like social class (see page 240) or ethnic origin
- other environmental factors, like cold weather and severe emotional stress.

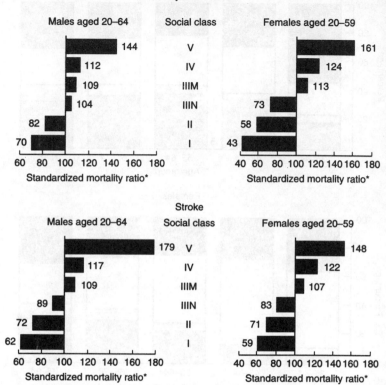

Figure 12.4 Variations in mortality by social class and sex, Great Britain 1979–1983. Standardized mortality ratio compares the mortality of a chosen group with that of a standard population; values >100 indicate higher mortality than average, values <100 indicate lower mortality. *Values are significant at the 1% level. Social classes by occupation: V, unskilled; IV, partly skilled; IIIM, skilled, manual; IIIN, skilled, non-manual; II, intermediate; I, professional. (Redrawn from COMA 46; Office of Population Censuses and Surveys. Mortality Statistics, HMSO, London, 1990.) Crown copyright is reproduced with the permission of the Controller of HMSO.

Over 200 risk factors have been found. Of these, the three modifiable factors have been found repeatedly to have a very strong association with increased risk are:

- raised blood pressure;
- raised plasma cholesterol, especially raised plasma low density lipoprotein (LDL, see page 77);
- cigarette smoking.

The known risk factors cannot, however, explain all the variations in CHD between people. The three major risk factors account for about

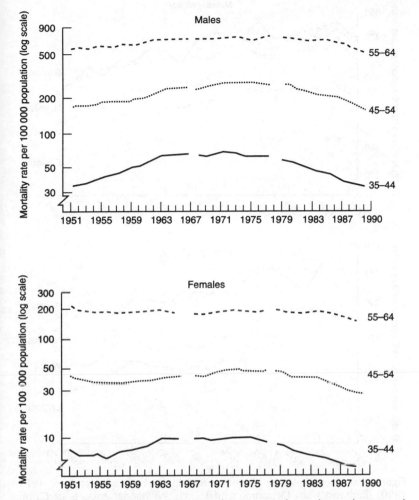

Figure 12.5 Standardized mortality rates for coronary heart disease by sex and age (35–64 years), England and Wales, 1950–1991. (Redrawn from Department of Health, *Nutritional Aspects of Cardiovascular Disease*, Report on Health and Social Subjects, no. 46, HMSO, London, 1994.) Crown copyright is reproduced with the permission of the Controller of HMSO.

50% of CHD occurrence. The conclusion must be that some factors are still unknown, and that these unknown factors would explain, for example, the lower rates of CHD in France compared with the UK, despite similar known risk factors (Garrow and James, 1993; Department of Health, 1994). Barker (1994) argues that events in fetal life may have an influence. Work on the Batemi and Masai people of Africa

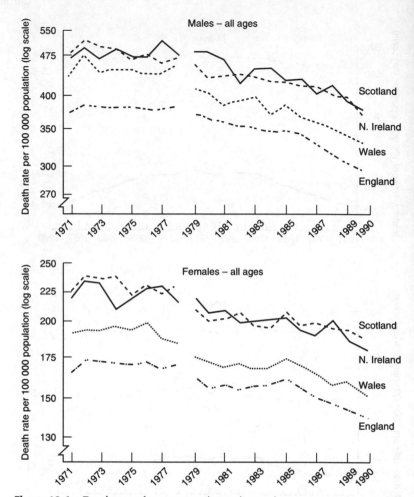

Figure 12.6 Death rates for coronary heart disease by country and sex, 1971–1990. (Redrawn from Department of Health, *Nutritional Aspects of Cardio-vascular Disease*, Report on Health and Social Subjects, no. 46, HMSO, London, 1994.) Crown copyright is reproduced with the permission of the Controller of HMSO.

shows how complex this subject is. The Masai eat up to 2000 mg of cholesterol a day and yet, on a diet of meat, blood and milk, maintain a very low *blood* cholesterol level of 3.5 mmol/l. A clue may be their use, as medicines and flavourings, of preparations from the barks of trees, which contain many substances, including saponins.

In a population with *one* risk factor, the increase in morbidity and mortality from CHD is not particularly high. With an increase in the number of risk factors, the increase in morbidity and mortality is

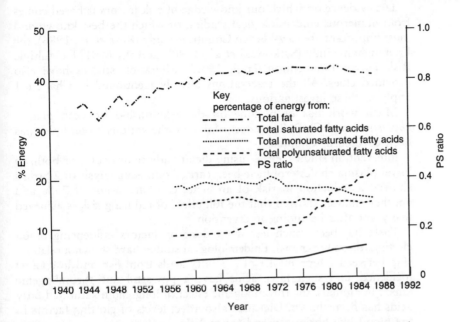

Figure 12.7   Trends in intake of fatty acids. PS ratio is the polyunsaturated: saturated fatty acid ratio. (Redrawn from Ministry of Agriculture, Fisheries and Food – Household Food Consumption and Expenditure, 1992; HMSO, London.)

multiplicative or synergistic (or, in layman's language, two plus two equals five or six).

BOX 12.2

Morbidity: the presence of disease
Mortality: death from a disease

BOX 12.3

RISK FACTORS FOR CORONARY HEART DISEASE (CHD)

Male, 45 years, non-smoker, low serum cholesterol: 7% chance of CHD in next 18 years
Male, 45 years, smoker, low serum cholesterol: 35% chance of CHD in next 18 years
Male, 45 years, smoker, glucose intolerance: 49% chance of CHD in next 18 years

From the Framingham Massachusetts study.

The evidence on which our knowledge of risk factors is based comes from numerous epidemiological studies, of which the best known and most important are Keys' Seven Countries Study (Keys *et al.*, 1986), the Framingham study (Sytkowski *et al.*, 1990), and the MRFIT (Multiple Risk Factor Intervention Trial, 1982). Migration studies have also provided clues. All the reservations already mentioned in Chapter 1 apply to these investigations.

Much work has been done on the relationship between *plasma cholesterol* and CHD. The effect of diet on the various blood lipids has been covered in Chapter 5.

Intervention studies, either using dietary advice or drugs, or both, to lower plasma cholesterol have been carried out. An analysis of 22 trials showed a reduction in risk of an acute coronary event of 23% and another analysis showed that the full effect of reducing risk is achieved five years after beginning intervention.

There has been much less work done on factors influencing blood clotting (thrombogenesis). Epidemiological studies have shown a relationship between a high intake of n-3 fatty acids from fish and low CHD incidence, and such fatty acids have a powerful anti-thrombogenic effect. In animals, the thrombogenic effect of long-chain saturated fatty acids has been shown. Diet may also affect levels of clotting factors in the blood like fibrinogen and factor VIIc.

Most of the work has been done on middle-aged men. Other population groups, with lower incidence of coronary heart disease, would require much larger numbers of subjects to show results. The general consensus is that it is likely that these results apply to other population groups.

Diet and risk

Dietary fat is important, through its influence on plasma cholesterol, as already noted in Chapter 5.

Saturated fats increase plasma cholesterol, PUFA (n-6 series) lowers it, as does replacing saturated fatty acids with oleic acid. Long-chain n-3 PUFA (oily fish) lower plasma triglycerides and *trans*-fatty acids (in some margarines) act like saturated fatty acids.

Dietary cholesterol has a small effect in raising dietary cholesterol, which varies considerably between individuals.

Soluble NSP causes a fall in plasma LDL cholesterol and in the levels of insulin and glucose after a meal.

Anti-oxidant nutrients are related to decreased risk of CHD, probably through the prevention of oxidation of LDL. Some people argue that anti-oxidant status is a major factor in CHD. The two theories (the lipid theory and the anti-oxidant theory) are not necessarily incompatible. The fact that in populations where the blood cholesterol averages less than 5 mmol/l, CHD is never a major problem, could be interpreted as showing that where there is less LDL available for oxidation, there will be less CHD.

Obesity is a risk factor.

Who should alter their diet?

Cardiovascular disease is so widespread in the UK that the dietary recommendations are aimed at the whole population. It is not possible to predict who will suffer. Everyone knows of exceptions where persons with no risk factors suffer premature CHD and others who smoke and eat a high fat diet remain healthy. But it is important to realize that they are exceptions to the general rule.

What about children? The recommendations of COMA 46 (Department of Health, 1994) is that the dietary recommendations do not apply before the age of two years, but apply in full from five years, with a flexible approach between these ages. There is not agreement over the question of the extent to which atherosclerosis begins in childhood. Fatty streaks in the arterial lining are seen in childhood, but they occur equally in populations with high and low risks of CHD and they are reversible. True atheromatous plaques first appear around puberty. There is the possibility of 'tracking' of risk factors, as there is for obesity. For example, 40% of children with the highest quartile for cholesterol will remain in this quartile in adulthood.

Diet control in the elderly? Rates of CHD and strokes rise sharply after the age of 65 years. The dietary recommendations apply to the elderly but care must be taken that adequate nutrient intake is achieved. This topic is also covered in Chapter 13.

Blood cholesterol: who should be tested?

The mean total blood cholesterol of a population is a good indicator of the prevalence and incidence of CHD. As already noted, no population with a low mean blood cholesterol of less than 5.0 mmol/l has a high incidence of CHD. In the UK, the mean cholesterol levels of men and women of all ages is high, just below 6 mmol/l. Less than one-third of the population has a blood cholesterol level of less than 5.0 mmol/l. So, we have a high level of susceptibility to atherosclerosis and CHD.

From the point of view of public health, it is important to know the changes, if any, in mean levels of blood cholesterol of the population.

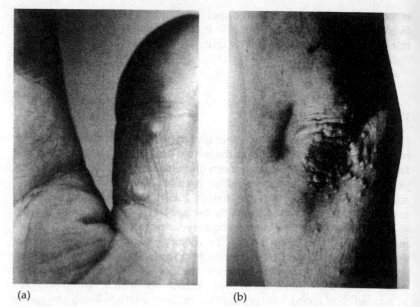

(a)   (b)

Figure 12.8 Tiny, wart-like outgrowths called xanthomata, usually on the thumb (a), just below the knee, and sometimes on the Achille's tendon and elbow (b) are diagnostic signs of hypercholesterolaemia. (Photographs courtesy of the Medical Illustration Department, Withington Hospital, Manchester.)

For the individual, there are many risk factors for CHD and no single factor is very much better than any other in predicting risk of CHD. High-risk categories, for whom, it may be argued, measurement of blood lipids is important, are:

- those with a diagnosis of CHD
- those with high scores on a multiple risk factor scoring system
- those with a strong family history of CHD, or hyperlipidaemia
- those with clinical signs of hyperlipidaemia (Figure 12.8)
- diabetic and hypertensive patients

Can atherosclerosis be reversed?

There is some evidence that this is possible. Workers of the University of California selected 48 patients who were randomly assigned to two groups, with one group following an optimal life-style programme. This programme included diet (no added fat, vegetarian, high in complex carbohydrates, less than 5 mg cholesterol/day, no caffeine and less than 2 units/day of alcohol), stress management (yoga, progressive relaxation, breathing techniques), smoking cessation, exercise and social support. After 15 months, in the optimal life-style group, LDL cholesterol had dropped by about 50% and angiograms showed reversal of blockages in the arteries. They found that the more life-style changes were made, the bigger the reversal (Ornish *et al.*, 1990). Such a programme would, of course, make a dramatic change to most people's lives.

STROKE AND HYPERTENSION

Hypertension or raised blood pressure (see also Chapter 7) increases the risk of CHD and stroke. An analysis of nine studies, involving 420 000 adults (largely men), showed a linear relationship between CHD and stroke incidence and diastolic blood pressure. This relationship was continuous across the range of blood pressures. That is, there was no threshold at which incidence sharply increased. To quantify the increased risk, it has been calculated that a 7.5 mmHg increase in diastolic pressure within the range 70–110 mmHg, was followed by a 29% increase in CHD risk and a 46% increase in stroke risk. This applied to both sexes and all ages.

Reducing blood pressure reduces the risk of stroke and of CHD.

BOX 12.4

> **Systolic** blood pressure: the highest point of blood pressure
> **Diastolic** blood pressure: the lowest point of blood pressure

The main dietary factors influencing blood pressure are sodium, potassium and calcium intakes, alcohol and obesity. There is evidence that sodium intakes in early life affect blood pressure (Eastwood *et al.*, 1992). Epidemiological studies have indicated a protective effect of adequate calcium intake against the development of high blood pressure (Eastwood *et al.*, 1992). The relationship between sodium and potassium intakes has already been mentioned (Chapter 7). An increase in the consumption of fruit and vegetables will increase potassium intake. Magnesium may also have a role but there is a lack of firm data.

1. Dietary guidelines for adults have been produced by WHO and by several expert committees. They all recommend a modification of fat intake, an increase in complex polysaccharides, maintenance of optimal body weight and avoidance of excessive alcohol consumption.   **Key points**

2. A high alcohol intake reduces nutritional status by influencing food choice, the digestion and absorption of nutrients and their transport, storage and excretion. The nutrients which may be affected are fat, fat-soluble vitamins, thiamin, folate, iron, magnesium and zinc. High alcohol intake is a risk factor for hypertension, CHD, and cancer of the oesophagus.

3. Long-term use of the oral contraceptive pill followed by repeated pregnancies may reduce folate status.

4. Obesity is common in adult life, often developing slowly (see Chapter 8).

5. Dietary factors are related to the incidence of some cancers, notably of the large bowel (fat, NSP), stomach, probably breast (fat) and prostate (fat). A high intake of fruit and vegetables is protective against cancers of the digestive and respiratory tracts.

6. Coronary heart disease (CHD) is a major cause of premature death in the UK. There are two main components, atherosclerosis and formation of a clot at an atherosclerotic site. Its cause is not known, but a number of risk factors have been found. Among these, hypertension and high blood cholesterol are important. The main dietary factors are fat intake (both type and amount), which influences blood cholesterol levels, and anti-oxidant status, which protects blood lipids from oxidation. Because CHD is widespread in the UK, it is recommended that all should modify their diet. An American group, adopting major dietary change and increasing exercise, decreasing alcohol consumption and not smoking, have shown reversal of atherosclerosis.

7. An increase in blood pressure with age is common in our society and there is a linear relationship between diastolic blood pressure and CHD and stroke. The dietary factors which may cause hypertension are alcohol intake, obesity and high salt intake. Calcium, potassium and magnesium are also implicated, being protective against hypertension.

The elderly 13

The aim of this chapter is to review the nutritional needs of the elderly and their nutritional status, to identify the risk factors for malnutrition and to suggest practical ways of preventing it.

The term elderly (or older people) is usually taken to mean women over 60 years and men over 65, that is, people of pensionable age. This definition covers a wide age range. The 'young elderly' may well be very healthy while the 'elderly elderly', over 75 years, are the group who are more likely to have problems of illness, disability and diet. The number of elderly people is increasing.

Note: in the rest of Europe the term elderly is defined as over 50 years and this should be borne in mind when reading the literature. The term 'older people' is often used now.

Recommendations and requirements

The age grouping for the Dietary Reference Values which includes the elderly is 50+ years. There was insufficient data on the particular requirements of the elderly as a group to justify separate groups for older people, although some studies suggest that the elderly have increased requirements for calcium, vitamin D and some of the B-complex vitamins. Certainly there is a need for more research.

The physical changes of ageing lead to decreased efficiency of the homeostatic mechanisms. Physical changes which may occur which affect nutrition are:

- decline in the senses of taste and smell;
- lack of teeth or unsatisfactory dentures;
- decreased salivary secretion;
- drug-induced loss of taste and dry mouth;
- hypochlorhydria (reduced secretion of hydrochloric acid in the stomach) affecting absorption of calcium, iron and vitamin B12;
- insensitivity to thirst;
- decline in renal function, affecting drug excretion and maintenance of water/electrolyte balance;

- the effect of medication, often long-term, on nutrient requirements and appetite;
- possible reduction in the efficiency of the immune system, making infections more frequent.

These physical changes occur along with social and economic changes, which may also affect diet.

In general, as people get older their dietary needs approach those of the very young; that is, they need a diet which is nutrient-dense, since energy requirements fall but nutrient requirements do not (Table 13.1). To ensure a good diet, it is essential that interest in food is maintained (Department of Health, 1992).

LRNIs and EARs (not given in the table below, which gives *daily* estimates) are available for thiamin (B1), riboflavin (B2), B6 and niacin. They are given in the COMA Report 41 (Department of Health, 1991), not as daily requirements, but either per 1000 kcal or per gram of dietary protein, as appropriate.

Table 13.1 Dietary Reference Values (quantity/day) for 50+ years). (From COMA 41, Department of Health, 1991) Crown copyright is reproduced with the permission of the Controller of HMSO.

	LRNI		EAR		RNI	
Nutrient	Female	Male	Female	Male	Female	Male
Protein (g)	–	–	37.2	42.6	46.5	53.3
B1 (mg)	–	–	–	–	0.8	0.9
B2 (mg)	0.8	0.8	0.9	1.0	1.1	1.3
Niacin (mg)	–	–	–	–	12	16
B6 (mg)	–	–	–	–	1.2	1.4
B12 (μg)	1.0	1.0	1.25	1.25	1.5	1.5
Folate (μg)	100	100	150	150	200	200
C (mg)	10	10	25	25	40	40
A (μg)	250	300	400	500	600	700
D (μg)	–	–	–	–	10*	10*
Calcium (mg)	400	400	525	525	700	700
Magnesium (mg)	150	190	200	250	270	300
Sodium	575	575	–	–	1600	1600
Potassium (mg)	2000	2000	–	–	3500	3500
Iron (mg)	4.7	4.7	6.7	6.7	8.7	8.7
Zinc (mg)	4.0	5.5	5.5	7.3	7.0	9.5
Copper (mg)	–	–	–	–	1.2	1.2
Selenium (μg)	40	40	–	–	60	75
Iodine (μg)	70	70	–	–	140	140

LRNI, Lower Reference Nutrient Intake.
EAR, Estimated Average Requirement.
RNI, Reference Nutrient Intake.
* After 65 years.

ENERGY

The limited survey data reveals a wide range of energy requirements. This is not surprising, since a fit and active retired person may be more active than when they were at work, while others, because of infirmity, may be chair- or bed-bound.

The gradual loss of lean body tissue with age reduces the basal metabolic requirements.

The lower the energy intake, the more important the quality of the diet (that is to say, its nutrient density) and the greater the risk of inadequate intakes.

NON-STARCH POLYSACCHARIDES (NSPs)

Constipation is common in the elderly. To alleviate this, increased intake of foods high in NSP is recommended but changes should be made gradually to avoid distension and flatulence (which even young people experience with a sudden change) as well as the possible reduction in the absorption of iron and calcium. No specific recommendations have been made for NSP for sub-groups in the COMA Report 41 (Department of Health, 1991).

FATS, SUGARS AND STARCHES

There is no evidence that the requirements of the elderly are any different from younger persons, but the dietary guidelines should be interpreted with common sense and moderation. At 84, say, would you deny yourself a cream cake or some chocolate in order to protect the state of your arteries?

Development of dental caries increases in old age. It is prevented by restricting the quantity and frequency of free sugars intake. Sugar-free chewing gum is helpful by promoting the flow of saliva.

PROTEIN

In proportion to the lean tissue mass, the DRVs for protein are higher than for young adults. But elderly people may avoid protein foods like meat because of their cost and texture. These foods are easily replaced by fish, cheese, eggs and milk, but the portions of cheese should not be very small, which is often the case. Peanut butter is a good protein food. A glass of milk at the main meal and plenty of milky drinks are a useful way of improving the diet of the elderly.

Table 13.2   Vitamin D content of foods (Davies and Dickerson, 1991)

Food	Quantity	Vitamin D content (μg)
Canned sardines	60 g (½ tin)	4.5
Canned salmon	60 g	8
Kipper	100 g	25
Canned pilchards	60 g	4.8
Canned tuna	60 g	3.5
Liver	50 g	0.3–0.7
Margarine	10 g	0.8
Butter	10 g	0.08
Egg, one, size 2	60 g	0.9
Cornflakes	30 g	0.9

Ovaltine (four heaped teaspoons) provides more than 20% of the RDA for vitamin D and for thiamin, riboflavin, niacin, B12.

VITAMINS

Vitamin D is the only vitamin where there is an increased recommendation for the elderly. The mean plasma level of a metabolite of vitamin D in a population over 75 years was found to be low and this was apparently due to inadequate exposure to the sun in summer (Lawson *et al.*, 1979). The vitamin D status of those in residential homes and hospitals is often low (Davies *et al.*, 1976). Kidney function declines with age and this results in less efficient production of the active substance (1,25-dihydroxy cholecalciferol) from vitamin D.

The panel on DRVs decided that dietary vitamin D, 10 μg, was essential for those over 65. The difficulty of supplying this without supplements can be seen from the amounts of the vitamin in average helpings of vitamin D-rich foods (Table 13.2).

It is easy to see the value of eating oily fish once or twice a week (for recipes, see pages 385–9) and that a supplement of vitamin D may be useful.

A good intake of the anti-oxidant vitamins is important. In addition to their other functions, recent work in the USA has shown a link between a high intake of anti-oxidant vitamins and reduced incidence of cataract.

MINERALS

The DRVs for minerals are the same for the 50+ group as for younger adults except that post-menopausal women have a lower requirement for iron than younger women. For the elderly elderly and particularly for those over 85 the salt restrictions which are generally advised are not suitable because of the risk of sodium depletion (Brown *et al.*, 1984).

The Report of the National Food Survey Committee (MAFF; annual reports) showed that the households of old-age pensioners which were sampled spent more on food than all groups except two (those were households with one or more earner in income group A and households without an earner in income group E1). In 1991 the average expenditure per person per week for OAPs was £13.65. The National Food Survey also gives a breakdown of food consumption by age group, including 65–74 and 75+. This shows a slightly lower expenditure by the older group. Not surprisingly therefore the nutrient intakes of OAP households were shown in this survey to be very good (Table 13.3), being mostly above the RNI, which is, after all, a generous estimate. But these figures refer to elderly people who live at home, probably the healthiest of this group. The diet of those in long-stay residential homes has not been surveyed.

It must be remembered that the elderly are a very heterogeneous group with widely differing states of health, income, living conditions and also age. Some other reports of nutrient intake and nutritional status in the elderly note a lower than average nutrient intake paralleling a lower energy intake. This lower nutrient intake is usually associated with lower serum and tissue nutrient levels, which respond to a diet improved by supplementation (Department of Health and Social Security, 1979; Davies, 1981).

The increased need for vitamin D and the low status of some groups has already been mentioned. A dietary survey of elderly people suffering from osteomalacia found that more than 50% had vitamin D intakes below 70 i.u./day and one, on a low-fat diet, had no measurable intake (Chalmers, 1991).

Ageing is associated with *increased illness* – some of which may be undiagnosed – and this may lead to malnutrition. Illness may result in

Nutrient intake and nutritional status in the elderly

Table 13.3 Nutritional value of household food as a percentage of Reference Nutrient Intake,1993, for OAPs. (From COMA report, 1993. Crown copyright is reproduced with the permission of the Controller of HMSO.)

Dietary component	RNI	Dietary component	RNI
Energy	95	Thiamin	156
Protein	130	Riboflavin	143
Calcium	121	Niacin equivalent	181
Iron	111	Vitamin B6	153
Zinc	100	Vitamin B12	349
Magnesium	82	Folate	125
Sodium	153	Vitamin C	118
Potassium	74	Vitamin A	215
		(retinol equivalent)	

long-term medication. Some drugs interfere with nutrient metabolism (see Chapter 5) and others may affect the sense of taste and appetite (Thomas, 1994). A relatively high alcohol intake, reported by some workers, may reduce nutrient intake by replacing some foods and may alter nutrient metabolism, particularly for some B vitamins and zinc and magnesium.

Risk factors for malnutrition

A number of workers have identified risk factors for malnutrition. Exton-Smith defined primary and secondary causes of malnutrition (Davies, 1981; Thomas, 1994) (Table 13.4).

A DHSS report identified social and medical factors which correlated with malnutrition. These were living alone, being housebound, no regular cooked meals, supplementary benefit, social class IV and V, low mental test score, depression, chronic bronchitis, emphysema, gastrectomy, poor dentition, difficulty in swallowing and alcoholism (Department of Health and Social Security, 1979).

Davies (1981) highlighted 10 main risk factors for individuals to identify those who need nutritional support. They are:

1. Fewer than five main meals, hot or cold, eaten in a week, that is, less than one main meal a day.
2. Very little milk consumed.
3. Virtual abstention from fruits and vegetables.
4. Wastage of food – even that supplied hot and ready to eat.
5. Long periods in the day without food or beverages.
6. Depression or loneliness.
7. Unexpected weight change, either a gain or loss (this is a more valuable index of risk than either obesity or underweight).
8. Shopping difficulties.
9. Poverty.
10. Indication in medical record of disabilities, including alcoholism.

The greater the number of risk factors found for an individual, the greater the risk of malnutrition. A Department of Health and Social

Table 13.4 Causes of malnutrition in the elderly

Primary causes	Secondary causes
Ignorance	Impaired appetite
Social isolation	Masticatory inefficiency
Physical disability	Malabsorption
Mental disturbance	Alcoholism
Iatrogenic disorder	Drugs
Poverty	Increased requirements

From Davies (1981).

Security survey showed that four or more risk factors make malnutrition very likely. The Department of Health recommends that assessment of nutritional status becomes a routine aspect of history-taking and physical examination of the elderly (Department of Health, 1992).

TYPES OF MALNUTRITION IN THE ELDERLY

As noted previously, surveys of the elderly show a wide range of nutrient intakes (Department of Health and Social Security, 1979; Davies, 1981). The nutrients which are most likely to be deficient are vitamin C, folate, riboflavin and other water-soluble vitamins, vitamin D, iron, potassium (in a diet rich in sugary foods), other trace elements and NSP. Of course an individual may adapt to low intakes or have a low requirement and so show no signs of deficiency, but depletion of body stores is likely. In this case sudden illness or accident may precipitate frank malnutrition.

In her survey, Davies (1981) found that foods supplying vitamin C were often avoided for a variety of reasons. Many found oranges too troublesome to peel, others complained that the acid in fruits stung their gums or lips, or thought that, being acid, they were bad for their rheumatism. Pips were a nuisance and often respondents drank orange or lemon squashes, not realizing that they did not necessarily contain vitamin C. Shopping difficulties sometimes led to over-long storage and some relied on meals on wheels for fruit and vegetables. The draw-back here is that the amount of heat-labile (that is, destroyed by heat) vitamins that are left in meals which are cooked in bulk and kept hot may be very small indeed. Davies found that nearly half the meals contained less than 5 mg vitamin C in total.

DEHYDRATION

Dehydration, due either to deficiency of water or of sodium, may result from almost any physical or mental illness in elderly people. About 75% of those admitted to hospital are dehydrated. It is easy to overlook because, when mild, the symptoms are non-specific, usually lethargy and confusion. Its recognition and treatment are important and aid recovery.

The most common cause of dehydration is decreased water intake. This is sometimes deliberate to prevent incontinence, or because of reduced thirst sensation or fear of drinking when, after a stroke, it causes choking. Diuretics are also an important cause.

Mild dehydration is easily overcome by drinking more fluid and regular drinks, whether thirsty or not, should be advised. More serious states require medical intervention (Scott, 1986).

THE EFFECT OF TEMPERATURE ON CARDIOVASCULAR MORTALITY

Deaths and hospital admissions for CHD and for stroke are higher in winter than in summer, the increase in mortality reaching 70% in some years. The reason for this is not clear; possible causes are an increase in blood pressure and a change in the blood clotting factors. The role of food in maintaining body temperature, both by increasing metabolic rate and by the hot food and drinks warming the body, is therefore important (Wilmshurst, 1994).

Practical ways to improve diet

There are a number of ways in which the diet of the elderly can be made adequate.

- By having appetizing food. Recommendations about nutrients need to be translated into suitable recipes. There are huge numbers of cookery books and leaflets. Davies (1972, 1979) has produced two useful recipe books especially for one or two persons. Appetizing food is the best way to stimulate appetite and interest in diet.
- Nutritional counselling, to help with the following suggestions and to dispel any disadvantageous dietary beliefs (like reducing fat intake without increasing starch intake).
- A good and acceptable meal pattern needs to be established, preferably by modifying the existing one.
- Help with shopping.
- Help with mobility (for example, a walking frame) or cooking aids.
- Help with meal provision, such as meals on wheels, luncheon clubs, home-helps, day hospital, day centres.
- Using nourishing convenience foods (some instant soups are low in nutrients, but drinks such as Complan, Build-Up, Fortimel, Fortisip, Fortify are useful and taste good).
- The addition of milk to the diet in cooking and drinks (milky coffee, hot chocolate, Marmite-flavoured milk).
- Increasing vitamin C intake with fruit juices, vitamin C tablets.
- Establishing an emergency food store cupboard (Box 13.1) in case of illness or bad weather (Gerontology Nutrition Unit).

AIDS FOR EATING

The infirmities of old age often make eating difficult and embarrassing. There are a number of aids to help which include the following (Vousden, 1986).

IDEAS FOR AN EMERGENCY STORE CUPBOARD

- UHT milk in cartons (keeps six months)
- Fruit juice in cartons
- Soups – canned or packets
- Meat or fish, canned
- Canned vegetables
- Canned milk puddings
- Marmite, other spreads
- Some sort of bread substitute, cream crackers, etc.

Cutlery

- Lightweight cutlery for those with poor grip or painful joints
- Long-handled cutlery for those with limited wrist or elbow movement
- Straps to fasten cutlery to paralysed hands
- Large handles for those whose grip is affected
- Use of Rubazote tubing on patient's own cutlery
- Rocking knife for single-handed use

Crockery

- Plates with special lip to prevent food sliding off
- Suction egg-cup which will stick to plate

Drinking aids

- Lightweight beaker
- Two-handled cup
- Flexi-straws or valved straws

Miscellaneous

- Arm-supports
- Non-slip mats to keep plates in position

Ideas for snacks, easy and cheap meals are given in Chapter 21. It is the *practical interpretation* of nutritional information into palatable, easily prepared meals which can be afforded, which enables a good diet to be eaten.

Feeding of the elderly in hospital is dealt with very well in Thomas (1994) and the effects of surgery on nutritional requirements is covered in Chapter 17.

Key points

1. The elderly are defined as those of pensionable age; that is, women over 60 years and men over 65 years. This group can be subdivided into the 'young elderly' and the over-75s, the 'elderly elderly'.

2. The top age range for Dietary Reference Values is 50+ years because there is not enough data to justify further subdivision. Additional vitamin D is advised for those over 65 years. The elderly have decreased homeostatic efficiency and more research on nutritional requirements is needed.

3. Nutritional status of the elderly in the National Food Survey is good, but those surveyed will be people living independently at home. Other surveys show wide ranges of nutrient intake. The nutrients likely to be deficient are water-soluble vitamins, vitamin D and some mineral elements.

4. Risk factors for malnutrition in the elderly have been identified. Primary factors are ignorance, social isolation, physical disability, mental disturbance, iatrogenic disorders and poverty. Secondary factors are impaired appetite, decreased ability to chew, malabsorption, alcoholism, drugs and increased requirements. Other suggestions of risk factors are given (Department of Health and Social Security, 1979; Davies, 1981). The larger the number of risk factors, the greater the risk of malnutrition.

5. Dehydration is a risk in the elderly, affecting a high proportion of hospital admissions. Cold weather causes an increase in morbidity and the warming effect of food is helpful.

6. Practical ways to improve the diet of the elderly are given, encompassing outside help, aids for cooking and eating, and nourishing, convenience foods. It is vitally important that an interest in food is maintained.

Ethnic groups 14

The aim of this chapter is to give an outline of the main food beliefs and habits of some ethnic groups in the UK, so that the health professional is able to take these into account when advising about food choice and dietary change.

Culture, which includes religious beliefs, affects food choice and therefore nutrition. Britain is a multicultural society and different ethnic groups have enriched the gastronomic scene with foods from, for example, the Indian subcontinent, from the Caribbean and from China.

The nutrient content of the diet is affected by food choice and restrictions (Table 14.1) and by cooking methods. If one staple food (for example, rice or wheat) predominates, then it affects the nutritional balance of the diet. Boiled white rice, for example, is low in thiamin (see Chapter 19). Today, a variety of foods is usually eaten, making the staple much less important nutritionally than when it is the major source of energy. An additional point to remember is that often people eat both traditional and European foods.

There are food tables for immigrant foods (*Immigrant Foods*, 1992).

When assessing diet, it is always worth enquiring about what drinks are usually taken with meals and as snacks. Some groups take sugary drinks which may add considerably to energy intake.

Table 14.1 Ethnic groups: permitted and prohibited foods (reproduced with permission from Henley, Asian Patients in Hospital and at Home, published by Oxford University Press, 1979)

Foods	Hindu (orthodox)	Hindu (unorthodox)	Sikh	Muslim
Alcohol	No	Yes	No(?)	No
Beef and offal	No	No	No	Yes, halal
Eggs	?	Yes	Yes	Yes
Fish – oily	No	No	Yes	Yes, if fins and scales
Fish – white	No	Yes	Yes	Yes, if fins and scales
Lamb and offal	No	Yes	Yes	Yes, halal
Poultry	No	Yes	Yes	Yes, halal
Pork and products	No	No	Rarely	No
Shellfish	No	?	Yes	No

South Asian diets   Several ethnic groups originate from South Asia, having different geographical origins and religions. The three main religions are Hinduism,
Islam and Sikhism. All influence diet (Henley, 1979).

HINDUS

Hindus believe in reincarnation: they revere life and strict Hindus are
vegetarians because they will not kill. The majority of Hindus in the UK
come originally from Gujarat on the north-west coast of India, and
their first language is Gujarati.

Most Hindus, then, are lacto-vegetarians; eggs are avoided because
they are seen as a source of life. Strict orthodox Hindus are vegans.
Less strict Hindus will eat lamb, poultry and fish. The cow is a sacred
animal and even the less strict Hindus will not eat beef.

At three major festivals, fasting is observed and devout Hindus may
fast one or two days each week, from dawn to sunset.

MUSLIMS (ISLAM)

The Muslim community in the UK came originally from Pakistan,
Bangladesh and East Africa. Lawful food is called Halal. It includes all
meats, except pork and its by-products. Meat must be killed in the
ritual way, by bleeding and Kosher meat is acceptable. Alcohol is
forbidden. Fish which has fins and scales may be eaten but not shellfish
or eels.

During Ramadam, in September, Muslims fast from dawn to sunset.
They get up early to eat a big meal and have another after sunset.
Pregnant, lactating and menstruating women, the old and children
under 12 are exempt.

SIKHS

Sikhs believe in a personal God and the signs of a Sikh man are uncut
hair, a special comb, a bangle and dagger. Most Sikhs in the UK
originate from the Punjab. Alcohol is forbidden but otherwise food
laws are a matter for the individual. Beef and pork are usually avoided.

'HOT' AND 'COLD' FOODS

Foods are classified as hot or cold, referring not to their temperature
but to their effects on the body. Hot foods are thought to increase body

temperature, and to stimulate emotions and activity. In the Hindu tradition, they are lentils, carrots, onions, eggplant, chilli, ginger, dates, eggs, meat, fish, tea, honey and brown sugar.

Cold foods are believed to reduce body temperature and to induce strength and cheerfulness. For Hindus they are cereals, chickpeas, green and red gram, all green leafy vegetables, potatoes, most other vegetables, all nuts, most fruits, milk and dairy products and white sugar.

Hot foods are restricted during pregnancy, and cold food during lactation.

The British Diabetic Association Diet Pack gives details of hot and cold foods (see References and further reading).

ASIAN FOODS

Some Asian foods are described in Chapter 20. Asian sweets, made from sugar, ghee, full-cream milk powder, nuts, flour and sweetened condensed milk are *highly* calorific.

ASIAN MEAL PATTERNS

As always, such summaries can only be generalizations. Breakfast is typically yoghurt with rice or chapattis or leftover curry and rice, or egg and bread or cereal with milk.

Main meals will include rice or chapattis, meat or fish for non-vegetarians, vegetable and pulse dishes, side salad, yoghurt. There may be less variety in the diet than for many Britons. Snacks are often deep-fried, like samosas and pakoras. In fact, a lot of oil or ghee is used in food preparation.

Many people eat a mixture of western and Asian foods.

ASIAN HEALTH PROBLEMS

Diabetes, CHD, obesity and osteomalacia and rickets are all more common in the Asian than the non-Asian population. A high intake of fat and sugary drinks may be contributory factors to some of these complaints. The increased requirements for vitamin D (see page 96) mean that supplements are desirable to prevent rickets and osteo-malacia.

Judaism has a system of laws some of which, the Kashrut, deal with food with the aim of maintaining health and hygiene. These laws are that   **Jewish diets**

- meat should be killed in the ritual or Kosher way
- only the flesh of animals which chew the cud and have cloven hooves should be eaten, so that pork and all pork products are forbidden
- chicken, duck, goose and turkey are allowed, but not birds of prey
- fish with scales and fins may be eaten, but not shellfish
- meat must not be cooked or served with milk or milk products. Orthodox Jews keep separate utensils for meat and milk. Interestingly, recent work has shown that milk inhibits the absorption of iron from a meal, so this law may be useful in maintaining iron status.

The degree to which these laws are kept varies between Orthodox and Reform Jews. The tradition of high standards of housekeeping, however, means that a lot of attention is paid to food provision (Rose, 1985).

Chinese diets   China is such a large country that to speak of the 'Chinese diet' is a gross generalization. For example, the staple may be either rice or wheat, according to area. The cooking methods are often quick, using the stir-fry technique, so reducing the loss of vitamin C. The use of ginger and garlic may be valuable for health as well as for flavour, according to recent reports.

YIN AND YANG

Foods are classified as 'hot' (yang) or 'cold' (yin) and these properties are thought to influence health. When giving dietary advice, this is an area which should be discussed. There is a lot of variation in the classification of foods (Table 14.2).

Table 14.2   Guidelines for the Chinese classification of foods. (reproduced with permission from Thomas, B., (ed) published by Blackwell Science Ltd, Oxford, 1994)

	'Cold foods'	'Neutral foods'	'Hot foods'
Food	Most fruit Vegetables Barley water Chinese herbal teas	White fish Rice bread Papaya Orange	Oily fish, meat Alcoholic drinks Ginger, spices Some fruit, e.g. mango, pineapples
Cooking method		Boiling Steaming Stir-frying	Deep frying Roasting

In pregnancy and illness this yin and yang are particularly important. Pregnancy is viewed as a 'hot' condition and so 'hot' foods, like red meat and fish may be reduced (Leeming and Huang Man-hui, 1983).

Monosodium glutamate, which enhances the flavours of a dish, is widely used. This increases sodium intake and may, in susceptible people, cause *Kwok's syndrome* or the *Chinese restaurant syndrome*. The symptoms are chest pain radiating to both arms, general weakness and palpitations.

In large towns, like Manchester, there may be Chinese Health Information Centres.

Afro-Caribbeans are people of African descent who come from the Caribbean islands, often from Jamaica. Many came to the UK in the 1950s and 1960s. Different islands have different eating habits, so, once again, Afro-Caribbeans are not a homogeneous group.

Afro-Caribbean diets

Starch comes form a variety of staples (rice, corn, oats and wheat) and from starchy fruits (green bananas, plantain, breadfruit, cassava, yam and sweet potato). A lot of pulses are eaten and yellow and dark green leafy vegetables are used in soups and stews. Callaloo is the name for spinach and may be used for all green vegetables. A lot of fish is eaten. All this makes for a healthy diet.

There has not been much research into health of the Afro-Caribbean community but obesity is a problem; possible contributory factors are a high fat intake from frying, using a lot of coconut cream in recipes and drinking sugary drinks. Salt intakes may be high from salt fish and salt pork.

Rastafarianism is a religious belief which is commonest among the Afro-Caribbean community. Rastafarians are often vegans (see page 270).

Rastafarianism

1. Culture, including religion, has a major effect on diet, through food choice, methods of cooking, meal planning and fasting.
2. People of South Asian descent usually belong to one of three main religions, Hinduism, Islam and Sikhism.
3. Hindus, believing in reincarnation, revere life. The strictest followers are therefore vegans, the less strict lacto-vegetarians while some eat lamb, poultry and fish, but never beef.
4. Muslims require meat to be killed in the ritual way, Halal. Kosher meat is acceptable. Alcohol is forbidden. Fish with fins and scales are acceptable but not shellfish. Ramadam is a prolonged fast, with children under 12 and pregnant women exempted.

Key points

5. Sikhs avoid alcohol and usually beef and pork, but otherwise individual dietary decisions are made.
6. Asian health problems include increased rates of diabetes mellitus, coronary heart disease, obesity, osteomalacia and rickets.
7. Judaism follows food laws laid down as the Kasrut. Meat must be Kosher, shellfish and pork are forbidden, and strict Jews do not eat meat and milk at the same meal.
8. The Chinese food patterns vary very much according to the area of origin. The diet is varied, foods are classified according to the yin and yang system. Sodium monoglutamate may be used and causes, in susceptible individuals, Kwok's syndrome.
9. The Afro-Caribbean community has a tradition of a varied diet, eating a lot of fish. There is comparatively little hard data. Obesity is common.

Vegetarianism 15

This chapter describes the various types of vegetarianism, and reviews the nutritional effects of these diets.

Vegetarian diets exclude, to a greater or lesser extent, animal foods. There are three main types: the common **lacto-ovo-vegetarianism**, which excludes animal flesh but includes animal products like milk and eggs, the less common **lacto-vegetarianism**, which also excludes eggs, and the least common, **veganism**, which excludes **all** food of animal origin.

Other types include **fruitarians** who eat only raw fruits, nuts and berries. **Macrobiotic diets** are based on brown rice, with fruits, vegetables and pulses. Tomatoes, potatoes and aubergines (the Solanaceae group) and processed foods are avoided and meat and fish are permitted only if they are hunted or wild.

In recent years the popularity of vegetarianism of all types has increased, particularly among the young, although precise estimates are difficult to obtain.

Types of vegetarianism

REASONS FOR VEGETARIANISM

There are many reasons why people become vegetarians. Some religions advocate vegetarianism; Hindus are lacto-vegetarians, Seventh-Day Adventists are lacto-ovo-vegetarians, and Rastafarians, vegans. Some people eat vegetarian diets for other ethical reasons, such as the avoidance of intensive animal-rearing methods. Others see vegetarianism as healthier than omnivorous eating.

Nutritional value of vegetarian diets

Like all the groups mentioned in this book, vegetarians are a heterogeneous group and their interpretation of the vegetarian diet equally diverse. The important question is how the dietary restrictions affect nutrient intake.

As Sanders and Reddy (1994) note in a very useful and comprehensive review, it is probably easier to select a balanced diet with meat than without it. Meat is an important source of protein, iron (in the form of haem iron, which is readily absorbed), thiamin, riboflavin, niacin, vitamins B12 and A. Fish has a similar composition, though it is less rich in iron, but oily fish is an excellent source of vitamin D. In a vegetarian diet, these nutrients must come from other sources.

Of course there are good and bad vegetarian diets, but vegetarians in general have been shown to have lower body weight, lower blood lipid levels, lower incidence of CHD, stroke and some cancers than the omnivorous population (Dwyer, 1991). These facts are due, no doubt, to a combination of the effects of diet and total life-style.

NUTRITIONAL STATUS OF VEGETARIANS

The groups at risk of dietary inadequacy are children and women of reproductive age. The risks are iron-deficiency anaemia, rickets, a low energy intake and, in vegans, vitamin B12 deficiency. The advantages of a well-planned vegetarian diet are high intakes of NSP and other complex carbohydrates and anti-oxidant nutrients.

PROTEIN IN VEGETARIAN DIETS

Lacto-ovo-vegetarians

Meat and fish are replaced by eggs, cheese, milk, nuts and soya protein. All of these, except for nuts, provide high-quality protein and will provide the B-group vitamins. Iron is not present in milk and its products to any useful extent although it is found in egg yolk. Soya protein, sold as textured vegetable protein, and Quorn, a protein produced from fungi may be enriched with vitamins. So in the lacto-ovo-vegetarian diet it is quite easy to replace meat and fish.

If a lot of whole milk and full-fat cheese is eaten, the diet would be high in saturated fat. But in fact, surveys of vegetarian diets have shown fat intakes slightly lower than in similar groups of omnivores (Thorogood et al., 1990). This is not surprising, since vegetarians are often concerned about health and diet and therefore take trouble to plan their meals carefully.

Vegans

The vegan diet is a good deal more limited than the lacto-ovo-vegetarian diet, relying entirely on plant proteins. The only plant proteins equal in quality to animal proteins are soya and Quorn.

Otherwise the protein of the diet must be met by a good *mix* of plant proteins, for example, pulses with wheat, rice with lentils, nuts with grains (see page 62). The present view is that, for adults, protein from two or more plant groups daily is likely to be adequate, but that for children, especially weanlings, two sources of protein at each meal is a sensible aim. Soya milk is especially useful for children. Surveys of vegans have shown adequate protein intakes (Sanders and Manning, 1992).

IRON AND IRON-DEFICIENCY ANAEMIA

The availability of iron is lower from plant foods than from meat and some groups show increased incidence of iron-deficiency. A number of investigations have shown:

- a higher incidence of iron-deficiency anaemia in the Asian vegetarian (especially rice-eaters) population in the UK, particularly among women and children, than among the general population. Serum ferritin concentrations were lower for Asian and 'ethical' vegetarian white women of child-bearing age compared with meat-eaters;
- an increased prevalence of iron-deficient anaemia in macrobiotic vegetarians;
- normal haemoglobin concentrations for Seventh-Day Adventists and 'ethical' vegans and lacto-ovo-vegetarians.

Vegan diets

Nutrients which might be deficient in a vegan diet are energy (it is a bulky diet), calcium (through reduced intake) and other minerals (due to reduced absorption from a diet high in NSP), and vitamins B12 and D.

As always, the groups at risk will be those with increased requirements, such as infants, children, pregnant and lactating women. Surveys of vegans have shown the following:

- fat intake at 30–35% of energy, with saturated fat at 5–7% of energy, but with a very high intake of linoleic acid. This intake can be reduced by the use of soya, rapeseed and olive oil products rather than the more usually advised corn, sunflower and safflower oils (Sanders and Manning, 1992);
- a high intake of carbohydrate and of dietary fibre.
- adequate iron intake, a similar incidence of iron-deficiency anaemia as omnivores but some evidence of low iron stores (Kelsay et al., 1988);
- adequate zinc intake, but a zinc status lower than for omnivores and inadequate plasma levels in a minority. A high intake of soya products may reduce the absorption of zinc;

- calcium intake has similarly been found to be adequate;
- vitamin B12 deficiency in adults was very rare but some signs of deficiency have been found in exclusively breast-fed infants. Some foods are fortified with B12 and a list is given in Thomas (1994). This is an area where vigilance is required and vegetarians may need to consider supplementing their diet with B12.

Thus, from the samples surveyed, the vegan diet seems to be adequate and in some respects, very good. Care is required over vitamin D provision for children and for pregnant and lactating women, where supplements are advised, and for calcium and vitamin B12.

Rastafarian and macrobiotic diets

Rastafarian and macrobiotic diets are the most restrictive vegetarian diets. Rastafarianism is a religion which includes dietary rules. Many Rastafarians are vegans, eating only 'ITAL' foods, which are those in a whole or natural state. Alcohol, tea and coffee are avoided. Rickets and protein—energy malnutrition (usually found only in developing countries) have been found in children following these diets.

Key points

1. There are three main types of vegetarianism, lacto-ovo-vegetarianism, which excludes meat and fish, lacto-vegetarianism, which excludes eggs as well, and veganism, which excludes all animal foods. Much less common are fruitarian diets, of raw fruits, nuts and berries, macrobiotic diets, of brown rice, fruits, vegetables and pulses and the Rastafarians, who are mainly vegans.
2. Reasons for vegetarianism may be religious, or for other ethical reasons, or for health. Fashion may be a deciding factor.
3. The choice of foods is important in determining whether the diet is good or bad. The risks are of iron deficiency, rickets and inadequate energy intake, and in vegans, vitamin B12 deficiency also. These risks are greatest for children and women of reproductive age. The more limited the diet, the greater the risk.
4. Iron-deficiency anaemia has been found to be increased in Asian vegetarians and those eating macrobiotic diets but not in Seventh-Day Adventists or 'ethical' vegans and lacto-ovo-vegetarians.
5. The advantages of well-planned vegetarian diets are high intakes of NSP, complex carbohydrates and anti-oxidant nutrients.

Low-income groups 16

The aim of this chapter is to define poverty, to review the problems those on low income have in obtaining a good diet, and to suggest practical ways in which these problems can be eased.

Definition and incidence of poverty

There are several definitions of poverty. The Policy Studies Institute (1994) classifies as poor households with children but no employed adult and people receiving income support. The Child Poverty Action Group, among others, draws the poverty line when income, after housing costs, is below 50% of the average. On this basis one in four people in the UK was living in poverty in 1993 and nearly one in three children. Single parents are among those most at risk; six out of ten lone parents are poor (Oppenheim, 1993).

The effect of poverty on diet and nutrition

It is not surprising that provision of food suffers in poverty; some items *must* be provided and paid for, but the amount of money spent on food is flexible and can be reduced to allow for more pressing demands.

There are other difficulties; the distance from the cheapest supermarkets for example may mean a choice between transport costs or using the more expensive local shops. The homeless and those in temporary accommodation have additional problems of poor or no facilities for food storage and preparation (Stitt *et al.*, 1994).

A number of surveys have shown that those with low incomes eat less well, in terms of palatability and nutrient intake, than the more affluent (Health Education Authority, 1989; Malseed, 1990). Up to 50% of income may be spent on food, the most important factors in choice being price, speed and ease of preparation, and family acceptability. Large amounts of convenience foods are eaten; fishfingers and burgers are popular because they are easy to cook, liked by children and relatively cheap. Most of the survey respondents were bored with their food and would have liked a greater variety including more lean meat, fruit, salad and cheese.

Table 16.1 Relative amounts of different foods eaten by low-income households compared with high-income households.

More	Less
Meat products	Cheese
Margarine	Carcass meat
Lard	Total meat
Sugar	Butter
Jam	Cooking oils
Potatoes	Fresh and frozen vegetables
Canned vegetables including baked beans	Fresh fruit
White bread	Wholemeal bread
Total bread	

Modified with permission from Thomas B, (ed) Manual of Dietetic Practice, published by Blackwell Science Ltd, Oxford, 1994

Table 16.2 Differences in fruit and vegetable consumption in Britain, 1991, ounces per person per week. (From COMA report, 1993. Crown copyright is reproduced with the permission of the Controller of HMSO.)

Food	Income group A (2 adults, 2 children	Income group D and E2 (2 adults, 2 children)
Potatoes	18.97	37.06
Fresh green vegetables	7.98	3.34
Other fresh vegetables	16.77	9.61
Processed vegetables	15.68	16.64
Fresh fruit	25.16	11.89
Other fruit/fruit products	16.20	5.52

Few surveys have been quantitative in the sense of analysing the amounts of foods eaten and estimating nutrient intake, but they give a vivid picture of the difficulties experienced. For example, 'I tend to run out the day before we are due to get paid. Towards the end of the fortnight we scrape through and manage on chips .... A few times when we've needed money to sort something out – like bills – I've gone without myself to feed the kids' (National Children's Home, 1991).

An analysis by MAFF compared low-income households with high-income households; their findings are summarized in Tables 16.1 and 16.2 (Thomas, 1994).

In addition, the National Food Survey (1993) found that low-income groups bought more canned soups and milk puddings than other groups (MAFF; annual reports).

These differences point to the probability that people on low incomes have a lower intake of vitamin C, beta-carotene, folate, vitamin E and zinc than the better-off.

Along with a poorer diet, it is well documented that the health of those on low incomes is less good than that of the affluent.

Many who are eligible for benefits do not claim them and this aspect should always be checked by health professionals.

Practical suggestions for eating on a low budget

It *is* possible to eat economically and well, but poverty often goes hand in hand with other problems and with low morale. The habits of thrift which were acceptable earlier in this century are no longer common. Many people lack cooking skills. But there are a number of practical ways in which diet and nutrition can be improved. Where such advice is acceptable, at least some of the suggestions given in this chapter may be of use.

The more difficult the situation, the more important it is to plan, to prioritize, and the harder it is to do this. The food provider of a household must first of all fill them up, second, provide what is liked and finally aim to get the necessary nutrient balance. The last thing on his or her mind will be to hit the target for energy from fat.

Everyone needs some luxuries and these may be hard to include. Home cooking is a solution but anxiety about fuel costs may be a hindrance. In fact, the cost of fuel for cooking is not large and is outweighed by the savings made compared with buying convenience foods. Unfortunately, to be really economical, some 'luxuries' like a microwave oven, a pressure cooker and a supply of herbs and spices are invaluable.

Today's emphasis on healthy eating does not always help. The constant message is that if you don't eat wholemeal bread and a lot of fruit and salads, you are not eating healthily. The truth is that there are a hundred-and-one ways of eating well and it is perfectly possible to do this without either wholemeal bread or fruit (substituting vegetables and pulses for example). Then the argument is used that calories are much cheaper from biscuits, say, than from fruit, so of course fruit is a bad choice for poor people. Of course biscuits are more calorific and no one, however well-off, would eat fruit as a source of calories. Its function in the diet is to provide nutrients other than energy, hence its value in a slimming diet. Of course there are better ways of obtaining calories than biscuits. But these views must add to a sense of deprivation.

SHOPPING

- Use a cheap supermarket if possible and buy own-brands. If it is at a distance, it may be possible to share a taxi with another person and do a big shop together.

- Fruit and vegetables are often cheaper at an open-air market, and even more so late on Saturday afternoon. But for those living alone, the more expensive supermarket fruit and vegetables, which may last longer, work out cheaper through less wastage. Some community dieticians have helped set up local cooperatives to buy fruit and vegetables in bulk with great success.

FOOD CHOICE AND COOKING

The closer the food is to its original state, the cheaper it will be. This means that it is cheaper to buy flour, margarine and sugar to make biscuits than to buy them. Of course this will not be acceptable to everybody. Cookery demonstrations with tasting sessions are useful. Colleges of Further Education and universities which have a department of Home Economics or Consumer Studies may be able to help.

- Bread: buy the cheapest or make your own, which is easy and a real luxury.
- Meat: liver and offal are very good value but not always popular. Some recipes are given on pages 362 and 382–3. Chicken liver paté (page 362) is easily made and a useful and nourishing spread. Mince is often very fatty and it may be cheaper to buy less of the leaner, more expensive mince. If a food processor is available, it is a good idea to buy stewing steak and mince it at home. It is excellent for burgers, extended with breadcrumbs (pages 361–2).
- Meat products: these are often popular because there is no worry about whether the meat will be tender and they are well-liked. Corned beef is a good buy.
- Fish: fresh herring and mackerel, and canned tuna, pilchards, and sardines are all good. Suggested recipes are on pages 385–8.
- Eggs: an excellent source of protein and are often cheapest at open-air markets.
- Cheese: buy the cheapest. Grate for use in sandwiches, it goes further.
- Pulses: baked beans are useful as an extra vegetable. Lentils can be used in soup, with spices (see page 00).
- Fruit and vegetables: use what is cheapest at the moment. If potatoes are expensive, use more rice and pasta. Canned and frozen fruit and vegetables are more or less equal nutritionally to fresh and may be cheaper. Root vegetables are useful; cook carrot and swede and mash together with a little butter or margarine. Home-grown produce from a garden or allotment gives the luxury of really fresh fruit and vegetables and the flavour and nutritive value are excellent. Home-grown parsley, sage, thyme, lemon balm, mint are

useful for flavourings. Stuffing made with fresh sage tastes entirely different from the packet variety.

FUEL ECONOMY

- Although it must be considered, people often worry unnecessarily about the fuel costs of cooking. They are, for the average household, less than 10% of total energy requirements.
- Average electricity consumption for a Sunday dinner for four is 2.56 units of electricity or 7.7 Kwh for gas. The cost is very small (about 12p in 1995) compared with the cost of the food. Heating up the oven and keeping it on for 30 minutes takes on average 0.7 units of electricity or at 150°C, 1.0 units at 190°C and 1.45 units at 240°C. It costs much more to heat up the oven than to keep it hot.
- So, when using the oven cook several things at once, for example, meat pie, apple pie, jam tarts, rice pudding or chicken plus jacket potatoes, bread and butter pudding.
- Make 'one saucepan' meals; for example, stew with plenty of vegetables (onions, carrots, beans, tinned tomatoes), adding potatoes or dumplings for the last 20 minutes of cooking.
- Make stir-fry meals (pages 370, 390). These use little fuel.
- Steam the vegetables for a meal over the boiling potatoes. This is especially valuable for a small household as small quantities of several vegetables can be cooked at once.
- Use a pressure-cooker or a microwave oven to decrease cooking time and save fuel. Pressure-cookers halve fuel consumption.
- Oven-baked jacket potatoes cook faster if a metal skewer is pushed through them; it conducts heat more quickly to the middle.
- It is cheaper to cook casseroles on the top of the stove than to use the oven for just one dish.
- It is cheaper to make toast using a toaster than the grill.

MEAL PLANS

One of the difficulties of a tight budget is that it is not possible to risk a failure. There is no room for wastage. So familiar foods are used like sausages, fish-fingers, burgers. These foods can be made into nutritious meals and need not always be served with chips. For example:

- Sausages (grill if possible), serve with jacket or mashed potato, fried onions (easy to do in a microwave oven, using a plastic margarine container with a pierced lid, adding a little fat or water), cabbage or baked beans. Serve with bread.

- Serve fish-fingers with baked beans and canned tomatoes for a very easy meal, or a green salad. Add potatoes or bread. As an alternative make fish cakes from canned pilchards and mashed potato (page 387). Most children like these and they are cheaper and more nutritious than fish-fingers.
- Roast chicken can be extended by serving with sage and onion or parsley and thyme stuffing (chop onion, added chopped herbs and breadcrumbs, mix with water and cook around chicken or fry gently in a small frying pan) and a lot of vegetables. Use bits of meat in a stir fry next day and then make the carcass into soup. Cover it with water, put in a couple of whole carrots and onions and cook for about 1 hour. Add some rice or pasta towards the end of cooking. Remove bones, take off any meat, chop up carrots and onions, return to pan and season.

Case studies   BERNADINE

Bernadine Lawrence (1989) fed her family of four on £28 a week in 1989. She baked her own bread and made her own breakfast cereals, spending one-and-a-half to two hours a day cooking. They ate a lot of vegetarian and pulse-based meals. This is an extreme case but it shows what can be done.

STUDENTS

Hattie and Alison eat healthily and cheaply as follows:

Breakfast: cereal and milk

Lunch: cheese and salad sandwiches.

Evening meals:

- Large helpings of spaghetti/other pasta/baked potato/rice with liver fried with onions and bacon
- Onion fried with bacon/ham/tuna plus vegetables in season, and a tin of tomatoes. Grated cheese on top
- Tinned soup plus lots of grated cheese
- Tin of mackerel in curry sauce
- Stir-fried vegetables with soy sauce
- Risotto made with vegetables and apple
- Spaghetti bolognaise with 'Vegemenu' instead of mince

'Luxury' meals:

- Chicken pieces with tomato sauce
- Pork casserole

Fast meals:

- Scrambled egg on toast
- Omelette
- Frozen pizza slice heated in microwave
- Breakfast cereals

Puddings:

- Fresh fruit, yoghurt, stewed apple with sultanas

OAPs

Joyce and Chris find that their best buy is a 4-lb chicken. They have this roasted on Sunday, with roast potatoes and parsnips (carrots when parsnips are expensive) and other vegetables. On Monday they have cold chicken, with salad and a jacket potato. The next day they strip the flesh and make a casserole adding any available vegetables, lentils, and so on. Finally they use the carcass to make stock for a soup. They find liver (without bacon, which makes it more expensive) a good meal.

MOTHER OF TEENAGE BOYS

Mary's problem is the boys' appetites. She uses a lot of bread and potatoes, baked beans and cornflakes. She bakes once a week, making a large batch of pastry and using it for a meat pie (using canned filling or mince, well flavoured with onion and herbs), an apple pie, a treacle tart and a cheese flan. This gives the basis for two main meals and the puddings for two more.

She adds dumplings to stews, serves Yorkshire pudding and gravy as a first course, and uses baked beans as an extra vegetable practically every day. A popular snack is a soft roll filled with home-made chips (a chip butty) with baked beans. A sandwich toaster makes fillings go further. For some meals she serves both roast and mashed potatoes.

For family meal plans, see Chapter 21.

1. Poverty, which may be defined in several ways, has a major effect on diet, because of lack of money, cooking facilities, access to the cheapest retail outlets. **Key points**
2. Surveys, both qualitative and quantitative, show that people find their diets limited and boring and that they sometimes have to go without food. Those on low incomes eat less cheese, carcass meat,

butter, cooking oils, fresh and frozen vegetables and fruit and wholemeal bread than those who are better off. They eat more total and white bread, more potatoes, canned vegetables, jam, sugar and meat products.

3. Practical suggestions for eating well on a low income are given. These include shopping at low-cost outlets and open-air markets, choosing the best value for bread, vegetables and meats, cooking from basic ingredients rather than buying convenience foods, and reducing fuel consumption by using the oven to cook a whole meal or using a steamer to cook several items.

4. Some case studies are given of students, old-age pensioners and a family.

Diabetes mellitus 17

The aim of this chapter is to describe briefly the two main types of diabetes mellitus, the symptoms and the role of diet in management of the disease.

Diabetes mellitus requires dietary modification, usually for the rest of the person's life, and advice is given initially by a dietician. There is an excellent chapter on this subject in Garrow and James (1993) and the British Diabetic Association has produced a lot of useful material.

Types of diabetes mellitus

TYPE I (INSULIN-DEPENDENT DIABETES MELLITUS, IDDM)

Formerly known as juvenile onset diabetes, type I diabetes mellitus usually begins in childhood or youth. There is pancreatic damage, often linked with viral infection, which is followed by autoimmune damage of the pancreas. People with particular blood groups and who have been bottle-fed are most susceptible (Garrow and James, 1993). There is *insulin deficiency*.

TYPE II (NON-INSULIN DEPENDENT DIABETES MELLITUS, NIDDM)

Formerly known as mature onset diabetes, the type II condition occurs commonly in middle or later life. It is associated with weight gain and over 75% of sufferers are overweight. There is a genetic predisposition. A low birth weight also results in a reduced ability of the pancreas to produce insulin.

There is *insulin resistance and a high pancreatic secretion of insulin* which nevertheless fails to maintain normal blood sugar.

OTHER TYPES

There are other, less common, types of diabetes mellitus which have various causes, namely pancreatic insufficiency, hormonal disturbance (as in Cushing's disease) and genetic abnormality (Garrow and James, 1993).

Functions of insulin

Insulin is produced by the beta-cells of the pancreatic islets of Langerhans. Insulin acts on most cells of the body, increasing the uptake of glucose and amino acids so stimulating synthesis of glycogen, fat and protein.

The effect of these actions is to lower blood glucose. Insulin secretion is mainly controlled by plasma glucose concentration (Lamb *et al.*, 1993).

Symptoms of diabetes mellitus

Typically the symptoms of IDDM are weight loss, thirst and increased urine production. NIDDM may be asymptomatic for some time; when the symptoms occur, they are thirst, increased urine and possibly pruritis vulvae and blurring of vision (Garrow and James, 1993).

COMPLICATIONS OF DIABETES MELLITUS

These are micro- and macro-vascular diseases which are proportional to the degree and duration of elevated blood glucose.

In *micro-vascular disease*, more common in type I diabetes, there are changes in the capillaries, namely thickening of the basement membrane and increased capillary permeability, which lead to haemorrhages and the blocking of the vessels. Blindness and kidney failure may result. Cataracts are also a complication.

The *macro-vascular disease*, more common in type II diabetes, is the development of atherosclerosis (see page 240), particularly in the peripheral arteries.

Cardiovascular disease is a major cause of death in both types of diabetes.

Dietary and nutritional requirements

AIMS

The combination of diet with insulin or hypoglycaemic drug therapy and the patient's level of activity aims to:

- control blood glucose within the normal range;
- prevent a rise in blood lipids;
- establish and maintain body weight in the optimal range.

Table 17.1 Summary of nutritional recommendations for diabetics. (Modified with permission from Thomas, B., Manual of Dietetic Practice, published by Blackwell Science Ltd, Oxford, 1994)

Energy source	To maintain BMI of about 22 (see page 156)
Carbohydrate, % energy	50–55%
Added sucrose or fructose	<25 g/day
Dietary fibre	30–35 g/day (see Chapter 2)
Total fat, % energy	30–35%
Saturated fatty acids, % energy	<10%
Monounsaturated fatty acids, % energy	10–15%
Polyunsaturated fatty acids, % energy	<10%
Protein, % energy	10–15%
Salt, normotensive	< 6 g
Salt, hypertensive	< 3 g
'Diabetic' foods	Avoid

Individual dietary assessment and counselling are necessary, usually given by a dietician, and individual characteristics and life-style must be considered.

The nutrition sub-committee of the British Diabetic Association have produced nutritional recommendations (Table 17.1).

You will see that the recommendations listed in Table 17.1 are very similar to those for the general population. The amount of dietary fibre is equivalent to 18–20 g NSP (COMA 41 recommendation is 18 g for the adult population). This similarity is valuable, since it means that special foods need not be eaten by the diabetic member of a household.

Energy

Ways of estimating energy requirements are given in COMA 41 (Report on Health and Social Subjects, 1991), Garrow and James (1993) and in Thomas (1994). Methods of slimming are given in Chapter 8. Weight reduction reduces the insulin resistance of type II diabetics and for some, very low-calorie diets may be useful for a few weeks, under supervision.

Carbohydrates

The different rates of absorption of various carbohydrates and the glycaemic index of foods are given in Chapter 3. For diabetics, the rate at which sugar enters the blood is important. Pulses are valuable as they are sources of soluble fibre which slows the rate of absorption of glucose.

Table 17.2 How to provide approximately 50% energy as carbohydrate in a diet giving 1600 kcal. (Modified with permission from Thomas, B, (ed) Manual of Dietetic Practice, published by Blackwell Science Ltd, Oxford, 1994)

Food	Amount
Branflakes	30 g
Semi-skimmed milk	½ pint (285 ml)
Wholemeal bread	Four medium slices
Fruit	Three pieces
Biscuits	Two
Potatoes	Three medium
Sweetcorn	Three tablespoons

An example of how to provide the necessary level of carbohydrate in a diet for 1800 kcal is given on pages 190–1 and for 1600 kcal in Table 17.2.

Sugars

Concentrated sources of sugar should be avoided (like confectionery, some desserts) but in other respects a normal diet can be eaten. Artificial sweeteners should be used for drinks, desserts and other suitable foods.

Fat

Reducing energy from fat is particularly important for diabetics because of their increased risk of developing coronary heat disease. The reduction of saturated fats is particularly important. Suggestions for doing this are given on page 80.

MEAL PATTERN

Three meals and three snacks is a sensible meal pattern to prevent hypoglycaemia and minimize insulin requirement. If this is not possible, then four meals a day should be the aim. Some ideas for snacks are given in Chapter 21, along with recipes for pulses. All meals and snacks should contain some carbohydrate.

ACTIVITY

Activity promotes the uptake of glucose by muscle cells and may help reduce insulin requirements. In this way it can improve overall health.

The main danger of exercise is *hypoglycaemia*. In the short term, extra carbohydrate may be needed to provide the energy for exercise. The necessary amount can be calculated from estimates of the energy cost of activity.

ILLNESS

Blood glucose tends to rise in illness and therefore insulin should be injected as usual and at least some carbohydrate should be eaten. Fluids should be increased to prevent dehydration.

Suitable drinks are Lucozade, fruit juices, Coca-Cola or Pepsi, milk and soup. Ice-cream, yoghurt, milk drinks like Horlicks, and glucose tablets will provide carbohydrate. A table of suitable amounts is available from the British Diabetic Association.

FOODS

It is even more important for a diabetic to follow the dietary guidelines than for a healthy person. Ways of reducing fat and salt and increasing NSP can be found in the relevant chapters. To eat a healthy diet means choosing whole cereals wherever possible and eating plenty of pulses, using them in salads or with tomato sauce, or adding baked beans as an extra vegetable. **Low-fat foods** should be chosen.

Fish, preferably oily fish, should be eaten twice a week. Some useful recipes are given in Chapter 21.

Alcohol inhibits the production of glucose from other substances in the body (gluconeogenesis) and therefore can increase the risk of hypoglycaemia. Diabetics should never drink and drive, two or three days a week should be alcohol-free and low-calorie mixers are recommended for spirits.

Special diabetic foods are no longer recommended since many are high in fat and many 'ordinary' foods are available in low-sugar versions.

HYPOGLYCAEMIA

The symptoms vary but include loss of energy, shakiness, weakness, dizziness, palpitations, blurred vision, confusion, irritability and aggression. Severe hypoglycaemia ends in loss of consciousness and convulsions.

Carbohydrate should be taken in the form of sugar, glucose, honey, jam, Lucozade and sugary fizzy drinks or orange juice. These quick-acting carbohydrate sources should be followed by a slower-acting carbohydrate food, like a sandwich, biscuits or banana.

Key points
1. There are two main types of diabetes mellitus. Insulin-dependent diabetes mellitus (IDDM) usually begins in youth and is caused by pancreatic damage; non-insulin-dependent diabetes mellitus (NIDDM) begins in middle age or later, is related to obesity and is caused by resistance of cells to insulin.
2. Insulin, produced by the pancreas, lowers the blood glucose by promoting its uptake by cells. It is essential in the control of blood glucose levels.
3. Symptoms are weight loss, thirst and increased urine production. The latter two are caused by the excretion of glucose in the urine. NIDDM may be asymptomatic for some time.
4. Dietary advice and control are essential to control blood glucose, prevent a rise in blood lipids and to optimize body weight.
5. The recommendations are the same as for the rest of the population (COMA 41) but are even more important.
6. Activity is good for general health but there is a risk of hypoglycaemia.
7. Illness tends to cause a rise in blood glucose and so insulin and some dietary carbohydrate are necessary. Suggestions of suitable foods are given.
8. Hypoglycaemia produces variable symptoms which include shakiness, weakness, palpitations, blurred vision, confusion and irritability.

Diet and nutrition in hospital 18

The aim of this chapter is to discuss the prevalence of malnutrition in hospital patients and its effects on recovery. Ways in which nutritional status may be assessed and methods of nutritional support are described, together with the cost benefits, thus raising awareness of the importance of nutrition in sick people. Hospital food policies and food provision are covered briefly.

Many hospital patients are malnourished and this delays their recovery. Such malnutrition is often not recognized, perhaps, as Lennard-Jones suggests because doctors and nurses are trained to focus on medical problems and not nutritional ones. This problem is discussed, clearly, concisely and comprehensively, in the report published by the King's Fund centre (Lennard-Jones, 1992). Detailed practical information is given in Thomas (1994).

It is vital that food in hospital either maintains, improves or, at least, minimizes the deterioration of the nutritional status of the patient. In doing so, recovery will be hastened.

The health service is a major supplier of food, as well as having an important role as educator, since in the UK more than 75% of the population attends a primary health unit each year.

Food policy

A food policy is a statement of intent about the provision of food and therefore affects the nutrition of the patients and staff of a hospital. Endorsed by the management, the food policy will be incorporated into the hospital's planning process.

Food policy documents will vary from hospital to hospital, but may cover the following points (Thomas, 1994):

- a review of the scientific evidence of the areas of nutrition relevant to the hospital population;
- the aims and objectives of the policy;
- the target group(s) within the population;
- dietary goals or aims for these groups;

- the interpretation of these goals into catering provision and delivery;
- time-scale for achievements;
- strategies for implementation;
- methods of monitoring and evaluation.

The hospital dieticians and health-promotion officers will have key roles in drawing up such a policy.

Overall, food policies for affluent industrialized countries aim to combat over-nutrition. While this is appropriate for hospital staff and for some patients, many sick people are at risk of *under-nutrition*, because of loss of appetite, difficulties in eating or increased requirements due to illness or injury, and it is essential that this risk is recognized. Individuals need advice which is based on the assessment of their particular needs and the variation between them is likely to be even greater than in the general population. This diversity, in age and pathology, makes optimal nutrition of every person a challenge.

Food provision   The process of providing food for a large institution involves a chain of people. One weak link, such as food being served cold instead of hot, is enough to affect the whole operation and reduce the quality of the diet which is eaten.

Health professionals have a role in observing what is eaten by patients, finding out what might suit them better and perhaps implementing small changes which nevertheless will greatly improve their well-being.

The provision of food for hospital staff is also important. In a recent correspondence about hospital nutrition in the *British Medical Journal* one letter noted that 'junior doctors are starving too', referring to the limited food available for on-call staff.

Patients   PREVALENCE OF MALNUTRITION

Malnutrition among hospital patients is common. Some will come into hospital in a malnourished state. A number of surveys have indicated the extent of this. In a multi-racial group of children, one in six showed stunting of growth and nearly as many were severely wasted (Moy *et al.*, 1990). Malnutrition has been shown among adults also, in this country, in the USA and Australia (Bistrian *et al.*, 1974; Zador and Truswell, 1987; McWhirter and Pennington, 1994).

Some patients will become malnourished while in hospital.

Surveys have found that only 10–15% of undernourished patients had both height and weight recorded (McWhirter and Pennington, 1994). At Napsbury Hospital a score sheet has been devised for assessing nutritional status in psychiatric patients (Table 18.1) and nearly 50% of the patients so assessed were at risk of malnutrition (Lock and Vald, 1994). An investigation of surgical patients showed 84 out of 206 malnourished, 37 seriously so, and most of the patients who had not eaten a normal meal for more than a week did not receive nutritional support although half were malnourished (Royce and Taylor, 1994).

This is obviously a field where research is needed.

CAUSES OF MALNUTRITION

Food intake may be reduced. There are many possible reasons for this. Handicaps such as arthritis, or muscle-wasting conditions may cause difficulties in preparing and eating foods. There may be loss of appetite, or food may be unsuitable for those with difficulties in chewing or swallowing or with sore mouths. Loss of interest in food is common, because of depression or chronic pain.

Nutrient requirements may be increased, as in surgery and infection.

Nutrient absorption may be reduced because of disorders of the gut or removal of part of the small intestine.

EFFECTS OF MALNUTRITION

Well-fed, healthy adults have reserves of nutrients so that a short period of undernourishment will have no ill-effects. But for those without stores and with increased requirements due to illness and for the very young, this period is much shorter. Premature babies survive only a few days without food, small sick children 2–3 weeks and adults about a month.

The effects of starvation are discussed in Chapter 8 and summarized as follows:

- There is loss of lean tissue and therefore of muscle strength. This means that cardiac output is reduced, recovery of mobility delayed, increasing the risk of thromboembolism and bedsores, and the respiratory muscles may be affected, impairing the ability to cough (Heymafiels *et al.*, 1978; Arora and Rochester, 1982).
- There may be impaired immune resistance to infection (Mainous *et al.*, 1991).
- The structure and function of the gut alters, increasing the possibility of entry of intestinal bacteria into the body (Mainous *et al.*, 1991).
- Psychological effects produce depression, anxiety, irritableness and apathy.

All these things will affect recovery.

NUTRITIONAL ASSESSMENT

This topic has been covered in Chapter 1, where the difficulties of such assessment were noted. In hospital, quick and simple methods are necessary. Lennard-Jones (1992) recommends that a note about each patient's nutritional status should be mandatory in medical and nursing admission records.

Body weight

This is a simple but important measurement. Patients should be weighed wearing light clothing and using accurate scales. The patient's weight and height should be recorded on admission and either compared with tables for optimal weight for height or the Body Mass Index calculated (see page 156). The presence of oedema should be noted.

Most patients should then be weighed regularly (for example, once or twice weekly) so that weight loss can be noted.

Dietary history

This is a useful tool (Thomas, 1994). As well as establishing the usual pattern of the diet, other questions which can be asked are :

- Has the recent diet been normal?
- Has there been chronic vomiting or diarrhoea?
- Has there been noticeable weight loss?
- What is his/her normal weight?
- Has there been increased fatigue? (Lennard-Jones, 1992)

The weighing of babies and young children is, of course, particularly important. Remember that the obese patient may lose muscle through not eating and still look overfed.

Physical signs

These may indicate frank malnutrition and are given in Thomas (1994).

The score sheet devised for use at Napsbury Hospital for elderly and psychiatric patients is shown in Table 18.1 (reproduced with permission from Thomas, B., (ed), Manual of Dietetic Practice, published by Blackwell Science Ltd, Oxford, 1994). There are a number of such score sheets available. This one aims to cover all aspects which may affect nutrition.

PATIENTS REQUIRING NUTRITIONAL SUPPORT

Lennard-Jones (1992) suggests that, for surgical patients, nutritional support is advisable for those who have lost more than 10% of body

Table 18.1 Nutritional assessment – score sheet (V. Vald, Napsbury Hospital)

Name .... Ward .... Age ....

BUILD/WEIGHT FOR HEIGHT

Height [ ]

Weight [ ]

Using Garrow Chart or Body Mass Index, is patient:

Average	0
Overweight	1
Underweight	3

Is there a history of recent (ie: in last three months) unwanted weight loss/gain? (If yes score)	2

EATING HABITS

3 Meals in a Day	0
1–2 Meals in a Day	1
Snacks only	2
Irregular	3

ACTIVITY

Ambulant	0
Walk/Help	1
Chairbound	2
Bedfast	3

ORAL STATE

Own Teeth	0
Denture – Top or Bottom Set	1
No Dentures or doesn't wear them	2
Dentures hurt	3
Rotten teeth Mouth, sore, dry Mouth, ulcerated Gum infection	3

SELF CARING

Self Caring	0
Needs Food Cut Up	2
Soft Diet	3
Needs to be Fed	3
Enteral Feeding	3

PAIN

No Pain	0
Intermittent Slight	1
Continuous Slight	2
Continuous Moderate	3
Continuous Acute	4

EATING DISORDERS

Anoraxia Nervosa	10
Bulimia Nervosa	10

DIET MODIFICATION

Diet Modification should be scored on first assessment only

Special Diet	2
Food Preferences eg: Ethics; Food allergy/Intolerance	2
On food substitutes without nutritional advice eg: Ensure Complan, Milk:	
1 week	1
2 weeks	2
Longer	3

MEDICATION

Taking medication which suppresses/increases appetite	3
Makes pt nauseated sick or distorts taste; Eg: Chemotherapy	3

PSYCHOLOGICAL

Alert	0
Apathetic	1
Confused/Anxious	2
Depressed/Paranoid	3
Withdrawn states	3
Dementia	3

PHYSICAL

Physical disability causing Abnormal Head/Neck/Body Positioning or Movement	4
Swallowing difficulties	4
Lack tongue movement	4
Nausea	3
Gut/Stomach Surgery	4
Constipation/Diarrhoea	4
Malabsorption symptoms affecting eating/breaking down of food	4

ADDITIONAL NUTRITION REQUIRED BECAUSE OF:

Sepsis	3
Catabolic Disease	3
Protein Losing Conditions such as: – Burns Pressure Sores, Fistulae, Major Trauma/surgery	3

TOTAL SCORE =

IS PATIENT NUTRITIONALLY AT RISK?

YES [ ] TICK   NO [ ] TICK

Signature .... Designation .... Date ....

weight in the three months before operation and who are not able to resume adequate oral intake for a week after the operation *and* for those who are not able to resume adequate oral intake within 10 days of operation.

Obviously, nutritional support is required by patients who are clearly malnourished and those who are shown to be at risk.

NUTRITIONAL SUPPORT

Where nutritional support is necessary a plan should be made by the medical, nursing and dietetic team and the situation should be regularly reviewed. Nutrition status can be improved in several ways.

Eating more

Getting the patient to eat more by providing suitable food, attractively served and perhaps more frequent small meals. This of course is easier said than done.

Diet fortification

Fortification of the ordinary diet can be done by adding skimmed milk powder to drinks, soups, mashed potato, and so on. Cream, butter or margarine and milk or evaporated milk can also be used. These adaptations are particularly useful for patients on puréed or liquidized diets.

Supplements

Sip feeds and nutritional supplements are available to supplement the diet or for use as total diet. They are available in sweet drinks, soups and puddings. Examples are Build Up, Build Up Soup, Complan, Complan Soup, and Fortimel. Full details of names, suppliers and composition are given in Thomas (1994).

Enteral tube feeds

These may be used where patients have a functioning gut but are either unable to swallow or cannot take sufficient food. Fine-bore nasogastric tubes are usually used. They are comfortable for patients and the feed can be given slowly and continuously day or night. Enteral tube feeding is relatively inexpensive and simple to administer. It can be carried out at home after suitable training.

THIS 'NUTRITIONALLY AT RISK SCORE' DOCUMENT HAS BEEN PRODUCED TO ASSIST NURSES IN IDENTIFYING PATIENTS WHO MAY BE NUTRITIONALLY AT RISK.

THIS FORM MUST BE COMPLETED WITH THE INVOLVEMENT OF THE PATIENT AND/OR CARER WHERE POSSIBLE.
THIS FORM MUST BE COMPLETED AND SIGNED BY AN ACCOUNTABLE NURSE.

DIRECTIONS FOR USE.

(I) WHEN TO USE

1: To be completed on admission of the patient.

2: To be completed on all patients.

3: To be reviewed at 'ward agreed' time intervals and when the risk factors change eg: taken off medication which suppresses appetite; having new dentures fitted etc.

4: The findings of this risk assessment are to be recorded in a care plan with intervention planned to reduce the risk. This should then be reviewed as specified in the care plan.

(II) HOW TO USE

1: Put a relevant number (could be more than one score per section).

2: Total score to establish if patient is 'at risk'.

    10+ = At Risk
    15+ = High Risk
    20+ = Very High Risk

3: If the Patient is identified as being 'at risk' ie: a score of 10 or over

    a) Inform responsible Medical Officer
    b) Refer to Dietitian
    c) Agree and set review date.

VV/LG
Nutrition & Dietetics 15.12.94. 6th Ed.

Patient Reassessment

DATE	NURSE SIGNATURE	SCORE

Table 18.2 Activity and injury factors for estimation of increases in basal energy requirements. (Reproduced with permission from Thomas, B., (ed), Manual of Dietetic Practice published by Blackwell Science Ltd, Oxford, 1994.)

Activity factors	
Patients confined to bed	× 1.2
Patients out of bed	× 1.3
Injury factors	
Minor surgery	× 1.20
Skeletal trauma	× 1.35
Major sepsis	× 1.60
Severe thermal burn	× 2.10

Tube feeding may also be done via a gastrostomy for long-term feeding or via a jejunostomy after major upper gastrointestinal surgery or hepatobiliary surgery.

For tube feeding the nutrient requirements of an individual must be calculated. If the individual is healthy with normal nutritional requirements, then the appropriate Dietary Reference Values are used. The effects of injury or illness must be taken into account and there are various equations and tables which help in this. Such estimates are the task of the dietician and the subject is covered in Thomas (1994).

An indication of the increased needs for energy in different states can be seen in Table 18.2.

Most dietetic departments have enteral feeding policies which cover all the major issues. Cooperation between dieticians and nurses is vital.

Total parenteral nutrition (TPN)

This is where nutrients are passed directly into a vein because it is impossible to maintain nutrition through the gut. Either a central or a peripheral vein is used.

TPN may be life-saving but it is expensive, and serious complications like sepsis, metabolic disorders and thrombophlebitis may occur. It must be closely monitored.

Requirements for energy, nitrogen, fluid, sodium and potassium are the same as for enteral nutrition. For some mineral and trace elements and vitamins, requirements are less because there is not the usual loss in absorption. Tables are available giving suggested daily intravenous intakes. Carbohydrates, fats and proteins are given in different forms from enteral nutrition because they are not first digested. Carbohydrate is given as glucose, fats as emulsions and amino acids are supplied instead of proteins.

NUTRITIONAL SUPPORT FOR BABIES AND CHILDREN

The necessity for good nutrition in babies and children is even greater than for adults, because of the extra demands of growth and their smaller reserves.

As well as the physical demands, psychological factors must be considered and food must be made attractive to the child. Often the advice for a healthy diet (low fat, high NSP and so on) must be reversed. Advice suitable for the overfed adult is not appropriate for the malnourished child.

EFFECTS OF NUTRITIONAL SUPPORT ON RECOVERY

Good nutrition benefits the patient. There are many studies in Britain and the USA showing that patients who are malnourished on admittance to hospital have a longer hospital stay, more complications and a greater risk of dying than similar patients who are well-nourished. This effect has been shown in surgical, medical and elderly patients.

Trials to show the benefits of nutritional support have shown variable results. A well-controlled trial requires the selected population to be homogeneous, the injury or illness clearly defined and of similar degree and few other factors which may also affect recovery (confounding variables).

Such a study on elderly patients with fractured neck of femur classified patients on admission as well-nourished, thin or very thin. The well-nourished patients were mobile in less than 50% of the time for the very thin group and there were fewer deaths. Randomly selected patients with evidence of malnutrition were supplemented with 1000 kcal (4.2 MJ) and 28 g protein overnight in a nasogastric feed, and they showed a significant decrease in the time taken to achieve mobility compared with the group who were not supplemented (Basto et al., 1983). Another study, giving a smaller supplement, produced similar results (Delmi et al., 1990).

In a study among elderly hospitalized patients, half were nutritionally supplemented with 400 kcal (1.7 MJ). Although the nutritional state of all the patients tended to deteriorate in hospital, this was less in the supplemented patients, who had a significantly lower mortality than the others (Larsson et al., 1990).

There have been a number of studies on the effect of nutritional support before and after operations. Some have shown advantages, others have not. But from the combined results it is clear that malnourished patients are likely to benefit from nutritional support, that this should be given long enough to have an effect, and that support should begin before surgery and continue afterwards.

Cost benefits of nutritional support

The potential for saving, based on shorter hospital stays and reduced complication rates, is very large. Some sample figures are given in Lennard-Jones' report (1992), and an estimate based on a five-day reduction in hospital stay for 10% of in-patients was £266 million at 1992 prices. This estimate took into account the cost of nutrients and their administration.

In conclusion, it is clear that nutritional status of patients is vitally important to optimize treatment and that it will save money.

Key points

1. Optimal nutrition in hospital patients has a significant beneficial effect on the rate of complications, rate of recovery and therefore hospital stay and mortality. This has been shown in well-designed studies of patients with fracture of neck of the femur and of the elderly.
2. All doctors and nurses should be aware of patients' nutritional status and Lennard-Jones (1992) recommends that a note of nutritional state be made for every patient.
3. A food policy for a hospital will identify aims for various groups within the hospital and how these can be implemented.
4. Food provision in a hospital is a complicated task, performed on a modest budget, and every link in the chain is important in providing patients with appetizing and nutritious food.
5. The prevalence of nutrition among patients should be identified by suitable methods (height and weight being useful and simple): it may be higher than is generally realized. This has been shown in studies of children, elderly, medical, surgical and psychiatric patients.
6. The cause of malnutrition is inadequate food intake, which may be caused by a variety of reasons. Requirements may be increased after surgery, injury or burns.
7. Undernutrition causes loss of lean tissue and therefore muscle weakness, a weakened immune system, changes in the gut which may lead to entry of bacteria into the body, and psychological changes like anxiety and depression.
8. Nutritional support may be effected by increasing food intake (more snacks, meals), fortifying the ordinary diet (with dried milk powder and so on), giving additional supplements (Complan, Fortisip, for example) or enteral feeding. Where the gut is not functional, total parenteral nutrition (TPN) through a peripheral or central vein may be life-saving, although expensive and with the

risk of serious complications like sepsis, metabolic imbalance, thromboembolism.

9. For enteral and total parenteral nutrition nutrient requirements must be estimated by a dietician. Babies and children have special requirements.

19 Adverse reactions to foods

The aim of this chapter is to provide information about the various types of adverse reactions to foods and to indicate their incidence, so as to give a balanced view of the relative importance of such reactions.

Adverse reactions to foods are not new but nowadays concern about them is often greater than the risk warrants. To quote Ryder, of MAFF, 'British food is varied, nutritious, of good quality and as safe as any in the world'.

On the other hand, food today is often eaten long after it has been produced and bacterial food poisoning is increasing. The food chain is the series of processes which start with food production, then continue through food processing, transportation, storage and retailing. These activities are often carried out in very large units so that contamination of food at one point may have widespread effects. The identification of hazards and their monitoring and control are necessary. The hazard analysis critical control point system (HACCP; Box 19.1) is necessary throughout the food chain.

BOX 19.1

HAZARD ANALYSIS CRITICAL CONTROL POINTS (HACCP)

The implementation of a HACCP system involves:

1. establishing a HACCP team;
2. constructing a flow chart of the operation;
3. identifying all the potential hazards;
4. identifying the critical control points, where preventative measures can be taken;
5. determining targets for each control point;
6. establishing a recording system.

While there is no need for people to be constantly worried about adverse effects from food, it is wise to be cautious. In Chapter 9 the nutritional benefits of variety in diet was emphasized. Variety also gives an in-built safety net. The more foods that are eaten, the less any one food will predominate and so the risk of a dangerous level of intake of any one harmful substance is reduced.

There are various types of adverse reactions to foods and they can be classified as follows:

- food poisoning from microbes;
- food poisoning from naturally occurring toxins;
- food poisoning from pollutants;
- food aversion, which may be psychological food intolerance or food avoidance;
- food intolerance, which includes:
  - allergy;
  - adverse effects of drugs (alcohol, caffeine and so on) in foods;
  - enzyme defects;
  - irritant and toxic effects;
  - fermentation of food residues;
  - other (Food Intolerance and Food Aversion, 1984).

Microbial food poisoning

Bacteria and moulds may enter foods from the air, from humans and from other sources. Some pathogens, mostly bacteria, cause illness, either by producing toxins in the body after they are eaten or through the toxins they produce in the food.

The incidence of bacterial food poisoning has been increasing in recent years (Figure 19.1).

Possible reasons for this increase are intensive food production, increased storage of food, both commercially and in the home, and the public demand for reduced use of 'chemicals', which results in the use of fewer preservatives in processed foods.

Some bacteria, like *Salmonella*, are present in the intestines of animals, particularly chicken and other intensively reared animals. Others, like staphylococci, are present in the nose and throat of people handling food, or are transferred from their fingers.

Whatever their source, bacteria multiply rapidly in the right conditions. They usually require warmth, moisture and a good food supply. Because reproduction is fast, a few hours is enough for very large numbers to be produced. Reproduction is slowed by cooling and most bacteria are killed by heating above boiling point.

So, to ensure that food is safe, it is important to *prevent contamination* wherever possible and then to *prevent multiplication* of microorganisms. This means hygienic food preparation and safe storage with food covered, kept cold and stored for the shortest possible time (Boxes 19.2 and 19.3).

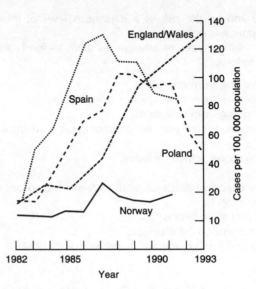

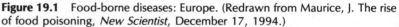

Figure 19.1   Food-borne diseases: Europe. (Redrawn from Maurice, J. The rise of food poisoning, *New Scientist*, December 17, 1994.)

BOX 19.2

It is estimated that 85% of domestic refrigerators are operating at too high a temperature for optimum storage of foods.

BOX 19.3

Cooked ham, for the picnic sandwiches, should not be cut on the chopping board which has just been used for raw chicken. The ham is not cooked again, so *Salmonella* from the chicken will not be killed by heating and may multiply and cause food poisoning.

As usual, the most vulnerable to food poisoning are the very young, the old and the sick. Good food hygiene is essential in the home and in all catering establishments.

BACTERIAL FOOD-BORNE DISEASE

Details of the common bacteria causing food poisoning are given in Table 19.1.

Table 19.1 Common bacteria causing food poisoning

Organism	Food sources	Killed by ...	Symptoms	Incubation period	Incidence
Salmonella	Raw meat and poultry, raw milk, eggs	Above 80°C Inhibited by acid	Diarrhoea, abdominal pain, fever, nausea, vomiting	6–36 hours	Very common form of food poisoning
Clostridium perfringens	Meats, poultry. dried foods, herbs, spices, vegetables	Extreme heat only Spores are heat-resistant	Diarrhoea, vomiting	8–22 hours	Fairly common, around 10% cases
Staphylococcus aureus	Cold foods (much handled during prepara-tion), dairy foods, especially if from raw milk	Toxin is stable to heat	Nausea, abdominal pain, vomiting, diarrhoea	2–6 hours	Not common
Bacillus cereus and others	Cereals, dried foods, dairy products, meat and meat products, herbs, spices, vegetables	Toxin and spores heat-resistant	Abdominal pain, nausea, vomiting, profuse watery diarrhoea	1–16 hours	Not common
Escherichia coli	Many raw foods, especially minced beef, beefburgers	Heat	Gastroenteritis	12–72 hours	Rare
Listeria monocytogenes	Meat, poultry, dairy products, vegetables, shellfish	Fairly resistant to heat	Mild influenza-like, meningitis, meningo-encephalitis	1–7 days	Very rare Pregnant women and the very young at risk
Campylobacter jejuni	Raw meat and poultry, raw milk, untreated water	Heat	As for salmonella	3 days, average	Very common

Sources of infection

Foods

There are some foods which hardly ever cause food poisoning, while others are always suspect (Table 19.2).

- **Safe foods**: *bread, flour, jams, pickles, fruits* and *fats* are usually safe because they do not provide the right conditions for bacteria to multiply. *Milk, ice-cream* and *canned foods* are safe, provided they

Table 19.2 Nine main reasons for food poisoning

1. Food prepared too far in advance and stored at room temperature.
2. Food cooled too slowly before being refrigerated.
3. Food not reheated to a temperature high enough to destroy food-poisoning bacteria.
4. Using cooked food contaminated with food-poisoning bacteria.
5. Undercooking food.
6. Not fully thawing frozen poultry.
7. Storing hot food below 63°C.
8. Contamination from infected food handlers.
9. Using of leftovers.

Modified from Sprenger, R.A. (1992)

are stored correctly, because they have been pasteurized or commercially sterilized.

- **Dried foods**: these may carry spores of the *Clostridium* and *Bacillus* groups which will become active when the food is hydrated. Herbs and spices often carry a heavy load but since they are usually added at the start of cooking, and often fried in fat, the bacteria are normally killed by heating.
- **Less-safe foods**: *frozen* or *chilled ready-to-eat foods* have usually received some heat treatment but they are unlikely to be sterile. Careful storage and use within the use-by date is important for the consumer.
- **Raw meats**: these are often contaminated with *Salmonella* and *Campylobacter*. For the consumer, proper storage and thorough cooking is important. Use of a chopping board solely for raw meat, or very thorough cleansing after use of an all-purpose one is important.
- **Eggs**: the contamination of eggs with *Salmonella* is well-known. Eggs should be thoroughly cooked before being eaten.
- **Cheeses**: these are mostly very safe but soft ripened cheese may contain *Listeria monocytogenes* and should be avoided by pregnant women.
- **Fish and shellfish**: these may be contaminated. Proper cooking is essential.
- **Fruits and vegetables**: in the UK, there is no problem, but if polluted water is used in their growing, then bacterial pathogens as well as viruses and parasites may be present and this is the hazard of eating salads in some countries.

How to know when a food is unsafe?

This is difficult and food may seem to be perfectly alright and yet be contaminated with food-poisoning bacteria. A handy guide, though, is to remember that a fresh food has its characteristic smell. As the food stales, this smell fades and so a cooked meat which no longer smells of 'meat' is old and it is best not to eat it. As a food decays more, unpleasant 'off' smells develop and the food can be seen to be bad. Always err on the side of caution.

Food poisoning from naturally occurring toxins

A number of foods contain toxins which, eaten in large enough amounts, will cause ill effects (Table 19.3). We all know that some fungi are poisonous. The fact that cyanide is present in almonds is not as well known, nor is it important. We don't eat enough almonds for the cyanide to be harmful and this applies to most other toxins in common foods.

The fear of 'additives' in foods, however, could more logically be directed towards some 'natural' foods. Certainly herbal teas should be used with caution since comfrey contains toxic alkaloids as may other, untested, herbal teas.

Table 19.3 Substances in some foods which may cause ill effects

Food	Active agent	Effects
Bananas	5-hydroxytryptamine	Effects on nervous system
Some cheese	Tyramine	Raises blood pressure; enhanced by monoamine oxidase inhibitors
Some fish, meat, cheese	Nitrosamines	? Cancer
Green potatoes	Solanine	Vomiting and diarrhoea

Adapted from Garrow, J.S. and James, W.P.T. (1993) (see Chapter 17).

Food poisoning from pollutants

Although surveillance of nutritional hazards in the UK is advanced, it is as well to remember that safety is relative rather than absolute and that our knowledge is incomplete in many ways.

Pesticides may be present in foods. Although farm workers are most at risk, residues in foods may be harmful. This area is monitored by MAFF.

There has also been concern about **antibiotics** used in animal feedstuffs. Such use is now illegal. There was in fact no evidence of direct harmful effects to humans but the danger is that strains of bacteria resistant to antibiotics might develop.

Oestrogens have been used in beef production but are now banned, although the amounts in meat were very small, smaller than in soya beans and eggs.

Radioactive fallout may yet be a problem, since there are recent reports of danger of another breakdown at Chernobyl.

Table 19.4   Examples of metal contaminants

Metal	Common sources	Effects
Aluminium	Used to purify water, in manufacture of cosmetics, medicines	Affects nervous system
Cadmium	Present in cigarette smoke, used in industrial processes	Fatigue, headache, vomiting, kidney failure
Chromium	Car manufacture	Lung cancer, kidney damage
Lead	Petrol, batteries	Damage to nervous system, bone marrow
Mercury	Industrial processes	Affects nervous system

Contaminants of soil, like **metals**, may enter the food chain (Table 19.4). One example was a high level of cadmium in Somerset where locally grown vegetables contained a dangerous level of the metal.

All this emphasizes the value of a varied diet, where no single food predominates, so that any hazard or contaminant will be eaten in small amounts only and therefore any harm minimized.

Food intolerance and aversion

Although food intolerance and aversion are serious and unpleasant to the few who are affected, they are much rarer than most people think. The raised public perception is probably because of the influence of publicity, the misattribution of genuine problems, and parents interpreting their children's normal behaviour as abnormal.

DEFINITIONS

Food intolerance is a reproducible, unpleasant reaction to a specific food or food ingredient and is not psychologically based (*Food Intolerance and Food Aversion*, 1984). It occurs even when the food is disguised and cannot be identified by the eater. Food intolerance may be caused by:

* enzyme defects, like lactase deficiency;
* pharmacological reactions, to caffeine or alcohol, for example;
* irritants and toxic substances. The mucous membranes of the mouth or bowel may be irritated from, say, highly spiced food. In some persons histamine release may be caused by some foods such as shellfish, strawberries and paw-paw, in a way that cannot yet be explained;
* allergic reaction;

- fermentation of food residues in the lower bowel, indirectly causing unpleasant effects;
- other mechanisms which are not yet identified.

Food allergy is a form of food intolerance where there is an abnormal immunological reaction to food (Box 19.4).

Food aversion includes **psychological avoidance**, when the subject avoids food for psychological reasons, triggered perhaps by having vomited after eating strawberries in childhood, and **psychological intolerance**, when an unpleasant physical reaction is caused by emotions associated with the food rather than the food itself. Psychological intolerance does not occur when the food is given in an unrecognizable form.

BOX 19.4

THE ALLERGIC RESPONSE

Foreign proteins which enter the blood stream may cause an allergic response. Normally, few proteins enter the body from the gut, because they are broken down by enzymes and because the cells present in the lining of the gut prevent such entry by the production of immunoglobulins.

The allergic response is caused by the reaction between the antibody and the antigen (foreign protein). There are four main types of allergic response.

Gastrointestinal defence mechanisms

The gut wall is protected from local immunological reactions in several ways:

- by the mucous coat;
- by the tight junctions between mucosal cells;
- by the immunological lymphoid tissues;
- by digestion of molecules;
- by the removal of substances through absorption and passage down the gut.

FOOD INTOLERANCE

Prevalence

Diagnosis is difficult and therefore accurate figures for prevalence are hard to come by. Food intolerance is *perceived* to be a problem by more than 20% of the population but in a careful study the actual prevalence in the population studied was less than 2% (MAFF, 1995).

Other estimates for the prevalence of food intolerance in children range from 0.3 to 20% (Food Intolerance and Food Aversion, 1984).

Symptoms of food intolerance

The symptoms of food intolerance may be eczema, urticaria, asthma, hyperactivity, migraine or abdominal pain. Allergic rhinitis and bronchitis may also occur and anaphylaxis may occur in severe allergic response.

Who suffers?

Food intolerance may be more common in childhood than in adult life. Genetic factors may play a part. It is well established that allergies of any type are more common in children with atopic parents and so this may hold for food allergy. Enzyme defects may also have a genetic component.

Which foods?

The most common foods causing food intolerance are wheat, eggs and milk. In adults they are milk, eggs, nuts, fish, chocolate and meat. Note that these are *not* processed foods or additives, as is commonly believed.

Often, intolerance lessens with age, but the allergy to nuts seems to be the exception to this (Hide, 1993).

Food intolerance caused by enzyme defects will relate to the particular substance, for example, lactose, which is affected.

Diagnosis

It is difficult to diagnose food intolerance and the only reliable way is by dietary investigation, which is time-consuming and demanding.

It is necessary to distinguish between the different types of food intolerance. The most common enzyme defect is *lactase deficiency* and if this is suspected, it is easily confirmed by tests on the stools for reducing substances (lactose is a reducing sugar).

Coeliac disease is a food-related disorder where there is sensitivity to gluten which produces a characteristic flattening of the mucosa of the small intestine, and this change is used for diagnosis.

For suspected *food allergy* there are two laboratory tests (the RAST or the radioallergosorbent test, and skin test), neither of which is very reliable. Other tests, like pulse testing, hair and nail tests and cytotoxic food tests, which may be promoted by private nutrition clinics, have not been proved to be reliable.

Dietary investigation

A dietician, in collaboration with a medically qualified colleague, would undertake the dietary investigation, and then advise patients about a maintenance diet. The dietary investigation seeks to identify the problem foods and then to test the hypothesis that food X causes the reaction with some type of food exclusion diet, followed by controlled reintroduction of foods.

Maintenance diet

The food(s) causing an adverse response must be avoided, although this will not necessarily be permanent. Children often grow out of their intolerance and foods can gradually be introduced.

One of the difficulties is that allergenic foods like nuts or soya flour are often found in unsuspected dishes. White bread often contains soya flour and peanuts may be in cakes, biscuits or desserts. Some bakers now have information about nuts in their products displayed.

COELIAC DISEASE OR GLUTEN ENTEROPATHY

Coeliac disease is a condition where the lining of the small intestine is damaged by gluten, a protein found in wheat, barley and rye. The villi become flattened and the absorptive capacity of the gut reduced so that children grow slowly and either lose, or fail to gain, weight.

The treatment is to avoid **gluten** in the diet. Unfortunately this means avoiding many foods. As well as the more obvious bread, cakes and biscuits, wheat flour is often used in processed foods. Gluten-free flour and bread are available.

It is thought that up to 12% of coeliacs may go undiagnosed, the condition being perceived as 'irritable bowel syndrome'.

CASE STUDIES

Veronica – self-diagnosis of intolerance

Now in her fifties, Veronica suffered from episodes of migraine headaches and nausea during her forties. During this time, as part of her work as a technician, she took part in a taste panel for soya cheese. She noticed she always felt ill afterwards. Realizing the prevalence of soya products in bread, ice-cream, cakes and similar foods, she began to read the labels carefully and to avoid soya. Her migraines have gone.

Recently, she was ill again after eating a frozen fruit strudel. Rescuing the packet from the dustbin, she found it contained a soya product.

Julia – an allergic response

Julia's problems stem from babyhood. She had eczema from birth. Breast-fed until eight months, she was given solids like baby rice and egg yolk from around six weeks, as was the practice 30 years ago. When offered fish, baby Julia closed her mouth and refused it. But where the prongs of the fork had touched her lips, weals appeared and remained for six hours. Fish was therefore avoided.

On Saturdays, the family usually had steak and kidney pie for lunch. Often, Julia, now a toddler, developed weals, poor breathing and swollen mucous membranes on Saturday afternoons. It seemed to be neither kidney, steak nor pastry. But Worcester sauce, added to the pie, contains anchovy essence and once this was avoided, steak and kidney pie was harmless. Once, the touch of her mother's finger, after she had handled fish, washed her hands, but not dried them, caused a weal on Julia. Julia is still allergic to fish.

As a toddler Julia rejected nuts. If she ate something containing nuts, she would say, 'my throat's scratchy'. Now, she is allergic to nuts, bananas, soya products (and has to be careful which bread she eats) and grass pollen.

Now grown-up, Julia's main difficulties are when she eats out and from the increasing use of nuts in food products. Her main reactions are weals, swollen mucous membranes and sometimes violent sickness and diarrhoea. She has required hospital treatment on several occasions.

Key points
1. Adverse reactions to foods may be due to one of several factors. These are food poisoning from microbes, naturally occurring toxins and pollutants: food aversion, which may be psychological; and food intolerance, which includes allergy, enzyme defects, pharmacological effects, irritants and intolerance of unknown cause.
2. Microbial food poisoning is increasing. Possible reasons are intensive food production, increased food storage, both commercial and domestic, and public demand for fewer additives, leading to reduced use of preservatives.
3. The two most common types of food poisoning are from *Campylobacter* (poultry) and *Salmonella* (poultry, eggs).

4. Naturally occurring toxins are present in many foods but are only dangerous if eaten in large amounts, which is not usually the case. Green potatoes contain a substance, solanine, and should not be eaten.

5. Pollutants in foods are under surveillance by MAFF. Residues of pesticides may be harmful. Antibiotics and oestrogens, both once fed to animals, are now banned. Radioactivity may yet be a hazard, from Chernobyl, for example. Metals, like lead, cadmium, may enter the food chain from the soil.

6. Food intolerance and aversion are comparatively rare. There are various forms and identification of the foods responsible may be difficult and time-consuming. A dietician would investigate many cases by dietary manipulation. The most common foods causing reactions are wheat, eggs and milk and not additives, as is commonly believed.

Part Three
Food and food products

Foods: their composition, labelling, storage and choice **20**

The aim of this chapter is to provide a reference source for information about labelling, and about the main nutritive characteristics of foods, and so to give a source of information for use in diet planning, and in answering questions about foods. It covers the relative nutritional values of fresh and processed foods, and deals with such vexed questions as 'health foods' and the use of additives. It is intended for reference rather than to be read straight through.

The choice of foods determines our nutrient intake and with the increased, and increasing, range available, knowledge of food products is more important than the knowledge of cookery.

Foods contain nutrients (proteins, fats, carbohydrates, vitamins and minerals) and a range of other substances some of which give flavour and colour.

    Samples of foods have been analysed for nutrients and the results published as food composition tables (Bender and Bender, 1986; Holland *et al.*, 1991). Numerous compilations of energy values exist. Useful as food tables are for dietary planning and analysis, these values are representative only. The composition of basic foods (like wheat, potatoes, beef) varies according to the particular species or type and the methods of production. For made-up dishes, recipes may vary considerably. So, these nutrient values may be a guide rather than accurate values. In general they are *most accurate* for the major components, proteins, carbohydrates, fats and hence energy, and *least accurate* for vitamins and minerals.

Food composition

LABELLING OF FOODS

The Food Labelling Regulations and their amendments state the requirements for food labelling. They are constantly updated. MAFF will supply information.

The label on a food must say *what the food is*, whether it is melon or sugar, say (Food Labelling Regulations, 1984; Byrne, 1993; MAFF, 1995). Labels on some fruits and vegetables must show the variety (for example, Desiree or King Edward potatoes). New foods must state clearly what they are: Choclac must be labelled as a hot chocolate drink and Coca-Cola as 'a soft drink with vegetable extracts'.

The name of a food may indicate a *flavour*. Strawberry, strawberry *flavour*, and a *picture of strawberries* means that the flavour comes mainly from *real strawberries*. *Strawberry flavour* means that a synthetic flavouring was used.

The label must also indicate a *particular type of processing*, as in *smoked* cheese or *dried* vegetables, although a common process like canning, which is obvious, is not indicated.

Ingredients

Labels on most pre-packed foods must include a complete list of ingredients, listed according to weight with the highest weight first. If water is added as an ingredient it must be listed, unless in a very small amount. Thus, a can of soup may have water as the first or second ingredient, a good indication that it is not an energy-dense food. The label on sliced ham may have water as its second ingredient, with the added information that it contains 'not more than 15% added water'. This system is useful but can be misleading. A pack of Mexican chicken (marinaded uncooked chicken joints) has a list of ingredients beginning 'chicken, sugar, modified starch...' but it is obvious that the amount of chicken is vastly in excess of all the other ingredients and it certainly is not rich in sugar.

Additives

Any additives must be shown on the ingredients list. They will be given by category and then by name (like citric acid) or by number. Numbers without an E denote additives which are controlled by the UK but not yet by the European Community; those prefixed by E are approved by the EEC. Details about additives are given on pages 342–352.

Nutritional labelling

The Ministry of Agriculture, Food and Fisheries (MAFF) has produced guidelines of nutritional labelling. At present these are voluntary unless a nutritional claim is made; this triggers the need for nutritional labelling. The amounts of nutrients must be given per 100 g (3.5 oz) of food *or* per portion if the packet contains less than 100 g. Two levels of labelling may be given. The minimum declaration is a 'Group 1' declaration, namely energy (kJ and kcal), protein, carbohydrate and fat. Group 2 requires energy (kJ and kcal), protein, carbohydrate, of which – sugars – g, fat, of which – saturates – g, fibre, and sodium. The Government recommends that Group 2 information is given on all foods, on a voluntary basis, as this gives consumers information on the key health-related nutrients (MAFF, 1995). The following nutrients may be included on a voluntary basis, but must be declared if a claim about them is made: sugars, polyols, starch, saturates, mono-unsaturates, polyunsaturates, cholesterol, fibre, sodium, vitamins, minerals.

These groups can lead to some rather odd labelling. Thus, fruit juice may be labelled for energy, protein, fat and carbohydrate, when in fact the consumer really wants to know its vitamin C content and perhaps its sugar level.

Datemarks

Best before is used on food which lasts a fairly long time. After this date it will not necessarily be dangerous, but will be past its best in terms of texture, flavour or nutritional value. A canned soup may have the month and year only (for example, 07–96), while a food which will stay at its best for less than three months will have the day and month, but not necessarily the year.

Use-by dates are put on perishable foods and mean that they must be cooked and eaten or frozen by that day. It is illegal to sell food after this date and potentially dangerous to eat it. This label has been extended, in some supermarkets, to foods like lettuce and it is certainly a safeguard against stale produce.

Other claims

- *Rich in or excellent for particular vitamins or minerals*: this can be used only when the quantity of the food that can reasonably be expected to be eaten in one day provides 50% of the RDA or RNI of that nutrient.
- *High in polyunsaturates*: this has a specific meaning and the actual amounts must appear on the label.
- *Low fat*: the official guideline is that such foods should have a total fat content of not more than 5 g fat per 100 g. But it is always wise to examine the label to see what the fat content actually is.
- *Low cholesterol*: this can only be used for foods which have less than 0.005% of cholesterol and if there is a claim about

polyunsaturates as well. This is not particularly useful since dietary cholesterol is not important for most people and for those for whom it is, the knowledge of which foods are very high in cholesterol is more valuable (see page 83).

- *Low calorie*: this may be used if there are less than 40 kcal in a serving and in 100 g or 100 ml.
- *Reduced calorie*: this may be used if there is less than 75% of the calories of comparable products.
- *Light or lite*: this may refer to calories, colour, taste, alcoholic strength and so on. In some drinks artificial sweeteners may replace sugar.
- *Diet*: this is similarly vague. Baked beans so labelled may have just as many calories as another 'ordinary' brand but be more expensive.
- *No added sugar*: this usually means that additional sucrose is not included but does not mean that the product is *necessarily* low in sugar. Natural sugar content may be high, or honey, syrup, or other sweet products may have been added.
- *Increased fibre*: the food must contain at least 25% more than a similar food *and* at least 3 g in either the reasonable daily intake of a food *or* in 100 g or 100 ml.

It is best to ignore these sorts of claims and look at the quantities of nutrients given on the label. A comparison of the labels on a brand of 'healthy' baked beans and the ordinary (unhealthy?) beans shows the following (values per 100 g):

	Healthy beans	Ordinary beans
Energy	65 kcal	85 kcal
Sugars	1.7 g	6.1 g
Fibre	3.7 g	7.6 g
Sodium	0.34 g	0.48 g

The difference in sugar content – 5 g – is a very small quantity, and the amount in an individual portion will be negligible.

Another brand of baked beans is labelled 50% less salt and 50% less added sugar. This vague claim (50% less than what?) is not, in my opinion, worth any extra expense.

Irradiation

This is a new permitted method of food preservation. Exposure to a low dose of ionizing radiation reduces the microorganisms present in foods and so increases shelf-life and safety (WHO, 1994). Suitable foods are poultry, seafood, spices, fruit and vegetables and irradiation is used at the moment on a limited commercial scale. There is loss of up to 20% of some vitamins, particularly thiamin and vitamin E. Irradiated food must be labelled as such or as treated with ionizing radiation.

A food can't claim to be 'reduced calorie' unless it is much lower in calories than the usual version.

When a product makes claims like these, it should back it up by giving the minimum amount either here where the claim is made or in the ingredients list.

Ingredients, including additives, are listed in descending order of weight at the time of their use in the preparation of the food. We can use the list to compare products for value, or to avoid ingredients we don't like.

Most additives must be listed, saying what their job is. The food company can use the name or the number (if the additive has been given one in the UK, with an 'E' if also agreed by the European Community). Both can be given.

If flavourings are used the packet must say, or give the names of each one. *They* don't have numbers.

This is where we can check what 'reduced calorie' amounts to. More companies are giving this information even if not making a claim.

Datemark must appear on the product.

Instructions for safe storage.

Name and address of the maker, packer or retailer, so we can write to them if we want.

The big **e** means that the average quantity must be accurate, but the weight of each pack may vary slightly.

Reduced Calorie

MAYONNAISE

made with fresh egg yolk

❀

INGREDIENTS

Water, soya oil, fresh egg yolk 7.5% (pasteurised), modified starch, spirit vinegar, sugar, mustard, red wine vinegar, salt, citric acid, stabiliser - carob gum, spices, preservative - potassium sorbate, natural flavourings.

CAN HELP SLIMMING OR WEIGHT CONTROL ONLY AS PART OF A CALORIE CONTROLLED DIET.

NUTRITIONAL INFORMATION

TYPICAL VALUES	Per 100ml	Tablespoon (15ml)
Energy	1205kJ / 288 kcal	181kJ / 43 kcal
Protein	1.7g	0.25g
Carbohydrate	9.0g	1.35g
Fat	27.0g	4.05g

Best before date on cap.
Once opened, store in refrigerator.
For best results use within one month of opening.
Contains less than half the calories of standard mayonnaise.

250ml **e**

Made in Wiltshire, England by the Manufacturer.
Full Address of Manufacturer.

Figure 20.1   From *Understanding Food Labels*, MAFF, 1995.

COMPLAINTS

First, go back to the shop where you bought the food. Further action requires going to the local authority which enforces food-labelling laws,that is the Trading Standards Department of the County Council or District Council.

Carbohydrate foods

These are the 'fillers', of medium energy density, between the watery vegetables and the high-energy fats. Ideally, we should get around one-third of our calories from starch, in foods that supply a good proportion of NSP and micronutrients. In general this aim is fulfilled by eating bread, potatoes and other cereals, particularly unrefined ones. The 'fancier' the food, as in cakes and biscuits, the more fat and sugar and the lower density of micronutrients. A good diet has a balance between plain and fancy.

FLOUR, BREAD AND OTHER CEREALS (Box 20.1)

BOX 20.1

FLOUR, BREAD AND OTHER CEREALS

Good for:

- starch;
- NSP (variable);
- protein;
- B-group vitamins;
- some minerals.

Low in:

- fat;
- fat-soluble vitamins;
- vitamin C.

Note that salt is used in most breads. The amount varies. For example, in one supermarket the cheapest white sliced bread has 0.5 g sodium per 100 g, two more expensive sliced breads have 0.7 g and 0.53 g per 100 g respectively, and a 'healthy eating' white sliced, 0.4 g per 100 g. Italian breads may have salt in the lower range, Pugliese at 0.4 g sodium per 100 g and Ciabatta, 0.4 g per 100 g, but this is not a great reduction. If you make your own bread, halving the amount of salt in the traditional recipe still produces a palatable loaf.

Bread and flour

Bread consumption, like flour purchases, has been falling for many years but bread still contributes on average 15% of our energy intake.

Bread (and wheat flour) are excellent foods. They are a good source of energy as starch, and the B vitamins, thiamin and nicotinic acid. Wholemeal bread has a higher level of non-starch polysaccharides (NSP, fibre) and a 'healthier image'. White flour loses some nutrients in processing but is fortified with calcium, iron, thiamin and nicotinic acid to make good these losses, so that white bread is equal to wholemeal except for NSP and is much the better source of calcium. Some white breads have added NSP. Brown bread has less NSP then wholemeal but more than white bread.

Bread is an excellent food for all age groups. McCance and Widdowson showed, in their work in German orphanages after the Second World War, that a children's diet where bread contributed 70% of the calories, enabled them to grow fast and to regain their health. So, *people should eat the bread they like and can afford.* Low in fat, bread is often generously spread with butter or margarine. But if it is eaten fresh, which is easier now that many supermarkets have in-store bakeries, it is so delicious this is not necessary. It can be cut thick and eaten with a meal or spread with jam or honey alone.

Storage: keep wrapped and cool. A few seconds in a microwave oven will improve stale bread and rolls.

Pitta bread

Very similar to ordinary white bread.

Chapatti

Less sodium and calcium than white bread. Energy value depends on whether made with fat or not. Unleavened (not raised with yeast).

West Indian bread

Similar to white bread but higher fat content and therefore higher energy value.

Poppadoms

Less moisture content than other breads and therefore more concentrated nutrients. Sodium content particularly high.

Self-raising flour

Raising agents are added and so this has a higher sodium content than plain flours.

Pasta

Pasta is made from wheat and therefore has a similar nutrient profile to bread. After cooking, it contains some resistant starch, which acts in the gut like NSP (see page 48). Wholewheat pasta has more NSP than white, takes longer to cook but has more flavour.

Rice

Rice has slightly less protein than bread and in white rice little thiamin or riboflavin remains. Rice contains no gluten and is therefore suitable for coeliacs. As a staple it is rather less nutritious than wheat, but has the reputation of being filling. **Brown rice** has more NSP, and higher potassium and magnesium contents than white.

Oats

Oats have similar protein content to wheat and more fat than most cereals. The NSP content is mainly of the soluble type, which has been shown to lower blood cholesterol.

Breakfast cereals

These are made from toasting, popping or otherwise treating maize, rice, oats and wheat. They are good foods, usually fortified with vitamins, and since they are commonly eaten with milk, supply a snack or meal lacking only in vitamin C.

- Vitamins: useful amounts of D, B1, B2, niacin, B6, folate, B12.
- Minerals: most cereals are a good source of iron, giving 15–20% adult RDA in a serving.
- Sugar: there are generous amounts in Frosties, Pop-tarts, and honey types, but most people need sugar to make cereals palatable, so whether these sweet varieties contain more than would normally be eaten depends on the individual. Oddly enough, All-Bran has more sugar than most non-sugared cereals.
- NSP: good sources are Shredded Wheat, Weetabix, All-Bran. Little in cornflakes, Rice Krispies.
- Sodium: low.
- Energy: little fat and light in weight, so not energy-dense; around 150 kcal (627 kJ) per serving.

Note: corn-flakes are one of the cheapest sources of nutrients and so are good for filling up hungry children.

Cakes and biscuits

Egg, fat and sugar are additional ingredients compared to bread dough. Therefore, as a source of micronutrients, cakes and biscuits are less beneficial than bread, but they *are* more energy dense. They have a place in the diet as attractive foods *but* as an 'extra' eaten at the end of a meal. Their palatability makes them a useful food when extra calories are required.

Potatoes and sweet potatoes

BOX 20.2

POTATOES AND SWEET POTATOES

Good for:

- starch
- NSP
- vitamin C.

Low in:

- fat
- protein.

Potatoes are an excellent cheap food, good for starch, NSP and vitamin C (highest in new potatoes, falling with storage) and iron. They contain no fat but the energy value and fat content are often increased in preparation, by roasting, mashing and chipping. Mashed potatoes are a good food for the young and grated cheese, dried milk and so on can be added to increase nutrient content.

Chips

For low-fat chips, use oven chips, or the recipe on page 392. To reduce the fat in ordinary chips, cut the chips thick or in thick circles. Drain on kitchen paper before serving. Chips have good vitamin C retention unless prepared a long time before cooking.

Storage of potatoes: in a cool dark place. Exposure to light makes potatoes go green and the compound formed (solanine) is toxic in large amounts.

Cassava

This is very low in protein, high in carbohydrate and low in vitamins except for vitamin C and folate.

Yams

These are also rich only in carbohydrate. There is some calcium, but only 3 mg vitamin C per average cooked serving.

Sugars

White granulated, white caster sugar

Sugar is the purest food available, in the sense that it contains only sucrose and nothing else. For this reason it is sometimes referred to as supplying 'empty calories'.

Brown sugars contain some colouring matter but otherwise are the same as white sugar.

Honey contains mainly sugars with some flavouring compounds. It has no special properties.

Golden syrup is a mixture of sugars.

Fruit and vegetables (other than potatoes)

Fruit and vegetables are the *protective* part of the diet, adding important micronutrients, namely carotenoids (or carotenes), the B group vitamins including folate, vitamin C, often iron and calcium, and NSP. They are bulky foods and low in fat and sodium. They contain many other substances, some of which are biologically active; it is thought that these may, along with carotenoids, be protective against some disease processes. They add flavour and texture to diet. Fruit is nearly always more expensive than vegetables.

BOX 20.3

FRUIT AND VEGETABLES

High in:

- water;
- NSP;
- carotenes (vitamin A);
- folate and small amounts of other B vitamins;
- vitamin C;
- potassium.

Low in:

- fat;
- energy;
- sodium.

To reduce vitamin loss from fruit and vegetables

Vitamin C, thiamin and folate are easily lost in storage, preparation and cooking. They are water-soluble and so will dissolve in cooking water and they are also destroyed by heat. Vitamin C is oxidized on exposure to air and by the enzyme, ascorbic acid oxidase, which is present in the cells of fruit and vegetables. This enzyme is released by chopping and cutting. To reduce loss to a minimum:

- use vegetables when fresh;
- tear leaves rather than cut;
- prepare just before cooking;
- cook in minimum water for the shortest possible time, *and don't use bicarbonate of soda* which destroys *all* vitamin C;
- do not keep hot.

In soups, the vitamin C will leach out into the water but will be eaten. Microwaving is good and so is steaming, especially for small helpings, when several vegetables can be steamed above the boiling potatoes.

Leaf vegetables

These include cabbage, Brussels sprouts, cauliflower, broccoli, lettuce. The greener the vegetable, the more carotenes present. Excellent food for all and especially slimmers.

Onions, garlic, leeks

As for green leafy vegetables, except they contain no carotenes. Garlic is claimed to lower blood cholesterol. *Celeriac* is rich in iron.

Cucumbers, courgettes, marrows

Very high in water but they add flavour, are excellent for slimmers. Courgettes good for vitamin C and folate.

Gourd (bitter/karela)

Fresh raw gourd is an excellent source of vitamin C and folate.

Tomatoes

Very good for carotenes and vitamin C. Canned tomatoes are a useful cheap food, good for vitamin C.

Peppers, green, yellow, red

Very good sources of vitamin C.

Fungi

Rich in potassium and phosphorus but not much else. Useful for flavour and texture but not important nutritionally.

Fruits

Citrus fruits and juices

Excellent for vitamin C. Whole fruit good for NSP. Sugars, largely fructose (sweeter but less cariogenic than sucrose). Skins of citrus fruits may be treated with preservatives such as sodium biphenyl-2-yl oxide (sodium orthophenylphenate) and then should not be eaten. The consumer has no way of knowing whether preservatives have been used except in Germany, where it is labelled.

Juices are a good source of vitamin C. The price reflects flavour and texture (there is a thickish sediment in some cheaper brands) more than vitamin content. Once opened the vitamin C content will begin to fall; they must be kept refrigerated (*Which?*, 1995).

Apples and pears

Less vitamin C than citrus fruits, and the level varies between different types. Pears less rich than apples. Apple skins may be treated with a variety of substances which may appear in apple juice.

Stone fruits

Moderate amounts of vitamin C. Peaches and apricots good for carotenes. Guavas are an excellent source of vitamin C (more than 170 mg per 100 g canned). Ortaniques and paw-paw (papaya) are also good.

Berries and black, red and white currants

Very good sources of vitamin C. Blackcurrants used for vitamin C-rich drink which is made at varying sugar levels. The high sugar variety should not be used in children's feeders.

Grapes

They are rich in sugar but low in vitamin C and NSP.

Banana

Differs from other fruits in that it contains starch and is therefore a useful energy source. Fairly low levels of carotene and vitamin C.

Kiwi fruit

A good source of vitamin C.

Buying, storage and preservation of fruits and vegetables

Buying: buy the freshest produce since this will last longer and should have the highest levels of vitamins. Some supermarkets label produce as staying fresh for a period of, say, a week. This is particularly useful for small households. Market produce is probably cheaper, may be fresh but from the cheapest stalls may not be. If it will be used immediately, then it is a good buy.

FRESH, FROZEN OR CANNED?

Fresh fruit and vegetables

When picked and eaten within a few hours, these have the best flavour of all as well as the highest vitamin content. However, a lot of 'fresh' vegetables are much older than this and their flavour and vitamin contents are reduced, according to the time which has elapsed since picking and the conditions in which they have been transported and stored. There are losses of vitamin C, thiamin and folate during cooking, as explained on page 323.

Canned fruit and vegetables

Canned fruit is more or less equal to fresh nutritionally. There is loss of thiamin, vitamin C and folate during processing but this may be no greater than in ordinary cooking and therefore canned foods may be used as alternatives. They may well be better than poorly cooked fresh, although rather lower in vitamin C than properly cooked fresh and frozen. Salt or sugar may be added; see the label. Water-soluble vitamins will have diffused into the liquid so it is sensible to use vegetables, juices in gravy. Canned vegetables are often cheaper than fresh or frozen. The main nutritional drawback of canned vegetables is the possible addition of salt and to fruit, of sugar.

Frozen fruit and vegetables

Again, these are just as good as many cooked fresh vegetables and fruits. A *Which?* report found them, on average, to be slightly higher in vitamin content than canned. If they have been kept at a constantly low temperature, then the losses of thiamin, vitamin C and folate are fairly small and after cooking they have similar or better values than fresh. Packs where the vegetables are stuck together may have thawed and been refrozen with adverse nutritional effects. After buying, frozen food should be kept cold and returned to a freezer as soon as possible.

Dried fruit and vegetables

Carbohydrates, fats, protein and minerals remain, but vitamin content is greatly reduced, vitamin C to zero.

Irradiated fruit and vegetables

These will be labelled to indicate the process. The effect on vitamins is to reduce some by about 20%.

Organic produce

This means it has been grown without the use of man-made fertilizers and pesticides. More expensive, there is little evidence of nutritional or flavour advantage. There should, however, be no risk of pesticide residues, *but* such residues may remain in soil for years and so traces may be present.

Storage of fresh fruit and vegetables: if possible in the cool and dark.

Protein foods   Protein provides the amino acids for the synthesis of new tissue and has the same energy value as starch and sugar.

MEAT

BOX 20.4

MEAT

Good for:

* protein;
* iron (well absorbed);
* B-group vitamins, especially B12.

but:

* may be high in saturated fat.

Note: frozen meat will, if properly stored, be equal to fresh meat nutritionally.

Red meats: beef, lamb, pork

Lean red meat is a very good food. Many people view red meats with suspicion because of their saturated fat content. The amount of fat varies enormously, according to the amount in the carcass and the way it is butchered and cooked. The fat in raw beef, lamb and pork varies from approximately 6 g per 100 g in lean cuts to 70 g per 100 g in fatty meat. The main contributor to the fat is the visible fat around the chop or joint and this can be removed before cooking or it may be lost during cooking, in grilling for example. There is some hidden fat present in the leanest meat. It may be cheaper to buy 'ordinary' meat and to trim off the visible fat than to pay possibly inflated prices for specially trimmed lean cuts. The fat content of mince varies enormously and in general, the cheaper the mince the higher the fat content. The fat can be reduced by first frying the mince gently and then pouring off the melted fat. To be certain of lean mince, buy braising or stewing steak and get the butcher to mince it for you or mince it yourself.

Red meat is a good source of high-quality protein, iron, zinc, copper and other trace elements. Sodium content is low, while potassium, phosphorus and magnesium are high. The B group vitamins, especially B12, are present.

Tenderized meat has been injected with a protein-digesting enzyme such as papain, which, by partially digesting some of the protein makes the product more tender and a cheaper meat more palatable.

BSE (bovine spongiform encephalopathy or 'mad cow disease')

This disease may be caused by a self-replicating protein. It is a disease of cattle, similar to scrapie in sheep. We do not know whether it can be transmitted to humans from meat, causing Creutzfeldt–Jakob disease (CJD), a spongiform encephalopathy. The available evidence is incomplete. (CJD has been transmitted to humans by injection of pituitary extracts for growth hormone from infected donors.)

However, positive precautions have been taken. BSE is a notifiable disease, and cattle tissues such as brain, spleen and the intestines, which might be likely replication sites for the BSE agent, have been banned from use by food manufacturers since November 1989 (Foodborne Illness, 1991).

White meats: chicken, turkey

There is less fat in these meats than in red meats, especially if the skin is removed. Skinned chicken contains 2–4 g fat per 100 g and with the skin, 17 g per 100 g. For turkey the values are 2 g per 100 g for flesh and 7 g per 100 g with skin. They also provide protein, B-group vitamins and the only difference from red meat is that they contain less iron. Note that water may be added to the carcass.

Offal

Offal is a cheap form of protein and is similar in fat content to lean meat. Liver and kidney are excellent sources of iron and the fat-soluble vitamins. The vitamin A content of some liver may be too high for safety for pregnant women and so liver should be avoided by them. Offal is not popular, although a boon for the hard-up. Some good recipes for liver are given on pages 362, 382.

Meat products

Mechanically recovered meat

This is the meat left on the bones after normal butchering, which is then stripped off by machine. The meat is forced through a sieve and appears as a paste which is used in pie and sausage fillings and in some canned meat balls. Nutritionally it is just the same as ordinary meat.

Reformed meat

Pieces of meat are 'joined' together by being rotated in a drum with a salt solution. This extracts some of the protein from the meat and the resultant protein solution binds the meat together when it is cooked. Again, it reduces the cost of the product without reducing nutritional quality and is used in meat pies, for example.

Bacon: variable fat content, high sodium.

Black pudding: high fat, energy, sodium, iron.

Corned beef: high fat (50% of energy), high sodium, good iron, B vitamins.

Ham: variable fat, high sodium. May have added water which affects texture.

Hamburgers: variable. Similar to minced beef with added rusk (carbohydrate). High fat. Salt often added. Home-made hamburgers are very good, see recipe page 361.

Paté: usually very high fat (for example, 65% of energy) although of course it may be eaten in fairly small amounts.

Pies: added fat and carbohydrate from pastry, variable amount of meat. But an average steak and kidney pie is a cheap main dish and eaten with plenty of vegetables is a good choice for economy.

Salami: high fat and sodium.

Sausages: made from finely ground meat (not less then 50% for beef and 65% for pork), soya or cereal rusk and a binder of some sort of protein, like egg, plasma, milk or soya. Fat content is very variable. Low fat (some 50% of fat of standard sausage) are available. They taste slightly less juicy but are perfectly acceptable.

Made-up dishes (chicken Kiev, lasagne)

The only way to know the ingredients is to read the label. There is absolutely no harm in using these occasionally, but for regular use high-fat types should not be chosen all the time. **Pot noodles**, etc. are relatively low in fat and not unwholesome, if unattractive to the adult palate.

Storage

All meat and meat products should be kept in a refrigerator until used. Mince should not be kept for more than 24 hours.

It is important that raw meat and cooked meat do not come into contact, when organisms present on raw meat might infect cooked meat, multiply and be eaten without being removed by cooking. In raw meat, cooking will greatly decrease any bacteria present. Raw meat should be stored on the bottom of the refrigerator, so that no drippage falls on foods below. Chopping boards should be very thoroughly cleaned after being used for raw meat or a separate one used.

FISH AND FISH PRODUCTS

BOX 20.5

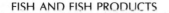

FISH AND FISH PRODUCTS

Good for:

- protein;
- iodine;
- low fat or PUFA fat;
- easy to chew and so good for very young and elderly.

Note: frozen fish is similar in nutrient value to fresh fish, although it may have less flavour. It is recommended that we eat fish twice weekly, including oily fish once. The popularity of fish has declined but some useful recipes are given on pages 385–390.

White fish

Cod, haddock, halibut, plaice, whiting, skate. These are low in fat, high in protein and iodine. Lower in B-group vitamins (except for B6) and iron than meat and higher in sodium.

Oily fish

Eels, herring, pilchards, salmon, sardines, sprats, trout, tuna, whitebait. Similar to white fish except that fat, high in polyunsaturates, is present along with the fat-soluble vitamins, and a higher level of water-soluble vitamins. The canned fish (tuna, sardines and pilchards) are a good cheap food and sardines on toast, tuna, sweetcorn and mayonnaise and pilchard fish cakes are all useful ways of serving them. Where the soft bones are eaten, calcium content is high. Tuna is often canned in soya oil.

Crustacea and molluscs

Mussels, oysters, scallops, crabs, shrimps, prawns, lobsters. Similar to other fish, low in fat but, except for cockles, oysters and scallops, high in cholesterol. Frozen prawns have a coating of ice which, if too thick, greatly increases the apparent cost.

Safety: if produced in polluted water, may be bacterially contaminated. Make sure they are fresh and properly cooked.

FISH PRODUCTS

Fish-fingers

The fish is cut from compressed slabs of frozen fish, either of one type or mixed. There is no legal minimum for fish content but this is almost certainly below 50%. The proportion of coating to fish varies. But a useful, cheap and acceptable food.

Taramasalata: this is cods' roe and therefore high in cholesterol and salt.

Preparation and storage

Cooking fish can make the kitchen smell. This can be avoided by cooking in a microwave oven, already arranged on the dinner plate. Excellent for sprats for example.

Storage: it is most important that fish is kept refrigerated or frozen. Fresh fish should be eaten as soon as possible.

EGGS

BOX 20.6

EGGS

Good for:

- protein;
- calcium;
- iron;
- vitamins A, D, B1 and B2.

but contain:

- some fat;
- cholesterol.

Care: eggs may be contaminated with the food-poisoning organism *Salmonella*, and therefore uncooked yolk should not be given to vulnerable groups like the young, elderly, the sick.

Eggs are graded according to size and are labelled to indicate production methods, *which do not affect nutritional values* although flavour may vary.

Most eggs are produced by the battery system. Barn eggs are produced by the deep-litter method, and range eggs are produced from hens which are allowed access to open space. True free-range eggs are not common but are sold by large supermarkets.

Test for freshness: when cracked the white around the yolk is thicker. In a stale egg all the white spreads flat.

Duck eggs

Similar in nutrient values to hens' eggs but are more likely to be contaminated with *Salmonella* and should always be well cooked.

Salted eggs

Not surprisingly, these eggs are very high in sodium.

MILK AND MILK PRODUCTS

Milk is an excellent food. It is useful for improving the nutritional value of the diet, for example by adding a glass of milk to a main meal or a snack for the elderly, ill or young. The fat is saturated but semi-

BOX 20.7

MILK AND MILK PRODUCTS

Good for:

- protein;
- calcium;
- B-group vitamins, including B12.

Fat (mainly saturated) content and fat-soluble vitamins depend on type.

---

skimmed and skimmed milks are now available and are useful for adults, providing a good range of nutrients. For decades milk has been regarded as a food for health and growth; now some see milk simply as a source of 'dangerous' saturated fats. This is unfortunate and there is a type of milk to suit every diet. It is *not essential* for a good diet, but it *is* a very good and cheap source of protein, calcium and other micronutrients.

Types of milk

Pasteurized: heated to 72°C for at least 15 seconds to kill harmful bacteria. Some loss of thiamin.

Sterilized: has more severe heat treatment, so that it can be kept for months unopened. The taste is altered and there is greater loss of B vitamins.

UHT (ultra-heat-treated): has been held at 130°C for 1 second. Long storage life when pack unopened and a fresher taste than sterilized.

Homogenized: the cream droplets have been broken up so that they do not rise to the top as cream but are evenly dispersed throughout the liquid.

- **Whole milk**: contains around 4% fat.
- **Semi-skimmed**: fat reduced by about half, therefore lower fat-soluble vitamins and calories.
- **Skimmed**: very little fat.
- **Flavoured milks**: a palatable way of drinking milk. A cheaper alternative is a home-made milk shake, made by adding drinking chocolate powder to cold milk and whisking.
- **Evaporated**: simply twice as concentrated as whole milk, with lower thiamin than pasteurized but may be enriched with vitamin D (some brands do not state this enrichment on the label). A very useful food for children and for the elderly and anyone who needs to enrich their diet. (See recipe for jelly whip on page 398.)

- **Condensed**: concentrated whole milk with added sugar.
- **Dried**: literally milk with the water removed. Its nutritional value is slightly reduced compared with fresh but it is a cheap food and for stringent economy can be used instead of fresh milk in cooking.
- **Goats' milk**: very similar to cows' milk. Fat is homogenized. May be useful for those who are intolerant of cows' milk. May not be pasteurized.
- **Soya milk**: compared with whole cows' milk, it has less protein (around 50%), very little calcium (about one-tenth of cows' milk), more iron (0.3 mg per 100 g), very little copper or zinc. The vitamin content is also very low but some brands (Plamil, Unisoy Gold) are fortified with vitamins D, riboflavin and B12. It is lactose-free.
- **Cream**: single cream contains about 18% fat, whipping cream about 39% fat and double cream about 48% fat. Used for its palatability, cream is also useful to increase the energy value of diets, for example for the frail elderly. Whipped or double cream will be made less fatty and will go further by folding in whipped egg white. Cream in pressurized containers is useful for finishing off desserts. Because it is aerated, a minimum is used.
- **Crème fraiche**: a cultured dairy cream, 30% fat, of which half is saturates.

BOX 20.8

CASE STUDY

Barbara and Noel, nearing retirement, use about 3 pints of milk a day, in drinks and milk puddings. By using a combination of skimmed and semi-skimmed milk, along with a fairly low-fat diet, they have reduced their fat intake, lost some weight and Noel's blood cholesterol has fallen. Barbara uses semi-skimmed or half and half semi- and skimmed milk for custard, skimmed for tea and coffee, and for things like parsley sauce and for rice pudding, ¾ pint of semi-skimmed and ½ pint of skimmed (to 3 tablespoons of rice). Milk used in this way is filling but not fattening.

Alternatives to cream

Fromage frais: made from fresh soft cheese, it has a variable fat content. Typical examples have between 5–8% fat only. Sold plain or flavoured. It is an excellent substitute for cream in puddings and desserts, sauces and gravies. Can be used as a dip with added herbs or alone as a dessert in the flavoured variety.

Yoghurt: made from milk which has been fermented by bacteria (*Lactobacillus bulgaricus*), so nutritionally it is similar to milk, except that lactose is reduced by the fermentation. There is only a trace of vitamin D in the unfortified type but some are fortified with the vitamin. A useful food for desserts.

Whipped evaporated milk: whisk chilled evaporated milk in liquidizer, food processor or with whisk, adding little lemon juice to thicken if liked. Good for children.

Smatana: a combination of cultured skimmed milk and single cream. Cheaper than double cream. Use in fruit fools, pavlovas, savoury dishes.

Modified cream: a blend of butter milk, vegetable oils and butter, with the single variety having 17 g fat per 100 ml, the whipping 33 g fat per 100 ml and the double type 43.3 g fat per 100 ml.

Ice-cream: ice-cream labelling seems to be less informative than for many foods. The main ingredients are milk, dried milk, butter fat or non-dairy fats, and sugar. Home-made ice-cream is not difficult and a recipe is given on page 402.

CHEESE

Cheese is made from milk by coagulating the protein to form a curd and then maturing this with suitable microbial cultures to produce a wide variety of cheeses. Cows' milk is commonly the starting point but goats' milk may be used.

Hard cheeses

Cheddar, Cheshire, Leicester, Edam, Gouda. A concentrated food with about one-third protein, one-third fat and one-third water. Rich in calcium, protein (obviously), calories, fat (though lower fat versions are available) vitamin A, and to a lesser extent the B group and in sodium. Of the hard cheeses, Edam is lowest in fat.

Store: wrapped in refrigerator.

Soft cheeses

Cottage cheese, cream cheese, feta, etc. These contain more water than hard cheeses and therefore are less nutrient-dense. Fat content varies between cream cheese (23%) and cottage cheese (less than 5%). They have a blander taste which can be enhanced by additions such as chives. Feta cheese (Greek) has a sodium content twice that of Cheddar.

Cheese analogues

These are made by blending milk protein with substances such as vegetables, oils and emulsifiers. They are used on some pizza toppings and cheeseburgers.

BOX 20.9

MIGRAINE SUFFERERS AND THOSE TAKING MONOAMINE OXIDASE INHIBITORS

The amino acid *tyramine* is present free (instead of bound in a protein as it is usually in foods) in cheese. This substance may cause migraine in some people and must be avoided by anyone on monoamine oxidase inhibitors, which are the older type drugs used for depression. There are newer drugs for which this prohibition does not apply. Tyramine is also found in *red wine*.

NON-ANIMAL PROTEIN FOODS

Soya products

The soya bean contains high-quality protein which is an excellent substitute for meat. It is available in several forms which equate with meat for protein and are low in fat.

TVP stands for *textured vegetable protein* made from soya. It is used in vegetable burgers, sausages, and ravioli and is also sold dry. Batchelors sell it under the brand name Beanfeast. It is a cheap alternative to meat.

Tofu or **bean curd** is the Japanese equivalent of cheese. It is sold fresh, has little taste but absorbs other flavours. There have been recent suggestions that it may be protective against breast cancers and research is proceeding on this. It is low in fat and in sodium, high in calcium but low in vitamins.

Other pulses (peas, beans, lentils)

Good for protein, NSP, starch, iron and calcium. Fresh (as in peas) contain some B vitamins, carotene and vitamin C. These are very useful foods and usually well-liked. Some people suffer from flatus, but otherwise to eat a pulse every day is a useful way to improve the diet. As a first course, butter beans in a tomato sauce is a good idea or a pulse can be served as a vegetable.

Lentils and rice, common in Indian cookery, give a very good combination of proteins.

Quorn is a mycoprotein produced from a fungus. It is sold as mince, chunks and in made-up dishes. It is more expensive than TVP and cheap cuts of meat. It is very low in fat (typically 3.2 g per 100 g), of which under 20% is saturated, has no cholesterol but some dietary fibre. Sodium is present at 0.1 g per helping.

Fats and oils   Fats and oils are the most energy-dense foods and add greatly to the palatability of food, whether by the mouth-feel of cream and butter or the crispness and smell of fried foods. The choice of fat hinges on taste, the polyunsaturated/saturated fat ratio, and for some people, cost.

BOX 20.10

EFFECT OF REUSING OIL FOR FRYING

At high temperatures fats and oils begin to decompose and gradually, with repeated heating, the colour darkens and the hazing point falls. At this point, or ideally before it, the fat or oil should be discarded

---

ANIMAL FATS

Mainly saturated fatty acids are present.

Butter: this is 82% fat, some vitamins A and D. May be salt-free or more commonly with added salt.

Ghee: this is clarified butter. It has a very low sodium content but otherwise is similar to butter. It may also be made from palm oil or other vegetable oils, which do not contain the vitamins A or D.

Lard: this is 99% pork fat, no vitamins, no sodium. There is a lard made from vegetable fat available and also a fat-reduced lard.

Suet: this is from cows, as for lard.

PLANT FATS

Oils

Oils are liquid at room temperature. They may be:

- monounsaturates – olive oil;
- polyunsaturated – corn, sunflower, safflower and rapeseed oils;
- mainly saturated – coconut oil.

To be sure of buying a largely polyunsaturated oil, choose those labelled corn, sunflower, safflower or rapeseed oil. Olive oil is nutritionally very good but expensive for general use. Often, the cheaper cooking oils are blended and may have a lower proportion of PUFA than the polyunsaturated oils. No vitamins A and D are present in any but plant oils are a good source of vitamin E.

Red palm oil: this is a very rich source of carotene.

Margarine: this is 81% fat, fortified with vitamins A and D. The amount of polyunsaturated fats present is variable. Not all margarines are necessarily high in polyunsaturates and therefore it is necessary to look at the label. *Trans* fatty acids may be present (see page 69).

Low-fat spreads: a variety are available with differing compositions. COMA report 46 *Nutritional Aspects of Cardiovascular Disease* (Department of Health, 1994) recommends their use instead of full-fat spreads. In a *Which?* survey, Sainsbury's County Light scored very well for palatability. Of course the point of their use is defeated if they are used *very* generously.

Water is lost in expired air, urine and sweat. It must be replaced to maintain homeostasis and dehydration is a serious hazard, especially to the very young and the very old. Thirst is the physiological signal that water is needed.

Drinks

WATER, TAP AND BOTTLED

Details of the composition of local tap water can be obtained from the supplier. There are limits imposed for certain substances like aluminium, nitrates and pesticides. Calcium and magnesium salts are present in hard water, to a degree which may be nutritionally beneficial. Rates of coronary heart disease are lower in hard water areas, although the reason for this is not known.

Lead is toxic and, although lead pipes have not been installed since 1976, in older houses some may still exist and lead salts may appear in the water. If this is suspected it is sensible to flush out water from the pipes by letting the tap run for a minute or two before using the water.

Bottled water has been a growth area with many brands now on the market. Carbonated or effervescent water has carbon dioxide present, either added or natural. Mineral waters will contain some mineral salts. If this includes sodium, then this seems an unwise choice, since most people consume too much of this element.

It is sensible to encourage children to drink water as opposed to fruit and soft drinks, which contain sugar.

SOFT DRINKS

Colas

Some are high in sugar and are acidic, and so are not good for the teeth. All contain caffeine (see below). They should come under the category of treats.

Fruit drinks

Most contain sugar (or sweeteners), variable amounts of macerated fruit and are acidic. Barley waters contain some starch. Some may have added vitamin C, others contain none. This is an area where the names of drinks are often misleading. Terms such as 'high juice' are meaningless. As an example of the variations, St Michael's Lite Orange Drink contains far fewer calories than St Michael's Orange Drink, and it also contains much more vitamin C (Which?, 1995).

Fruit juices

See page 324.

Tea, coffee, cocoa

All contain caffeine, with most in coffee, followed by tea and cocoa. Caffeine is a stimulant and does, in some people, cause increased heart rate and restlessness. It can prevent feelings of fatigue.

Tea adds fluoride to the diet but reduces the absorption of iron. It is difficult to predict the importance of this in an individual's diet.

Cocoa is the most useful of the three nutritionally, containing iron, as well as usually being made with milk. It contains sodium.

Alcohol

Alcohol (that is, ethyl alcohol) depresses the activity of the brain, in small amounts giving a feeling of well-being, and in larger amounts loss of mental and physical control and finally death. Excessive drinking leads to risk of liver damage, oesophageal and pancreatic cancer, inflammation of the stomach lining, obesity, impaired sexual function, and long-term brain and nerve damage.

Nutrients from alcohol: energy from all types, iron from wine (white or red), and riboflavin and nicotinic acid from beers. Spirits contain no vitamins or minerals.

Table 20.1   The alcohol content of drinks

Spirits	cl	% Alcohol	Units in 1 pub measure (24 ml)	Units in 1 bottle
Crème de Cassis	50	15	0.4	7.5
Advocaat	70	17	0.4	12
Campari	70	25	0.6	18
Pimms	70	25	0.6	18
Tia Maria	70	26.5	0.6	18
Orange Napoleon Liqueur	70	30	0.7	21
Vodka	70	37.5	0.9	26
Gin	70	37.5	0.9	26
White Rum	70	37.5	0.9	26
Whisky	70	40	1.0	28
Malt Whisky	70	40	1.0	28
Brandy	70	40	1.0	28
Rum	70	40	1.0	28
Cointreau	70	40	1.0	28
Drambuie	70	40	1.0	28
Grand Marnier	70	40	1.0	28

Cream liqueurs	cl	% Alcohol	Units in 1 glass (50 ml)	Units in 1 bottle
Chocolate Cream Liqueur	70	17	0.9	12
Irish Cream Liqueur	70	17	0.9	12
Swiss Chocolate Cream Liqueur	70	17	0.9	12

Units: 1 unit is 10 ml pure alcohol. So, a drink labelled 4% alcohol will have 4 ml alcohol in 100 ml and one unit (10 ms) in 250 ml (Table 20.1).

Sauces and relishes

Bottled sauces, especially tomato sauce, are much loved by the British, particularly children. They are made from fruits and vegetables in an acid syrup. They are relatively high in salt, but they increase the palatability of many dull foods.

Salad cream and mayonnaise

Salad cream is made from vinegar, starch and gums and is low in fat. Mayonnaise has a high fat content and used generously on, say, jacket potato instead of butter, may add a similar amount of fat. Low-fat versions are available.

Table 20.1   Continued

These are typical examples of alcoholic strength. The % alcohol may change very slightly from one vintage to another.

Table wine	cl	% Alcohol	Units in 1 glass (125 ml) ¹⁄₆ bottle)	Units in 1 bottle
Alcohol Free	75	0	0	0
Moscatino	75	3	0.4	2
Lambrusco Light	75	3	0.4	2
Vino Spumante	75	6.5	0.8	5
Spatlese	75	7.5	0.9	6
Lambrusco	75	8.0	1.0	6
Piesporter	75	9	1.1	7
Vinho Verde	75	9	1.1	7
Liebfraumilch	75	9.5	1.2	7
Sancerre	75	11	1.3	8
Soave	75	11.5	1.4	9
Frascati	75	12	1.5	9
Sélection Chardonnay	75	12	1.5	9
Australian Shiraz Cabernet	75	12.5	1.5	9
Premières Côtes de Bordeaux	75	13	1.6	10
Californian Cabernet Sauvignon	75	13	1.6	10

Fortified wines	cl	% Alcohol	Units in 1 glass (50 ml)	Units in 1 bottle
Sanatogen	70	14.5	0.7	10
Martini	75	14.7	0.7	11
Cinzano	75	14.7	0.7	11
Dubonnet	75	14.7	0.7	11
British Cream Sherry	75	15.5	0.8	12
Fino	75	16	0.8	12
Noilly Prat	75	17	0.9	13
Oloroso Sherry	75	17.5	0.9	13
Ruby Port	75	20	1.0	15

Snack foods

Snack foods are not intended to be a major part of anyone's diet but to provide pleasure as a treat, at parties, between meals and so on. Many processed snack foods are made from wheat or potato starch, which are often extruded and flash fried, having a fairly high fat and salt content. However, they are sold in small weights for occasional consumption. As David Conning notes they 'are often criticized as if they were intended to be a major component of the diet. No snack, whatever its depiction as a "healthy" foodstuff, could be regarded as other than

Table 20.1 Continued

Beer/Lager	ml	% Alcohol	Units of alcohol – can or bottle or glass
Kaliber	300	0.05	0.02
Low alcohol lager	330	0.5	0.2
Low alcohol bitter	440	0.5	0.2
Swan Light	330	0.9	0.3
Tennent's LA	330	1.0	0.3
Mackeson	275	3.0	0.8
Bitter	500	3.0	1.5
Lager	500	3.3	1.7
Ruddles Best Bitter	440	3.8	1.7
Labatts lager	440	4.0	1.8
McEwan's lager	440	4.0	1.8
Stella Artois	440	5.0	2.2
French lager	250	5.0	1.3
Diat Pils	440	6.2	2.7
Kestrel Super	440	9.5	4.2
Gold Label	275	10.9	3.0
Cider			
Low alcohol	330	1.0	0.3
Medium sweet	440	3.5	1.5
Blackthorn	440	5.0	2.2
Babycham Sweet	100	6.0	0.6
Vintage	284	7.2	2.0
White cider	275	8.2	2.3

Modified from 'Sensible Drinking', J. Sainsbury plc, London.

incidental to the main diet'. A typical 30 g bag of potato crisps contains 8.2 g fat (about ½ teaspoon), of which less than 50% is saturated fat, 0.6 g sodium and 147 kcal (615 kJ). As always, it is the *amount eaten* that matters. One bag of crisps is fine, six or so a day is not and some children may eat as many as this.

CONVENIENCE FOODS

There has been a steady increase in the consumption of convenience foods for some years. In 1993, 35% of the average food bill was spent on canned, frozen, ready meals and other convenience foods, compared with 25% in 1973 and 27% in 1983. (The National Food Survey gives a list of foods included in this definition.) Much of this increase is due to a large increase in take-away meals brought home, rather than straightforward canned and frozen products.

The nutritional contribution to the diet of convenience foods is better than is often thought. On average such foods provided, in 1993, 28% of total calories, 37% NSP, 25% polyunsaturated fatty acids and a higher proportion of iron (42%), magnesium, thiamin, potassium, niacin, B6, folate and vitamin C (43%) than of energy. They provided comparatively little calcium or retinol. Convenience forms of meats and cereals were almost as important sources of iron as the more traditional foods.

Convenience foods also contributed 26% of the total saturated fatty acids, 23% of cholesterol and 36% of non-milk-extrinsic sugar.

Health foods   There has been marked growth in health food shops, selling a variety of products. There is no such thing as a 'health food' for, as we have seen, any food eaten in excess may unbalance the diet. There is no need for special foods to eat well, simply a sensible food choice and combinations.

FUNCTIONAL FOODS

Functional foods may well be the next growth area in food marketing. They are foods manufactured to provide a stated amount of a nutrient or NSP and so can be eaten to improve a person's diet.

Additives   Additives are flavours, preservatives, emulsifiers and stabilizers, colourings, sweeteners, anti-oxidants and flour improvers which are added to foods. They may be acids, gelling agents or anti-foaming agents and they are valuable in increasing the safety of food in terms of keeping quality and its palatability. Additives are rigorously tested for their safety for human consumption but a minority of persons may be sensitive or intolerant to some. This matter is discussed on page 304.

Many permitted additives have been given a number. An E number means that it has been approved by the European Community as well as by UK authorities. The number of the additive, or the name, or both may be used on the label. An E number does not necessarily indicate an *artificial* compound. E101 is the vitamin riboflavin for example.

The claim that 'no artificial colours and preservatives' are used is a result of the public's suspicion of additives as a whole. This strategy is not always advantageous for the consumer. A minority of people may be intolerant of particular natural colours, which replace synthetic ones, and a reduction in the use of preservatives may mean an increase in food spoilage. There are around 3500 additives used by food manufacturers. A list of additive numbers and the substances to which they refer is given in Table 20.2.

WHAT IS THE AVERAGE INTAKE OF ADDITIVES?

The Ministry of Agriculture, Fisheries and Food (MAFF) carries out estimates of dietary intakes of food additives as part of the risk assessment and regulatory evaluation of additives. To find the average intake per head of population, estimates of the total amount of each additive used by the food industry were obtained and the totals divided by the UK population. These *per capita* (per head) intake estimates show that the overall additive intake of the UK population is 2.9 kg per person per year or 8 g per person per day. Most of this is made up of a few widely used additives; these are modified starches (2.2 g per day), E330 citric acid (1.1 g per day) and E150 caramel (0.6 g per day). Modified starch is a product of starch, which has been altered in such a way that its properties are different from ordinary starch. Citric acid is a mild acid which is present in many natural foods, like citrus fruits. Caramel is a breakdown product of sugar, which has been used as a flavouring and colouring for centuries, as in caramel custard or gravy browning.

The intake of other additives was found, in most cases, to be less than 0.1 g/day.

ACCEPTABLE DAILY INTAKES (ADIs)

ADIs for food additives have been determined by two government committees. When dietary intakes of additives were compared with these ADIs, only five had intakes greater than 10% of their ADI. These were sulphur dioxide and the sulphites (E220–227), sodium nitrite (E250), benzoic acid and the benzoates (E210–212), erythrosine (E217) and annatto, bixin and norbixin (E106b). None of these were consumed over 50% of the ADI.

Of course, average intakes hide individual variations but these results show, overall, that there is no need for great concern. Once more, the advantage of variety in diet is clear, since it reduces the likelihood of an excessive amount of any one additive.

To sum up, the easiest way to know what you are eating is to buy the raw materials, the basic foods, and cook them in the traditional way. But it is perfectly possible to eat well and healthily using prepared foods by adopting a wise pattern and choosing sensibly. There are so many attractive foods on the market and while it might not be wise to eat

Table 20.2   Food additives currently allowed in food in the UK. They are listed in groups to give an example of the types of food in which they may be found. The examples are not the only food in which an additive is used, but merely give an idea of where they might be found. When shopping, additives can be found on this list first by looking for its category, such as colour or preservative, and then looking for its number.

Antioxidants
Stop fatty foods from going rancid and protect fat-soluble vitamins from the harmful effects of oxidation.

E300	L-ascorbic acid – *fruit drinks; also used to improve flour and bread dough*
E301	sodium L-ascorbate
E302	calcium L-ascorbate
E304	6-0-palmitoyl-L-ascorbic acid (ascorbyl palmitate) – *scotch eggs*
E306	extracts of natural origin rich in tocopherols – *vegetable oils*
E307	synthetic alpha-tocopherol – *cereal-based baby foods*
E308	synthetic gamma-tocopherol
E309	synthetic delta-tocopherol
E310	propyl gallate – *vegetable oils; chewing gum*
E311	octyl gallate
E312	dodecyl gallate
E320	butylated hydroxyanisole (BHA) – *soup mixes; cheese spread*
E321	butylated hydroxytoluene (BHT) – *chewing gum*
	diphenylamine
	ethoxyquin – *used to prevent 'scald' (a discolouration) on apples and pears*

Colours
Make food more colourful, compensate for colour lost in processing.

E100	Curcumin – *flour confectionery, margarine*
E101	Riboflavin – *sauces*
E101a	Riboflavin-5'-phosphate
E102	Tartrazine – *soft drinks*
E104	Quinoline yellow
E110	Sunset Yellow FCF – *biscuits*
E120	Cochineal – *alcoholic drinks*
E122	Carmoisine
E123	Amaranth
E124	Ponceau 4R – *dessert mixes*
E127	Erythrosine BS – *glacé cherries*
128	Red 2G – *sausages*
E131	Patent Blue V
E132	Indigo Carmine
133	Brilliant Blue FCF – *canned vegetables*
E140	Chlorophyll
E141	Copper complexes of chlorophyll and chlorophyllins
E142	Green S – *pastilles*
E150	Caramel – *beer, soft drinks, sauces, gravy browning*
E151	Black PN
E153	Carbon Black (vegetable carbon) – *liquorice*
E154	Brown FK – *kippers*
155	Brown HT – *chocolate cake*
E160(a)	*alpha*-carotene; *beta*-carotene; *gamma*-carotene – *margarine, soft drinks*
E160(b)	annatto; bixin; norbixin – *crisps*

Table 20.2 Continued

Preservatives
Protect against microbes which cause spoilage and food poisoning. They also
increase storage life of foods.

E200 sorbic acid – *soft drinks; fruit yoghurt; processed cheese slices*
E201 sodium sorbate
E202 potassium sorbate
E203 calcium sorbate – *frozen pizza; flour confectionery*
E210 benzoic acid
E211 sodium benzoate
E212 potassium benzoate
E213 calcium benzoate
E214 ethyl 4-hydroxybenzoate (ethyl para-hydroxybenzoate)
E215 ethyl 4-hydroxybenzoate, sodium salt (sodium ethyl para-hydroxybenzoate)
E216 propyl 4-hydroxybenzoate (propyl para-hydroxybenzoate)
E217 propyl 4-hydroxybenzoate, sodium salt (sodium propyl para-
      hydroxybenzoate
E218 methyl 4-hydroxybenzoate (methyl para-hydroxybenzoate)
E219 methyl 4-hydroxybenzoate, sodium salt (sodium methyl para-
      hydroxybenzoate) – *beer, jam, salad cream, soft drinks, fruit pulp,
      fruit-based pie fillings, marinated herring and mackerel*
E220 sulphur dioxide
E221 sodium sulphite
E222 sodium hydrogen sulphite (sodium bisulphite)
E223 sodium metabisulphite
E224 potassium metabisulphite
E226 calcium sulphite
E227 calcium hydrogen sulphite (calcium bisulphite) – *dried fruit, dehydrated
      vegetables, fruit juices and syrups, sausages, fruit-based dairy desserts,
      cider, beer and wine; also used to prevent browning of raw peeled
      potatoes and to condition biscuit doughs*
E228 potassium bisulphite – *wines*
E230 biphenyl (diphenyl)
E231 2-hydroxybiphenyl (orthophenylphenol)
E232 sodium biphenyl-2-yl oxide (sodium orthophenylphenate) – *surface
      treatment of citrus fruit*
E233 2-(thiazol-4-yl) benzimidazole (thiabendazole) – *surface treatment of bananas*
234   nisin – *cheese, clotted cream*
E239 hexamine (hexamethylenetetramine) – *marinated herring and mackerel*
E249 potassium nitrite
E250 sodium nitrite
E251 sodium nitrate
E252 potassium nitrate – *bacon, ham, cured meats, corned beef and some cheeses*
E280 propionic acid
E281 sodium propionate
E282 calcium propionate
E283 potassium propionate – *bread and flour confectionery, Christmas
      pudding*

Table 20.2   Continued

433	polyoxyethylene (20) sorbitan mono-oleate (Polysorbate 80)
434	polyoxyethylene (20) sorbitan monopalmitate (Polysorbate 40)
435	polyoxyethylene (20) sorbitan monostearate (Polysorbate 60)
436	polyoxyethylene (20) sorbitan tristearate (Polysorbate 65) – *bakery products; confectionery creams*
E440	(i) pectin
E440	(ii) amidated pectin
	pectin extract – *jams and preserves*
442	ammonium phosphatides – *cocoa and chocolate products*
E460	(i) microcrystalline cellulose – *grated cheese*
E461	methylcellulose – *low fat spreads*
E463	hydroxypropylcellulose
E464	hydroxypropylmethylcellulose – *edible ices*
E465	ethylmethylcellulose – *gateaux*
E466	carboxymethylcellulose, sodium salt (CMC) – *jelly; gateaux*
E470	sodium, potassium and calcium salts of fatty acids – *cake mixes*
E471	mono-and di-glycerides of fatty acids – *frozen desserts*
E472(a)	acetic acid esters of mono- and di-glycerides of fatty acids – *mousse mixes*
E472(b)	lactic acid esters of mono- and di-glycerides of fatty acids – *dessert topping*
E472(c)	citric acid esters of mono- and di-glycerides of fatty acids – *continental sausages*
E472(d)	tartaric acid esters of mono- and di-glycerides of fatty acids
E472(e)	mono- and diacetyltartaric acid esters of mono- and di-glycerides of fatty acids – *bread; frozen pizza*
E472(f)	mixed acetic and tartaric acid esters of mono- and di-glycerides of fatty acids
E473	sucrose esters of fatty acids
E474	sucroglycerides – *edible ices*
E475	polyglycerol esters of fatty acids – *cakes and gateaux*
E476	polyglycerol esters of polycondensed fatty acids of castor oil (polyglycerol polyricinoleate) – *chocolate-flavour coatings for cakes*
E477	propane-1, 2-diol esters of fatty acids – *instant desserts*
E481	sodium stearoyl-2-lactylate – *bread, cakes and biscuits*
E482	calcium stearoyl-2-lactylate – *gravy granules*
E483	stearyl tartrate
491	sorbitan monostearate
492	sorbitan tristearate
493	sorbitan monolaurate
494	sorbitan mono-oleate
495	sorbitan monopalmitate – *cake mixes*
	extract of quillaia – *used in soft drinks to promote foam*
	oxidatively polymerised soya bean oil
	polyglycerol esters of dimerised fatty acids of soya bean oil – *emulsions used to grease bakery tins*

Table 20.2   Continued

E160(c)	capsanthin; paprika extract
E160(d)	lycopene
E160(e)	*beta*-apo-8'-carotenal
E160(f)	ethyl ester of *beta*-apo-8'-carotenoic acid
E161(a)	Flavoxanthin
E161(b)	Lutein
E161(c)	Cryptoxanthin
E161(d)	Rubixanthin
E161(e)	Violaxanthin
E161(f)	Rhodoxanthin
E161(g)	Canthaxanthin
E162	Beetroot Red (betanin) – *ice-cream, liquorice*
E163	Anthocyanins – *yoghurt*
E171	Titanium dioxide – *sweets*
E172	iron oxides; iron hydroxides
E173	Aluminium
E174	Silver
E175	Gold – *cake decorations*
E180	Pigment Rubine (lithol rubine BK)

Emulsifiers and Stabilisers
Enable oils and fats to mix with water in foods; add to smoothness and creaminess of texture; retard baked goods going stale.

E322	lecithins – *low fat spreads; chocolate*
E400	alginic acid – *ice-cream; soft cheese*
E401	sodium alginate *cake mixes*
E402	potassium alginate
E403	ammonium alginate
E404	calcium alginate
E405	propane-1, 2-diol alginate (propylene glycol alginate) – *salad dressings; cottage cheese*
E406	agar – *ice-cream*
E407	carrageenan – *quick setting jelly mixes; milk shakes*
E410	locust bean gum (carob gum) – *salad cream*
E412	guar gum – *packet soups and meringue mixes*
E413	tragacanth – *salad dressings; processed cheese*
E414	gum arabic (acacia) – *confectionery*
E415	xanthan gum – *sweet pickle; coleslaw*
416	karaya gum – *soft cheese; brown sauce*
432	polyoxyethylene (20) sorbitan monolaurate (Polysorbate 20)
E460	alpha-cellulose (powdered cellulose) – *slimming bread*

Sweeteners
There are two types of sweeteners – intense sweeteners and bulk sweeteners. Intense sweeteners have a sweetness many times that of sugar and are therefore used at very low levels. They are marked with * in the following list. Bulk

Table 20.2   Continued

sweeteners have about the same sweetness as sugar and are used at the same sort of levels as sugar.

	*acesulfame potassium – *canned foods, soft drinks, table-top sweeteners*
	*aspartame – *soft drinks, yogurts, dessert and drink mixes, sweetening tablets*
	hydrogenated glucose syrup
	isomalt
	lactitol
E421	mannitol – *sugar-free confectionery*
	*saccharin
	*sodium saccharin
	*calcium saccharin – *soft drinks, cider, sweetening tablets, table-top sweeteners*
E420	sorbitol; sorbitol syrup – *sugar-free confectionery, jams for diabetics*
	*thaumatin – *table-top sweeteners, yogurt*
	xylitol – *sugar-free chewing gum*

Others

Acids, anti-caking agents, anti-foaming agents, bases, buffers, bulking agents, firm-
ing agents, flavour modifiers, flour improvers, glazing agents, humectants, liquid freezants, packaging gases, propellants, release agents, sequestrants and solvents.

E170	calcium carbonate – *base, firming agent, release agent, diluent*
E260	acetic acid
E261	potassium acetate
E262	sodium hydrogen diacetate
262	sodium acetate – *acid/acidity regulators (buffers) used in pickles, salad cream and bread; they contribute to flavour and provide protection against mould growth*
E263	calcium acetate – *firming agent; also provides calcium which is useful in quick-set jelly mix*
E270	lactic acid – *acid/flavouring protects against mould growth; salad dressing, soft margarine*
E290	carbon dioxide – *carbonating agent/packaging gas and propellant; used in fizzy drinks*
296	DL-malic acid; L-malic acid
297	fumaric acid – *acid/flavouring; used in soft drinks, sweets, biscuits, dessert mixes and pie fillings*
E325	sodium lactate – *buffer, humectant; used in jams, preserves sweets, flour, confectionery*
E326	potassium lactate – *buffer; jams, preserves and jellies*
E327	calcium lactate – *buffer, firming agent; canned fruit, pie filling*
E330	citric acid
E331	sodium dihydrogen citrate (monosodium citrate); disodium citrate; trisodium citrate
E332	potassium dihydrogen citrate (monopotassium citrate); tripotassium citrate

Table 20.2   Continued

E333	monocalcium citrate; dicalcium citrate; tricalcium citrate – *acid/flavourings, buffers, sequestrants, emulsifying salts (calcium salts are firming agents); used in soft drinks, jams, preserves, sweets, UHT cream, processed cheese, canned fruit, dessert mixes, ice-cream*
E334	L-(+)-tartaric acid
E335	monosodium L-(+)-tartrate; disodium L-(+)-tartrate
E336	monopotassium L-(+)-tartrate (cream of tartar); dipotassium L-(+)-tartrate
E337	potassium sodium L-(+)-tartrate – *acid/flavourings, buffers, emulsifying salts, sequestrants; used in soft drinks, biscuit creams and fillings, sweets, jams, dessert mixes and processed cheese*
E338	orthophosphoric acid (phosphoric acid) – *acid/flavourings; soft drinks, cocoa*
E339	sodium dihydrogen orthophosphate; disodium hydrogen orthophosphate, trisodium orthophosphate
E340	potassium dihydrogen orthophosphate; dipotassium hydrogen orthophosphate; tripotassium orthophosphate – *buffers, sequestrants, emulsifying salts; used in dessert mixes, non-dairy creamers, processed cheese*
E341	calcium tetrahydrogen diorthophosphate; calcium hydrogen orthophosphate; tricalcium diorthophosphate – *firming agent, anti-caking agent, raising agent; cake mixes, baking powder, dessert mixes*
350	sodium malate; sodium hydrogen malate
351	potassium malate – *buffers, humectants; used in jams, sweets, cakes, biscuits*
352	calcium malate; calcium hydrogen malate – *firming agent in processed fruit and vegetables*
353	metatartaric acid – *sequestrant used in wine*
355	adipic acid – *buffer/flavouring; sweets, synthetic cream desserts*
363	succinic acid – *buffer/flavouring; dry foods and beverage mixes*
370	1,4-heptonolactone – *acid, sequestrant; dried soups, instant desserts*
375	nicotinic acid – *colour stabiliser; bread, flour, breakfast cereals*
380	triammonium citrate – *buffer, emulsifying salt; processed cheese*
381	ammonium ferric citrate – *bread*
385	calcium disodium ethylenediamine-NNN'N'-tetra-acetate (calcium disodium EDTA) – *sequestrant; canned shellfish*
E422	glycerol – *humectant, solvent; cake icing, confectionery*
432	polyoxyethylene (20) sorbitan monolaurate (Polysorbate 20)
E450(a)	disodium dihydrogen diphosphate; trisodium diphosphate; tetrasodium diphosphate; tetrapotassium diphosphate
E450(b)	pentasodium triphosphate; pentapotassium triphosphate
E450(c)	sodium polyphosphates, potassium polyphosphates – *buffers, sequestrants, emulsifying salts, stabilisers, texturisers – raising agents; used in whipping cream, fish and meat products, bread, processed cheese, canned vegetables*
500	sodium carbonate; sodium hydrogen carbonate (bicarbonate of soda); sodium sesquicarbonate
501	potassium carbonate; potassium hydrogen carbonate – *bases, aerating agents, diluents; used in jams, jellies, self-raising flour, wine, cocoa*

Table 20.2 Continued

503	ammonium carbonate; ammonium hydrogen carbonate – *buffer, aerating agent; cocoa, biscuits*
504	magnesium carbonate – *base, anti-caking agent; wafer biscuits, icing sugar*
507	hydrochloric acid
508	potassium chloride – *gelling agent, salt substitute; table salt replacement*
509	calcium chloride – *firming agent in canned fruit and vegetables*
510	ammonium chloride – *yeast food in bread*
513	sulphuric acid
514	sodium sulphate – *diluent for colours*
515	potassium sulphate – *salt substitute*
516	calcium sulphate – *firming agent and yeast food; bread*
518	magnesium sulphate – *firming agent*
524	sodium hydroxide – *base; cocoa, jams and sweets*
525	potassium hydroxide – *base; sweets*
526	calcium hydroxide – *firming agent; sweets*
527	ammonium hydroxide – *diluent and solvent for food colours; base; cocoa*
528	magnesium hydroxide – *base; sweets*
529	calcium oxide – *base; sweets*
530	magnesium oxide – *anti-caking agent; cocoa products*
535	sodium ferrocyanide
536	potassium ferrocyanide – *anti-caking agents in salt; crystallisation aids in wine*
540	dicalcium diphosphate – *buffer, neutralising agent; cheese*
541	sodium aluminium phosphate – *acid, raising agent; cake mixes, self-raising flour, biscuits*
542	edible bone phosphate – *anti-caking agent*
544	calcium polyphosphates – *emulsifyng salt; processed cheese*
545	ammonium polyphosphates – *emulsifier, texturiser; frozen chicken*
551	silicon dioxide (silica) – *anti-caking agent; skimmed milk powder, sweeteners*
552	calcium silicate – *anti-caking agent, release agent; icing sugar, sweets*
553(a)	magnesium silicate synthetic; magnesium trisilicate – *anti-caking agent; sugar confectionery*
553(b)	talc – *release agent; tabletted confectionery*
554	aluminium sodium silicate
556	aluminium calcium silicate
558	bentonite
559	kaolin – *anti-caking agents*
572	magnesium stearate – *emulsifier, release agent; confectionery*
575	D-glucono-1, 5-lactone (glucono delta-lactone) – *acid, sequestrant; cake mixes, continental sausages*
576	sodium gluconate
577	potassium gluconate – *sequestrants*
578	calcium gluconate – *buffer, firming agent, sequestrant; jams, dessert mixes*
620	L-glutamic acid
621	sodium hydrogen L-glutamate (monosodium glutamate; MSG)
622	potassium hydrogen L-glutamate (monopotassium glutamate)

Table 20.2 Continued

623	calcium dihydrogen di-L-glutamate (calcium glutamate)
627	guanosine 5'-disodium phosphate (sodium guanylate)
631	inosine 5'-disodium phosphate (sodium inosinate)
635	sodium 5'-ribonucleotide – *flavour enhancers used in savoury foods and snacks, soups, sauces and meat products*
900	dimethylpolysiloxane – *anti-foaming agent*
901	beeswax
903	carnauba wax – *glazing agents used in sugar and chocolate confectionery*
904	shellac – *glazing agent used to wax apples*
905	mineral hydrocarbons – *glazing/coating agent used to prevent dried fruit sticking together*
907	refined microcrystalline wax – *release agent; chewing gum*
920	L-cysteine hydrochloride
925	chlorine
926	chlorine dioxide
927	azodicarbonamide – *flour improvers; cake and biscuit doughs*
	aluminium potassium sulphate – *firming agent; chocolate-coated cherries*
	2-aminoethanol – *base; caustic lye used to peel vegetables*
	ammonium dihydrogen orthophosphate; diammonium hydrogen othophosphate – *buffer, yeast food*
	ammonium sulphate – *yeast food*
	butyl stearate – *releasing agent*
	calcium heptonate – *firming agent, sequestrant; prepared fruit and vegetables*
	calcium phytate – *sequestrant; wine*
	dichlorodifluoromethane – *propellant and liquid freezant used to freeze food by immersion*
	diethyl ether – *solvent*
	disodium dihydrogen ethylenediamine-NNN'N'-tetra-acetate (disodium dihydrogen EDTA) – *sequestrant; brandy*
	ethanol (ethylalcohol)
	ethyl acetate
	glycerol mono-acetate (monoacetin)
	glycerol di-acetate (diacetin)
	gylcerol tri-acetate (triacetin) – *solvents used to dilute and carry food colours and flavourings*
	glycine – *sequestrant, buffer*
	hydrogen
	nitrogen – *packaging gases*
	nitrous oxide – *propellant used in aerosol packs of whipped cream*
	octadecylammonium acetate – *anti-caking agent in yeast foods used in bread*
	oxygen – *packaging gas*
	oxystearin – *sequestrant, fat crystallisation inhibitor; salad cream*
	polydextrose – *bulking agent; reduced and low calorie foods*
	propan-1, 2-diol (propylene glycol)
	propan-2-ol (isopropyl alcohol) – *solvents used to dilute colours and flavourings*
	sodium heptonate – *sequestrant; edible oils*
	spermaceti
	sperm oil – *release agents*
	tannic acid – *flavouring, clarifying agent; beer, wine and cider*

Modified from A Guide from the Food Safety Directorate, MAFF, 1994.

some of them frequently and regularly, there is no harm at all in a modest intake.

Special foods   PROPRIETARY ENERGY AND NUTRIENT SUPPLEMENTS

There are a large number of such supplements on the market. They include drinks like Complan and Build-Up which are based on milk protein and fortified with vitamins and minerals. Available in several flavours, they are often useful for the frail elderly. Others, like Caloreen and Polycal, provide carbohydrate as an energy supplement.

The market changes rapidly and therefore tables of composition quickly become out-of-date. Thomas (1994) provides such a table for guidance, but it is always wise to check the label.

Meals and recipes 21

However much we know about nutrient requirements, what we want is food which is good to eat. The aim of this chapter is to provide menu plans and recipes so that advice about diets can be practical as possible. The number of cookery articles and books published are testimony to the fact that everyone likes a good recipe or a new idea, and ways to improve diets are probably better received if given in a practical way.

The recipes here are favourites of mine or my friends. In general, salt has been omitted wherever there is enough flavour from other ingredients. When vegetable oil is given, it is best to choose a polyunsaturated oil, as it is also for margarine. When using mayonnaise, it is sensible to use the low-fat variety in most cases. Occasionally, butter is the recommended fat. A little butter sometimes improves the flavour of a dish a lot, and 25 g in a four-person dish is hardly excessive.

Abbreviations: tsp = teaspoon
                  tbsp = tablespoon
Conversions: 1 oz = 28 g, but 25 g is often used for convenience
                  1 pint (pt) = 600 ml

THE IMPORTANCE OF BREAKFAST

Breakfasts

Breakfast *is* important, especially for children who eat fairly early in the evening and therefore have a long time without food before next morning. Breakfast has been shown to improve work performance, both physical and intellectual. Most research has been on children and teenagers, but there have been some reports of work on adults. It has shown that breakfast makes a significant contribution to the total diet, that, if breakfast is missed, the nutrient deficit is not made up later in the day, and that missing breakfast affected children's school work in the morning and the work performance, both physical and mental, of adults (Malnutrition, Learning and Behaviour, 1976; Morgan *et al.*, 1981; Morgan and Zabik, 1984; The Roper Organization, 1986; Sommerville and O'Reagan, 1993).

The problem for most people is balancing an extra five minutes in bed with time for breakfast but there are a lot of quick breakfasts which are nutritionally sound.

IDEAS FOR BREAKFAST

Fruit

It is useful to include some fruit or fruit juice at breakfast time. It helps to increase intake towards the proposed average of 5–6 helpings of fruit and vegetables a day.

Suggestions

1. Mix canned or fresh grapefruit (if using fresh, add orange juice or a light sugar syrup, about 50 g or 2 tablespoons of sugar dissolved in ½ pint water to the mix) with canned mandarin oranges. For small households, keep in bowl in fridge, eating some every day.
2. Mix some fruit with cereal, for example banana, prunes, canned or fresh peaches, strawberries or raspberries in season. Can add yoghurt or fromage frais instead of milk.
3. People living alone may find it more practical to buy individual cartons of fruit juice rather than the litre size, which inevitably deteriorates with keeping.

Case study

Derek Tangye, author of the *Minack Chronicles*, now living alone, has a small can of fruit for breakfast every day. It is easy, provides energy for the morning and a useful addition to micronutrient intake.

Cereals and porridge

These are useful sources of nutrients, and so is the milk taken with them.

Apricot whirl, for a special breakfast

50 g (2 oz) crunchy oat cereal
50 g (2 oz) dried apricots (the no-need-to-soak variety)
100 ml (⅕ pt) unsweetened orange juice
¼ tsp ground ginger
175 ml low-fat yoghurt

1. Divide the crunchy oat cereal between two sundae glasses.
2. Simmer the apricots and ginger in the orange juice. Purée and leave to cool.
3. Mix half the apricot purée with the yoghurt and pour over the oat mixture.
4. Swirl the remaining purée into the mixture, using a cocktail stick.
5. Chill for 30 minutes.

Porridge

This is especially quick if a microwave oven is used. Most packets give a recipe. A typical one is this.

50 g (2 oz) Scotts Piper oatmeal
300 ml (½ pt) water (or half water, half milk)

1. Put in a large bowl. Do not cover.
2. Cook at full power for 3½–4 minutes, stir briskly, and cook for another 3½–4 minutes. Stir and serve.

This gives one generous or two small portions.

Toast

Cut the bread thickly. Alternatives to butter/margarine and marmalade are lemon curd (easy to make at home, good source of vitamin C, some butter but less than if used alone as a spread), Marmite, peanut butter.

Muffins

Blueberry muffins (from *Make a Meal of It*, National Dairy Council).

150 g (5 oz) plain flour
1 tbsp baking powder
50 g (2 oz) porridge oats
50 g (2 oz) light muscavado sugar
1 egg
175 ml (¼ pt) semi-skimmed milk
3 tbsp corn or sunflower oil
100 g (4 oz) fresh or frozen blueberries, defrosted, or dried fruit, like sultanas)

1. Beat all the ingredients except blueberries until smooth.
2. Fold in the blueberries, spoon into lightly greased, 12-hole, deep muffin tin.
3. Bake at 220°C, Gas Mark 7 for 15 minutes or until well risen and golden brown.

Serve immediately.

Cooked foods

For those with high energy requirements add, to fruit and cereal, poached egg on toast, baked beans on toast, bacon (3 minutes on kitchen paper in the microwave) and tomato, mushrooms on toast.

No time to stop

Everyone has overslept, or had to rush the children to school with no time for breakfast. For an emergency, 'portable porridge' in the form of flapjack (recipe page 396) is high in energy. Eaten with a banana, it makes a good breakfast for a child when there's no time for anything else.

Liquid breakfasts

Honey and grapefruit milk shake

568 ml (1 pt) cool semi-skimmed milk
568 ml (1 pt) grapefruit juice
30 ml (2 tbsp) clear honey
1 egg white

Whisk all ingredients together till thick and frothy.
Serves 4–6

Orange refresher

This can be made in a low-fat version or with full fat ingredients for the young and elderly.

450 ml (¾ pt) fresh milk
150 ml (¼ pt) orange juice
1 individual carton orange yoghurt

Mix the ingredients and whisk.
Serves 2

Inexpensive luxury

Use packs of 'ready to cook' rolls, which cook in 7 minutes and are cheaper than buying fresh. Cook bacon in oven at same time.

Stocks and soups   STOCKS

Stock is often required in recipes. It really does improve the flavour of soups and casseroles *and* reduces the amount of salt necessary. Stock cubes can be used but they are usually high in salt. For this reason, I have included details about stock, which is really very easy to make.

Stock is made from the bones and flesh of meat, poultry or fish with added root vegetables, carrot, onion, celery sticks, and herbs. Avoid turnips as the flavour is too strong, also potatoes, which make the stock cloudy. Herbs used for flavouring are bay leaf, thyme and parsley, or a bouquet garni can be used. Carcasses from roasted birds and bones from cooked joints are also used for stock. Although most people don't make stock and think it a lengthy process, in fact it is very easy. I always make stock from chicken bones, or the remains of a shoulder of lamb, even if I don't bother to add vegetables. Cover the bones and chopped vegetables with water, bring to the boil and simmer gently for an hour or so. **Keep refrigerated** or **freeze** in cartons.

SOUPS

Soups are useful as a light meal, as a first course and as a low-calorie snack. They are also a good way to increase the amount of vegetables eaten. Soup and a main course is often a better combination than a main course and a pudding. The general method is to fry fresh vegetables gently in a little fat to add flavour, add stock and herbs and simmer until everything is cooked. There are hundreds of possible combinations of flavours and ingredients and soup-making is much easier than many people think. There is no need to be absolutely exact in the amount of ingredients used. A smooth soup is easily produced using a liquidizer or food processor.

Minestrone

This is an excellent soup which, with bread, will make a good meal for a toddler or young child and a useful snack for adults. The ingredients of minestrone can be varied to make use of what is in the refrigerator and store cupboard or according to the season. If cooked vegetables are to be used, they should be added 10 minutes before the end. Including celery really does improve the flavour. A typical recipe is:

50 g (2 oz) each of carrot, celery, potato, leek, onion, cabbage
400 g (14 oz) canned tomatoes or 225 g (½ lb) tomatoes
2 rashers bacon, diced
400 g (14 oz) can butter beans
100 g (4 oz) peas
900 ml (2 pt) water
100 g (4 oz) macaroni (small pieces)
bouquet garni
large clove garlic
1 tbsp chopped parsley

50–75 g (2–3 oz) grated cheese for each three helpings
37 g (1½ oz) margarine or oil

Serves 4–6

1. Dice all vegetables except the cabbage which should be shredded.
2. Fry in the margarine or oil until just colouring.
3. Crush garlic and add to the vegetables.
4. Add boiling stock or water to vegetables in pan. Add bacon, bouquet garni, macaroni, tomatoes and shredded cabbage.
5. Simmer for 20 minutes.
6. Add a little seasoning if necessary. Simmer for a further 10 minutes.
7. Add chopped parsley and stir.
8. Serve with a bowl of grated cheese.

Lentil soup

100 g (4 oz) red lentils
1 litre (2 pt) stock
75 g (3 oz) lean bacon, chopped *or* boil a bacon joint and use the water as stock for the soup
1 onion, skinned and diced
400 g (14 oz) can tomatoes
2 carrots, peeled and diced
450 g (1 lb) potatoes peeled and diced
2 sticks celery, scraped and chopped
25 g (1 oz) margarine or oil

Serves 4–6

1. Heat fat in pan. Add onions, carrots and celery and fry gently for 4–5 minutes.
2. Add the remaining ingredients and simmer gently for 30–35 minutes, stirring occasionally until lentils are soft and the vegetables are cooked.
3. If you like a very smooth soup, liquidize or whizz in a food processor.

Jewish chicken soup (from Michelle Guiness's book *A Little Kosher Seasoning*)

It is folklore that every Jewish mother believes that her chicken soup will cure all ills, and it is an easy way to cook a chicken and make a good soup at the same time.

Serves 6

1 boiling fowl, including giblets
1½ litres (3 pt) water
1 onion
2 carrots
3 celery stalks
1 leek
1 parsnip
salt and pepper

1. Put chicken, salt and pepper into a large pan, cover with the water, bring to boil. Add all the other ingredients and simmer for at least 3 hours.
2. Remove chicken and vegetables. Use the chicken for sandwiches, salads, etc. and discard the vegetables except the carrot.
3. Store the soup in the refrigerator overnight. Next day, remove any fat, reheat, adding egg noodles if liked and the chopped carrot. It is not necessary to keep the soup overnight but it improves the flavour.

Weight Watchers' vegetable soup

Recommended as a low-calorie snack or as part of a meal.

90 g (3 oz) onion, chopped
1 clove garlic, put through garlic press or finely chopped
180 g (6 oz) cabbage, finely shredded
90 g (3 oz) carrot, thinly sliced
90 g (3 oz) tomato, skinned and chopped
1 tsp parsley
Good pinch salt, mixed herbs, pepper
450 ml (¾ pt) water
1 vegetable stock cube

Serves 2

1. In a large saucepan, combine all the ingredients. Cover and cook over a moderate heat until vegetables are soft, about 20 minutes.
2. Using a slotted spoon, remove about (90 g) 3 oz vegetables from the saucepan and set aside. In two batches, puree remaining soup in a blender. Return puréed mixture to saucepan, add reserved vegetables and heat.

Chicken and bean sprout soup

1 tbsp oil
225 g (9 oz) can bean sprouts
1 onion
225 g (9 oz) cooked chicken
50 g (2 oz) cucumber

1 litre (2 pt) chicken stock
100 g (4 oz) mushrooms
1 tbsp soy sauce
2 carrots
1 tbsp plain flour

Serves 4–6

1. Wash all vegetables and peel. Chop onion. Cut carrots into 1″ lengths, then ⅛″ (25 × 3 mm) slices lengthwise and across into narrow sticks. Cut cucumber into dice and slice mushrooms finely. Drain bean sprouts.
2. Cut the cooked chicken into small dice.
3. Heat oil in a saucepan and cook the onion gently for 2–3 minutes until soft. Stir in flour and cook for a few minutes over low heat.
4. Add chicken stock, bring to the boil and add cooked chicken, soy sauce and carrots. Simmer for 10 minutes.
5. Add bean sprouts, cucumber and mushrooms. Cook for a further 5 minutes and serve very hot.

Leek and potato soup

This is quick and easy, tastes good, makes a lot of soup and is very cheap.

800 g (2 lb) leeks
800 g (2 lb) potatoes
25 g (1 oz) butter or oil
1½ litres (3 pt) stock
300 ml (½ pt) milk
Chopped chives

Serves 4–6

1. Slice the leeks (after washing well) and potatoes.
2. Melt the butter or heat the oil in a large saucepan or pressure-cooker, add the leeks and cook gently, with the lid on, for a few minutes, stirring occasionally.
3. Add the potatoes and the stock and cook for 30 minutes or for 5 minutes in a pressure-cooker.
4. Liquidize, return to the pan, add the milk, heat, season and serve garnished with chopped chives.

For a richer soup (and a higher fat content) single cream can be used instead of milk.

Quick meals and snacks

Jacket potatoes

Jacket potatoes a good source of starch, along with NSP and other nutrients. Although some people prefer the crisp outside of potatoes cooked in a conventional oven, the convenience of a few minutes in a microwave oven is hard to beat. Good varieties of potato for baking are Maris Piper, King Edward, Desiree, Cara and Pentland Squire.

1. Wash and scrub potato and prick all over.
2. Brush with oil if liked. It makes them look much more appetizing.
3. Cook in a conventional oven at 220°C, Gas Mark 7, for 1 hour or 170°C, Gas Mark 3 for 2–2½ hours. In a microwave oven approximate times are 5–6 minutes for one potato, 8–10 minutes for two potatoes and 15–18 minutes for four potatoes. They should be turned once during cooking.

Toasted sandwiches

Toasted sandwiches are a good, nourishing snack. With wholemeal bread or NSP-enriched white, they are rich in NSP and starch and relatively low in fat, depending on the filling. The following suggested fillings are suitable for both jacket potatoes and toasted sandwiches.

Fillings

1. Edam or Double Gloucester cheese, grated and mixed with finely chopped onion or chives.
2. Cheddar cheese, grated and mixed with chopped pineapple.
3. Lancashire cheese, grated and mixed with onion and tomato.
4. Stir-fried mixed vegetables (peppers, mushrooms and beansprouts), mixed with grated cheese.
5. Diced red pepper, sweetcorn and grated cheese.
6. Sardines and tomato.
7. Tuna and sweetcorn, with low-fat mayonnaise if liked.
8. For jacket potato only: gently cook two chicken livers in oil, add chopped onion, mushroom, tomato and stock and cook gently. Thicken with flour or cornflour.

Beefburgers

By using lean minced beef, these hamburgers are low fat and quick to make. Someone living alone can make just one or two burgers.

455 g (1 lb) minced beef (often leaner if you buy some stewing or braising steak and mince it in a food processor)
1 tbsp chopped fresh parsley (optional)
1 clove garlic, crushed (optional)
1 egg
4 tbsp breadcrumbs
2 tbsp vegetable oil
stock
4 fresh bread rolls or baps

1. Mix beef, parsley, garlic and breadcrumbs.
2. Add egg and enough stock to bind ingredients together. Roll mixture into a sausage shape.
3. Cut across roll in ¾" (20 mm) slices and shape each slice into a burger.
4. Heat oil in frying pan and cook burgers for 4–5 minutes on each side until golden brown, or grill.
5. Drain on crumpled absorbent kitchen paper and place in halved bread rolls or baps.

Serve with mixed salads.

Chopped liver

This is a Jewish recipe from Michelle Guiness *A Little Kosher Seasoning*.

200 g grilled chicken livers
1 medium onion
2 hard-boiled eggs (optional)
2 tbsp margarine or oil
Pinch of salt, pepper, cinnamon, ground ginger

1. Fry the chopped onion in the fat until golden, then add the other ingredients, put through a mincer or give a quick whizz in a food processor and mix well.
2. Serve cold with bread as a first course.

Chicken liver pâté

This is a cheap sandwich filling, good for iron and vitamins A and D.

250 g (8 oz) chicken livers
25 g (1 oz) margarine
1 small onion, finely chopped
1 clove garlic, crushed
Mixed herbs, salt, pepper
1 tbsp tomato paste
1 tbsp milk or cream

1. Remove the green part from the livers, fry gently in margarine until they change colour.
2. Add onion, garlic, seasoning and cook for 5 minutes.
3. Cool, add tomato paste and milk.
4. Purée in a blender or press through a sieve. Chill.

Pizza baps

4 large baps
2 large tomatoes
1 tbsp olive oil

8 anchovy fillets
1 large onion
170 g (6 oz) Mozzarella or Double Gloucester cheese
60 g (2 oz) button mushrooms
Marjoram (to taste)

Serves 2–4

1. Slice baps in half and brush surfaces with oil.
2. Slice onion thinly and cook slowly in 1 tbsp oil until soft.
3. Slice mushrooms and add to the onion and cook for another 2 minutes.
4. Slice the tomatoes ¼″ (6 mm) thick and place on top of the bap halves. Sprinkle with a little marjoram or oregano.
5. Spoon the onion and mushroom mixture on top and cover with the cheese, thinly sliced.
6. Halve the anchovy fillets and arrange in a cross pattern on top of the cheese.
7. Bake the baps in the centre of a pre-heated oven to 180°C, Gas Mark 4, for 10–15 minutes or until cheese is a golden colour. Serve with a green salad.

Gerry's instant pizza

This is even quicker than the previous recipe.
1 packet wholemeal pitta bread
400 g (14 oz) can chopped tomatoes
A little margarine
300 g (12 oz) grated Cheddar cheese
1 finely chopped onion
2 tsp oregano

1. Place the six pitta bread slices on two baking trays. (It can be used straight from the freezer.)
2. Spread each piece with margarine and spoon out the chopped tomatoes onto them.
3. Add the onions and oregano, plus salt and pepper to taste.
4. Grate the cheese directly on top of the tomatoes. Decorate with olives and/or anchovies if wished.
5. Cook in the oven, 200°C, Gas Mark 5–6, for about 10 minutes. Serve with salad.

Fried savoury rice

225 g (8 oz) long-grain brown rice
600 ml (1 pt) stock
2 tbsp oil
75 g (3 oz) button mushrooms, sliced

3 eggs
4 spring onions, chopped
175 g (6 oz) cooked meat
2 shredded lettuce leaves
1 tbsp soy sauce

Serves 3–4

1. Cook rice, covered, for about 15–20 minutes in boiling water or stock. Rinse in cold water and drain thoroughly.
2. Cut meat into thin strips.
3. Heat oil in a large pan over medium heat. Beat eggs, pour into pan and cook, stirring with a spoon until eggs are beginning to set.
4. Stir in cooked rice, meat, vegetables and soy sauce. Cook, stirring constantly, until all the ingredients are heated through. Serve hot with peas or green beans.

Sweetcorn and bacon potatoes

450 g (1 lb) potatoes, peeled and par-boiled
225 g (8 oz) lean bacon, rind removed and chopped
1 large onion, peeled and chopped
340 g can of corn kernels
3 eggs

Serves 2–4

1. Slice potatoes and place in the bottom of a greased pie dish.
2. Fry onion and bacon lightly until cooked. Add sweetcorn.
3. Cover potatoes with bacon mixture and pour lightly beaten eggs over the top.
4. Bake at 190°C, Gas Mark 5, for 30 minutes until set and lightly browned. Serve with a salad or green vegetables.

Main meals   Variety is an important factor in making food attractive. Some dishes, liver for example, are enjoyed occasionally but are not acceptable too often. Many mothers, finding that their fussy child likes fish-fingers, give them so often that the child (and everyone else) becomes quite fed up with them.

Planning weekly meals is probably less common nowadays than it used to be, but it is a real help to the meal provider especially when time is short. A weekly rotation suits some households but a four-

Table 21.1 Planning weekly meals

	Week 1	Week 2	Week 3	Week 4
Sunday	Roast lamb	Roast pork	Roast chicken	Roast beef
Monday	Moussaka	Sweet and sour pork, fried rice, stir-fried vegetables	Chinese chicken	Shepherd's pie
Tuesday	Spaghetti Bolognaise	Quick pasta	Tuna pasta salad	Lasagne
Wednesday	Chicken joint, jacket potato, salad	Chilli con carne, jacket potato, salad	Mixed grill, salad, jacket potato	Cold meats, jacket potato, salad
Thursday	Fish cakes, broccoli, tomatoes, mushrooms	Mackerel in foil, vegetables, crusty bread	Poached cod with shrimp sauce	Sweet soused herrings, vegetables, crusty bread
Friday	Grilled gammon, chips, baked beans	Egg, chips, baked beans	Pork casserole	Mixed grill, vegetables, chips
Saturday	Pizza	Chicken casserole	Hamburgers in rolls, potato salad, salads	Kleftiko lamb

Table 21.2 Quick meals for the weekdays

Monday	Quick pasta	Fresh fruit
Tuesday	Myra's chicken	Yoghurt
Wednesday	Mackerel in foil (or microwave)	Fruit salad
Thursday	Mixed grill, jacket potato	Fruit loaf and banana
Friday	Soup	Gerry's instant pizza and green salad

weekly plan, based on a common pattern, for example, roast on Sunday, leftovers on Monday, pasta on Tuesday, and so on, is useful and prevents boredom.

The plans given in Tables 21. 1 and 21. 2 are fairly economical. They can easily be made more luxurious.

CHICKEN DISHES

Chicken flesh has little fat, most of which lies under the skin, so wherever possible skin chicken joints before use.

Myra's chicken: low-fat, quick and easy

This recipe, from my friend and colleague Myra, is the easiest and nicest chicken dish I know.

4 skinned chicken joints
1 (400 g) jar apricot or peach chutney
½ (90 g) jar French mustard
1 tsp ground cumin
1 tsp curry powder
2 tbsp water

Serves 4

1. Mix all ingredients except the chicken. Pour over the chicken joints.
2. Cook in the oven at 180°C, Gas Mark 4, for 30 minutes or until the chicken is cooked. Serve with rice or potatoes, and, say, cabbage and courgettes.

Chicken with apricot sauce

This is nearly as easy but less spicy, and includes a good deal of fruit in the sauce. To reduce the fat, the chicken could be cooked in the sauce instead of being fried first.

4 boned and skinned chicken breasts
1 medium onion, finely chopped
25 g (1 oz) butter or oil
200 g (8 oz) dried apricots, cooked with a little water, and puréed in a food processor
300 ml (½ pt) chicken stock
pepper

Serves 4

1. Melt the butter in a large frying pan or heavy saucepan and fry the chicken on both sides until cooked.
2. Soften onions, then stir in the apricots, chicken stock and pepper.
3. Simmer gently for about 10 minutes, adding the chicken at the end to heat it through.
4. Serve with a salad, and rice, jacket potato or crusty bread.

Chicken casserole

This is a good meal in itself, although another vegetable could be served with it. Good for families with young children. For one or two, use half and freeze the rest for another day.

1400 g (3 lb) chicken or chicken joints
450 g (1 lb) potatoes
60 g (2 oz) streaky bacon
400 g (14 oz) can tomatoes
2 large onions
bouquet garni
2 sticks celery
2 tbsp oil
100 g (¼ lb) mushrooms
chicken stock
1 small turnip or parsnip
parsley for garnish

Serves 4–6

1. Joint the chicken into 6–8 pieces and wipe clean. Remove skin to reduce fat.
2. Remove rind from bacon and cut into small pieces.
3. Peel and slice onions, scrub and slice celery, trim and slice mushrooms, wash and peel turnips or parsnips and cut into quarters, then into slices.
4. Heat the oil in a large pan. Add the bacon, onions and celery. Cook slowly over a low heat for 3 minutes, add mushrooms and cook for a further 2 minutes.
5. Tip the pan to draw the fat to one side. Remove vegetables and bacon with a perforated spoon and spread over base of a large casserole.
6. Fry the chicken pieces in the fat left in the pan, until they are slightly brown, adding a little more fat if necessary. Remove from pan and place on the bed of vegetables.
7. Scrape or peel potatoes and cut into 1″ (25 mm) pieces. Peel and cut turnips, or parsnips into fairly small pieces. Add these together with the canned tomatoes and bouquet garni to the casserole.
8. Add chicken stock to bring the level of moisture to just below the surface.
9. Season with freshly ground pepper and cover with kitchen foil before securing the lid, to prevent escape of steam.
10. Cook on the middle shelf at 150°C, Gas Mark 3, for about 1½ hours, or until chicken is tender.
11. Sprinkle with a little grated orange rind and chopped parsley before serving and serve in the casserole.

Quick chicken marengo

This is very quick and inexpensive to prepare, and to cook, using a pressure cooker, and it tastes good.

4 skinned chicken joints
1 tbsp oil
1 sliced onion
1 crushed clove of garlic
400 g can tomatoes
300 ml (½ pt) of chicken stock
¼ tsp thyme
bayleaf
100 g (4 oz) button mushrooms
salt and pepper

Serves 4

1. Cook the onion gently in the oil. Add all the ingredients and either cook in a pressure cooker for 7 minutes at high pressure or in the oven, 180°C, Gas Mark 4, for 1 hour.
2. At the end, mix 1 tbsp of flour with cold water to a thin paste, add a little of the liquid, mix and return it all to the pan or casserole. Mix well, cook for another few minutes to thicken the sauce and serve.

Chicken with savoury rice

1 stick celery
1 tbsp oil
1 medium-size onion
1 medium-size carrot
¼ tsp each of paprika, dried sage, marjoram and rosemary
1 green pepper
600 ml (1 pt) hot chicken stock
1 clove garlic
100 g (4 oz) brown rice
2 rashers streaky bacon
2 tbsp soya sauce
seasoning
4 whole portions cooked chicken (these could come from the chicken in Jewish chicken soup)
slices of green pepper rings for garnish
paprika

Serves 4

1. Peel and chop the vegetables, crush garlic.
2. Remove rind from bacon and cut into narrow strips. Cook bacon slowly in oil, add chopped vegetables and fry gently until onion is golden and the celery is tender. Stir in herbs. If very low-fat dish required, leave out the frying stage.

3. Wash rice under running water and drain. Add to the ingredients in pan. Stir in well and heat gently with the vegetables.
4. Stirring slowly add seasoning, soy sauce and stock. Bring to the boil and continue cooking for 10 minutes.
5. Place cooked chicken portions on top of rice mixture. Lower heat and cover. Simmer slowly until the rice has absorbed all the liquid. When cooked the rice should be tender, light and dry.
6. Lift chicken joints on to hot plate. Stir rice and pile on a hot serving dish. Place chicken joints on top. Garnish with thin slices of green pepper and a little paprika.

Note: if chicken pieces are small, stir into the rice mixture at stage 5.

Chicken and ham pasta

Easy to eat, suitable for the very young and elderly.

225 g (8 oz) cooked chicken
25 g (1 oz) plain flour
100 g (4 oz) cooked ham or fried bacon
300 ml (½ pt) chicken stock
350 g (12 oz) pasta in small shapes, e.g. shells
1 tsp French mustard
1 tbsp oil
1 lemon
1 clove garlic
150 ml (¼ pt) crème fraiche or low-fat yoghurt
1 onion
chopped parsley
100 g (4 oz) button mushrooms

Serves 3–4

1. Add pasta to boiling water in a large pan and simmer for 10–12 minutes until just tender and floating to the surface.
2. Cut chicken into dice, chop ham.
3. Wash mushrooms, parsley and lemon. Peel and chop onion, dry parsley and chop. Grate rind of lemon and squeeze out juice.
4. Heat oil in frying pan, add crushed garlic and onion. Cook slowly to soften, about 2–3 minutes, and add flour. Heat, stirring, for 1 minute.
5. Remove from heat and gradually add stock. Return to heat, add mushrooms, stir and cook until sauce has thickened.
6. Add mustard, lemon rind and juice and crème fraiche.
7. Stir well, add chicken and heat gently for 5 minutes.
8. Drain pasta. Pour 1 tbsp oil into the warm pan, return pasta and turn it in the oil to coat pasta and prevent pieces sticking together.
9. Serve in a shallow dish with chicken sauce poured over. Sprinkle with chopped parsley to garnish.

Chicken curry with rice

Cooked or raw chicken can be used for this mild curry.

4 chicken portions
1 tbsp desiccated coconut
1 tbsp vegetable oil
1 large cooking apple, e.g. Bramley
1 onion
25 g (1 oz) raisins or sultanas
1 carrot
1 tbsp chutney
1 tomato
500 ml (¾ pt) chicken stock
2 tsp mild curry powder
1 tbsp plain flour

Serves 4

1. Peel and chop onion, carrot, and apple. Cut tomato in half, remove seeds and chop.
2. Heat oil in saucepan and fry chicken pieces for 4–5 minutes each side over a low heat until slightly brown. Remove from pan and keep warm.
3. Add chopped onion and carrot. Fry slowly until onion is slightly coloured, add curry powder and flour and stir over gentle heat.
4. Add stock, stir and bring to the boil. Add chicken joints and stir in chopped apple, raisins and chutney and coconut.
5. Cover and simmer for 30 minutes until chicken is tender and juices from chicken run clear.
6. Serve with boiled brown rice.

Note: if cooked chicken portions are used for this recipe, leave out stage 2 and add chicken joints at stage 5 after the sauce has been simmering for 15 minutes, then gently heat the chicken joints for 10–15 minutes.

TURKEY DISHES

Turkey and ginger stir-fry

Stir-fries are very quick, use little fuel, can be adapted to many different ingredients and are easy to do for one or two. This one is especially rich in vitamin C.

1 tbsp vegetable oil
2 small (about 100 g, 4 oz) turkey fillets cut into thin strips

piece of root ginger, about ¾" (2 cm) long, peeled and chopped finely
½ each of a red, yellow and green pepper
75 g (3 oz) beansprouts
3–4 spring onions, quartered
1 tsp cornflour
2 tbsp vinegar
2 tbsp soy sauce
4 tbsp water
1 tbsp honey
pepper

Serves 2

1. Mix cornflour and water to a paste, and add honey, vinegar and
    soy sauce (this is the 'soy mix').
2. Heat the oil in a wok or deep frying pan.
3. Add turkey strips and ginger. Fry for 2–3 minutes until browned.
4. Stir in the peppers, spring onions and beansprouts and stir-fry for
    2–3 minutes.
5. Add the soy mix, bring to the boil, stirring. Check seasoning.
6. Serve with rice or noodles.

LAMB DISHES

Moussaka

This a good way of using up cooked lamb. Aubergines are sometimes
expensive and potatoes can be substituted.

2 medium aubergines or 1 aubergine and 1 large potato
25 g (1 oz) flour
25 g (1 oz) butter or margarine
1 large onion
300 ml (½ pt) milk
3 tbsp oil
1 egg
2 tsp tomato purée
28 g (1 oz) Cheddar cheese, grated
225 g (8 oz) can tomatoes
200 g (½ lb) cooked and minced lamb
150 ml (¼ pt) stock
pepper and cinnamon to taste

Serves 3–4

1. Slice aubergines thinly. (Many recipes advise sprinkling with salt, leaving and then washing and draining. This removes any bitter taste, but I usually don't bother and it works well.)
2. Peel, slice and chop onions. Heat 1 dessertspoon of oil in a pan and cook onions gently until soft, about 5 minutes, covering pan with lid.
3. Add tomato purée, canned tomatoes and stock. Season with pepper and a little cinnamon. Bring this mixture to the boil and simmer until liquid is slightly reduced.
4. Add cooked minced lamb and mix in well. Heat until just simmering.
5. Fry aubergine slices in 2 tbsp oil in batches until golden on both sides and drain on absorbent paper *or* cook in a microwave oven until softened. In this case, no oil is required.
6. Arrange a layer of aubergine slices in the bottom of a large fireproof dish or casserole, then add a layer of mince, then repeat with alternate layers of aubergine and mince until everything is incorporated, finishing with a layer of aubergine
7. For the topping, melt butter in a pan over low heat and stir in the flour.
8. Cook very gently for 1 minute then gradually blend in the milk, stirring continuously.
9. Bring to the boil and simmer for 1–2 minutes.
10. Draw the pan off the heat and allow to cool slightly. Add beaten egg and grated cheese and mix well.
11. Spoon the sauce over the moussaka. Place in the centre of a pre-heated oven and bake at 180°C, Gas Mark 4, until hot and brown in colour.

Ragoût of lamb with butter beans

A filling family meal which adds a pulse to the diet and has a good vegetable content.

4 lean lamb chump chops
25 g (1 oz) margarine or oil
2 onions, chopped
4 carrots, diced
2 turnips, peeled and diced
25 g (8 oz) can tomatoes or fresh tomatoes
bouquet garni
stock
1 400 g can butter beans, drained
1 tbsp parsley

Serves 4

1. Trim all fat from chops.
2. Heat fat in frying pan and lightly brown chops. Drain and place in casserole. This improves the flavour but can be omitted.
3. Add vegetables and bouquet garni to the chops. Cover with stock.
4. Cover and cook at 180°C, Gas Mark 4, for 1½ hours.
5. Add butter beans and cook for a further 30 minutes.
6. Serve sprinkled with chopped parsley.

Kleftiko lamb

This is an imitation of the popular Greek dish. It is extremely easy to do and can be cooked slowly in the oven (with a rice pudding perhaps) or more quickly in a microwave oven.

4 'roasting' lamb chops
4 large old potatoes
sprig rosemary
2 onions
stock or stock cube

Serves 4

1. Put the chops in a flattish dish, sprinkling with rosemary and a crumbled stock cube and a few tablespoons of water or stock. Tuck pieces of onion between the chops.
2. Peel and halve the potatoes, cover with boiling water and leave for a few minutes.
3. Cover the meat with the potatoes and then cover all with foil or, if the microwave oven is used, with cling-film or a lid.
4. Cook in a very slow oven for 2–3 hours or about 30–40 minutes at half power in a microwave oven. At the end the meat should be falling off the bones and the potatoes very soft. Serve with a green vegetable and a pulse.

Mixed grill

This is a quick and easy meal which makes a pleasant change. It can be as expensive or as cheap as needed according to the choice of meats. For economy, the lamb cutlets are omitted.

4 lamb cutlets, ½–1" (15–25 mm) thick
4 lambs kidneys
30 g (1 oz) butter
4 small sausages
4 rashers back bacon
8 mushrooms
4 medium-sized halved tomatoes
30 g (1 oz) melted butter or oil
watercress

Serves 4

1. Trim off surplus fat from cutlets. Remove skin and core from kidneys. Brush cutlets and kidneys with butter or oil.
2. Prick sausages with fork.
3. Peel mushrooms and brush with butter or oil on both sides.
4. If liked, flatten rashers of bacon with blade of knife, cut in half if long, and form into rolls.
5. Brush tomatoes with butter or oil.
6. Grill the tomatoes and kidneys, first on skin side then the cut side. Grill the bacon until crisp, then grill the mushrooms. Remove from pan when cooked and keep warm. Place cutlets in grill and cook under very hot grill for 3 seconds. Withdraw from grill and brush with oil or butter. Add sausages and continue cooking for 2½–3½ minutes. Turn meat and repeat process for the second side. Lamb should not be served underdone, just a very pale pink inside.
7. Serve with watercress to garnish, jacket potatoes and a salad. Traditionally maître d'hôtel butter is served on the cutlet. (Mix butter with chopped parsley and lemon juice.)

BEEF DISHES

Spaghetti bolognaise

An old stand-by but it is a useful dish. You can use leftover cooked beef or lamb, or mince or soya protein.

300 g (12 oz) minced raw beef or 200 g (8 oz) cooked lamb or beef, minced
1 level tbsp flour
1 tsp chopped parsley
1 onion
¼ tsp mixed herbs or bouquet garni
1 garlic clove
2 level tsp tomato purée
100 g (4 oz) mushrooms
meat stock
400 g (14 oz) can tomatoes
black pepper
1 tbsp oil
225–340 g (8–12 oz) spaghetti

Serves 3–4

1. Prepare vegetables. Peel and finely chop onions and garlic. Trim mushrooms and slice thinly.

2. Heat oil in large frying pan, add onion and cook gently on low heat until tender, with pan covered. (Miss out this stage for very low-fat dish and go on to stage 5.)
3. Add garlic and mushrooms and cook for a few minutes.
4. When raw beef is used, move onion to one side of pan, add the raw mince at this stage and cook for a few minutes, turning the meat in the pan continuously. Drain off any fat.
5. Add flour and stir well, then add tomatoes with juice, seasoning, herbs and tomato purée.
6. Bring to the boil, adding stock if necessary to make a smooth sauce.
7. Lower heat and simmer gently for 40–45 minutes adding more stock if required to keep the sauce fluid.

Note: when cooked meat left over from a joint is used for this recipe omit stage 4 and proceed as follows:

5. Add flour, stir well, then add tomatoes with juice, seasoning, herbs and tomato purée.
6. Bring to the boil, add stock if necessary to make a smooth sauce.
7. Lower heat and simmer gently for 5 minutes.
8. Check consistency, add cooked meat and simmer for 5–10 minutes to re-heat thoroughly.

About 15 minutes before the sauce is ready put the spaghetti in a large pan of boiling water. Bring back to the boil and cook for 12 minutes or until just firm to the bite. Drain before piling onto a hot serving dish. Pour the sauce over the spaghetti. Sprinkle with chopped parsley. Serve with grated cheese.

Meat and vegetable casserole
This is a comforting and easy dish for winter. The proportions of meat and vegetables can be altered as liked.

900 g (2 lb) middle neck of lamb or 600 g (1½ lb) chuck steak
2 onions, medium sized
450 g (1 lb) potatoes
2 sticks celery
2 tsp tomato purée
1 turnip or parsnip
2 carrots
black pepper
50 g (2 oz) mushrooms
bouquet garni or ½ tsp mixed herbs
stock

Serves 4

1. Wipe meat and remove any fat and gristle. Cut meat into small even pieces and toss in seasoned flour.
2. Cut some small potatoes in half and retain for top of casserole.
3. Cut the rest of the potatoes, carrots, celery and parsnip into slices ¼" (6 mm) thick. Cut onion and turnip into quarters and then into slices ¼" (6 mm) thick. Mix all these vegetables in a bowl and sprinkle with herbs.
4. Arrange vegetables and meat in layers in a large casserole, beginning with mixed vegetables and ending with halved potatoes on top.
5. Add about ½ pt stock until it almost reaches the top.
6. Cover with greased greaseproof paper and a tight-fitting lid.
7. Cook slowly in an oven at 180°C, Gas Mark 4, for about 3 hours.
8. Remove lid and paper 30 minutes before serving. Raise the oven heat to 200°C, Gas Mark 6 and put the casserole near top of oven so that the potatoes will brown slightly on top. Serve in the casserole with a green vegetable and a pulse.

Shepherd's pie

This is a very tasty version of an old favourite.

350 g (12 oz) roast lamb or beef
250 ml (½ pt) good gravy from joint or 250 ml (½ pt) stock
1 medium-sized onion
1 level tbsp tomato purée
4 mushrooms, finely chopped
1 tsp Worcester sauce
1 tbsp oil

Top of pie:
500 g (1 lb) hot cooked potatoes
25 g (1 oz) butter or margarine, melted in 2 tbsp hot milk
1 egg (optional)
nutmeg

Serves 3–4

1. Remove skin, gristle and fat from meat. Mince meat; the quickest way is in a food processor. A slice of bread can be included here.
2. Chop onion and cook slowly in oil until soft. Add chopped mushrooms and cook for 1–2 minutes. Add gravy, tomato purée and Worcester sauce, stirring well.
3. Add minced meat and heat slowly in the gravy.
4. Sieve or mash the hot potatoes till smooth. Heat milk and butter in pan and add potatoes. Mix well. Add egg and beat vigorously over gentle heat until potato leaves sides of pan and is light and soft.

5. Heat the meat and gravy to almost boiling before pouring into hot pie dish.
6. Pile potatoes on top and spread smoothly with knife dipped in milk.
7. Bake at 200°C, Gas Mark 6, for 20–30 minutes. Grill top slightly if not brown enough.

Serve with two vegetables.

Note: if gravy is insufficient, add 1 tbsp flour to onion at stage 3. Stir until it browns slightly. Add 250 ml (½ pt) stock using bouillon cube if necessary. Bring to the boil and proceed with remainder of recipe.

Lasagne

225 g (8 oz) lean minced meat
225 g (8 oz) oven-ready lasagne verdi
60 g (2 oz) ham or bacon chopped (optional)
1 tbsp olive oil
25 g (1 oz) parmesan cheese for top
1 clove garlic
1 onion
85 g (3 oz) butter, margarine or oil
1 carrot
85 g (3 oz) plain flour
400 g (14 oz) can tomatoes
¼ nutmeg
2 tbsp tomato purée
300 ml (½ pt) stock

For white sauce:
85 g (3 oz) margarine
85 g (3 oz) plain flour
1½ pt milk
nutmeg

Serves 3–4

1. Chop the onion and carrot small.
2. Heat oil in large pan. Fry chopped bacon over low heat until fat runs out. Add onion, crushed garlic and carrot. Fry gently for 4–5 minutes.
3. Add mince, stir in well, fry for 3–4 minutes stirring continuously until meat is brown.
4. Add canned tomatoes, tomato purée and stock, stir well, cover with lid and simmer gently for 30 minutes.
5. Remove lid and simmer for 10–15 minutes further to reduce if necessary.

6. Make the white sauce. Melt butter, add flour and stir for 1 minute over low heat. Remove from heat and gradually stir in milk. Bring to the boil, stirring until thick. Add a pinch of grated nutmeg and pepper.
7. Cover base of the prepared dish with one-quarter of the pasta sauce, then one-quarter of the white sauce and a single layer of the lasagne on top. Repeat these layers until all the ingredients are used, finishing with the white sauce. Sprinkle the parmesan cheese on top.
8. Bake in a pre-heated oven at 190°C, Gas Mark 5, for 20–25 minutes until top is crisp and brown. Serve from the dish accompanied by a green salad.

Note: the dish can be prepared well in advance and kept refrigerated or frozen. If leftover meat is used, leave out stage 4 and add cooked, minced meat at stage 6.

Tzimmis

This is a Jewish dish (from Michelle Guiness *A Little Kosher Seasoning*). It is a sweet stew, which is quickly prepared and then left to cook for 4 hours. It uses a cheap cut of meat and a lot of the fat is removed.

1 kg (2 lb) carrots
700 g (1½ lb) potatoes
1 kg (2 lb) beef brisket joint
4 tbsp golden syrup
1 tbsp cornflour
1 tsp salt
pepper

Serves 6

1. Trim fat from meat and cut into cubes. Peel and chop carrots. Put meat and carrots, with 2 tbsp of golden syrup into casserole. Barely cover with hot water, bring to boil and simmer for 2 hours.
2. Allow to cool and remove any fat. Peel and cut the potatoes into large cubes. Mix the cornflour to a thin paste with a little water and add to the casserole, mixing well. Put potatoes into casserole, add water until they are just submerged, add the remaining syrup and seasoning. Cover and cook very slowly for 3 hours when it should be a deep golden colour. Dumplings can be added if liked.

Chilli con carne

450 g (1 lb) lean minced beef
2 onions

1 clove garlic
400 g (14 oz) can tomatoes
1 tsp chilli powder or 1 finely chopped chilli pepper
400 g (14 oz) can red kidney beans
1 tbsp vegetable oil
1 tbsp tomato purée
1 cooking apple

1. Prepare vegetables. Peel and thinly slice onions, crush garlic. If using fresh chilli pepper, remove all seeds and chop pepper finely. Peel and chop apple.
2. Heat oil in a heat-proof dish or pan over low heat and cook onions until soft.
3. Add mince and fry, stirring occasionally until the meat has browned, about 5 minutes.
4. Add canned tomatoes, tomato purée and apple and stir in well.
5. Drain red kidney beans and add to the mince. Stir and season to taste with chilli.
6. Bring to the boil. Reduce heat to low, cover with well-fitting lid and simmer on top of the stove for 45 minutes, or in the centre of a pre-heated oven at 150°C, Gas Mark 2, for 1 hour. Add a little stock if necessary to keep the mixture moist. Taste the sauce before serving, if too hot, add a little yoghurt or fromage frais.

Serve with jacket potatoes and salad.

PORK DISHES

Chinese-style fried pork

This is delicious.

250 g (8 oz) pork fillet
1 piece fresh root ginger
2 tbsp soy sauce
1 tsp brown sugar
2 tbsp cider or stock
200 ml ($\frac{1}{3}$ pt) water
1 leek
2 tbsp white wine vinegar
2 carrots, medium size
2 tsp cornflour
1 green pepper
50 g (2 oz) sunflower seeds
150 g (6 oz) peas

150–250 g (6–8 oz) brown rice
1 tbsp oil
paprika

Serves 3–4

1. Cut pork across the grain into thin strips, 1½″ (40 mm) long and
    place in a shallow dish. Mix soy sauce and cider or stock. Pour
    over meat to cover and leave to marinate for 1 hour.
2. Cut leek and carrots into thin strips about 1½″ (40 mm) long.
    Grate root ginger. Cut pepper in half, remove seeds and cut pepper
    into thin strips.
3. Heat oil in a large pan or wok. Fry sunflower seeds until slightly
    brown, stirring constantly. Drain and keep warm. Remove meat
    from marinade and place in the pan. Fry until brown, stirring
    constantly.
4. Remove meat and keep warm. If using wok, push meat up the sides
    of pan. Place leek, carrots and grated ginger in pan. Fry, stirring
    constantly for 3–4 minutes.
5. Add meat, pepper, water, sugar and marinade. Stir and allow to
    simmer for 10 minutes. Add peas and heat for about 1 minute.
6. Blend vinegar and cornflour together. Add to pan and stir
    constantly until sauce thickens. Pour into a shallow dish and
    sprinkle sunflower seeds on top.
7. Serve with boiled brown long-grain rice with a little paprika
    sprinkled on top.

Boiled rice:
Allow 600 ml (1 pt) liquid to each 80 g (3 oz) rice.
Put water into a large pan, bring to the boil and add rice. Boil rapidly
for 12–15 minutes or until soft. To test the rice, squeeze a grain
between thumb and forefinger. When cooked the centre will be soft.
Drain the rice in a sieve and rinse under hot water. Return to pan and
toss in a little butter or oil. Cover pan for a few minutes to dry rice,
shaking the pan occasionally. Alternatively, dry rice in a slow oven.

Sweet and sour pork

A pork joint is often a very good buy and this is a nice way of using up
the leftovers, or of using cubed pork.

700 g (1½ lb) lean pork cut into ¾″ (20 mm) dice, or, use cooked
    pork from joint cut into ¾″ (20 mm) dice and omit stage 1 in recipe
1 level tbsp cornflour
1 tbsp oil
2 tbsp soy sauce
1 green pepper cut into strips 1″ long and ½″ wide (25 × 10 mm)

Sauce:
1 tbsp cornflour
2 tbsp caster sugar
2 tbsp white vinegar
2 tbsp fresh orange juice
1½ tbsp soy sauce
1½ level tbsp tomato purée
1½ tbsp cider or stock

Serves 3–4

1. Toss the diced pork in 1 tbsp cornflour. Heat oil in pan and fry pork cubes for 4–5 minutes turning often, until pale brown. Pour the remaining oil into a separate pan.
2. Add 2 tbsp soy sauce to the pork, stir over low heat for 2 minutes.
3. Heat remaining oil from stage 1 in separate pan, add green pepper cut into strips and stir fry for 1½ minutes over moderate heat.
4. To make the sauce, blend cornflour with 2 tbsp cold water in a bowl. Add rest of sauce ingredients and mix well until smooth.
5. Add sauce mixture to the green pepper strips and stir continuously over moderate heat until sauce thickens and becomes translucent. Add more liquid if necessary.
6. Add pork cubes and heat in the sauce, stirring for 2 minutes.
7. Serve with fried rice and stir-fried vegetables.

Fried rice:
115 g (4 oz) long-grain brown rice
2 rashers streaky bacon
1 onion
30 g (1 oz) butter or oil
300 ml (½ pt) chicken stock
black pepper

1. Wash rice thoroughly under running water.
2. Remove rind and cut bacon into small pieces.
3. Peel onions and chop finely.
4. Fry the bacon over low heat in a dry pan until the fat runs. Add butter or oil, rice and onion. Continue frying until the onion is transparent and the rice faintly coloured.
5. Pour 300 ml (½ pt) stock over the rice and cook over moderate heat until all liquid is absorbed. Stir occasionally and add more stock as required until the rice is just tender – after about 20 minutes. Season to taste.

Pork casserole

An easy one-pot dish which can be served with red cabbage and peas, say.

1 kg (2 lb) potatoes, peeled and thinly sliced
450 g (1 lb) cooking apples, peeled, cored and cut into rings
1 can condensed cream of mushroom soup
4 pork chops
4 tbsp stock or water
2 tbsp chopped parsley
4 tbsp soured cream

Serves 4

1. Place a layer of sliced potatoes in a greased oven-proof dish.
2. Cover with the apple rings.
3. Mix soup, soured cream and stock. Pour over the apples. Arrange a layer of overlapping potato slices on top.
4. Heat a little oil in a frying pan, brown the pork chops quickly. (Omit for low-fat diets.) Place on top of the potato layer.
5. Cover with greaseproof paper then a lid or a piece of aluminium foil.
6. Cook at 190°C, Gas Mark 5, for 1–1¼ hours.

Serve sprinkled with the parsley.

Quick pasta dish

This is very quick and can be made in 15 minutes. It makes a light meal which can be served with salad.

1 jar creamy pesto sauce
4 rashers bacon
200 g (8 oz) pasta
Parmesan cheese, or Cheddar for economy

Serves 3–4

1. Cook the pasta in boiling water for 8–10 minutes.
2. Grill the bacon and cut into dice.
3. Warm the pesto sauce and mix with the bacon and pasta. Serve with parmesan cheese and a green salad.

LIVER DISH

Liver with orange

This dish is cheap, and very high in nutrients, especially iron. The orange diminishes the slightly bitter taste of some liver and adds vitamin C.

200 g (8 oz) lambs' liver
2 tbsp flour
good pinch of pepper, dry mustard, cayenne pepper
50 g (2 oz) margarine, butter or oil
1 onion, sliced
2 cloves garlic, crushed
5 tbsp red wine, optional
5 tbsp stock or 10 tbsp stock or stock cube and water
1 tbsp chopped fresh parsley and thyme (or 1 tsp dried herbs)
1 orange, with peel, thinly sliced

Serves 2–3

1. Mix seasonings with flour and coat liver.
2. In half the fat, fry onion and garlic until soft and golden brown.
3. Remove and fry liver for 3–4 minutes on each side.
4. Add wine, stock, herbs and simmer for 1–2 minutes.
5. Cook orange in rest of fat to slightly brown it, use to garnish liver.

VEGETARIAN DISHES

Chilli bean pot

This recipe is from Sainsbury's *Whole Food Cooking*.

250 g (8 oz) red kidney beans
125 g (4 oz) blackeye beans
125 g (4 oz) chick peas
2 onions, chopped
1 clove garlic, pressed
2 tbsp hot chilli powder (adjust to taste)
2 400 g (14 oz) cans chopped tomatoes
½ tsp caraway seeds
150 ml (¼ pt) vegetable stock (or stock cube)
1 green pepper, chopped
125 g (4 oz) mushrooms, chopped
1 tbsp oil

Serves 4

1. Cover the beans with cold water, in a large pan, bring to the boil and boil hard for 10 minutes, then cover and simmer for about 45 minutes until fairly soft. Drain well and rinse.
2. At a convenient moment during stage 1, prepare the rest of the mixture by heating the oil in the pan, adding the onion and garlic and frying until softened. Add the chilli powder, tomatoes, caraway seed,

stock and green pepper. Bring to the boil as the beans get ready. Add the softened, drained and rinsed beans from stage 1.

3. Simmer for 25 minutes, add the mushrooms, pepper to taste and cook for about 10 minutes until all ingredients are tender.
4. To serve, decorate with a swirl of natural yoghurt and a pinch of paprika.

Vegetable gratin

225 g (8 oz) red lentils
2 leeks, sliced
2 carrots, chopped
1 turnip, chopped
1 parsnip, grated
400 g (14 oz) passata (type of tomato sauce)
1 tbsp chopped parsley
1 tbsp chopped sage
1 tbsp chopped thyme
½ tsp mustard
100 g (4 oz) Cheddar cheese

Serves 3–4

1. Put lentils, leeks and carrots in a saucepan. Cover with water and bring to the boil. Simmer for 10 minutes until vegetables are tender.
2. Add parsnip and turnip and cook for 2–3 minutes. Drain.
3. Stir in passata, herbs and mustard. Mix well.
4. Put in an oven-proof dish and top with cheese.
5. Bake for 15–20 minutes until cheese is golden brown.
   Serve immediately.

Mixed vegetable stew

This low-calorie, low-fat vegetarian dish, using tofu for protein, is from Weight Watchers.

2 tsp vegetable oil
2 leeks, sliced
2 tbsp tomato purée
1 clove garlic, crushed
1 tbsp basil
1 small (227 g/8 oz) can chopped tomatoes
60 g (2 oz) split red lentils
270 g (9 oz) firm tofu, diced
60 g (2 oz) mushrooms, diced or sliced
150 ml (¼ pt) water or vegetable stock
2 tbsp soy sauce
pepper

Serves 2

1. Heat the oil in a saucepan, add the leeks and stir-fry for 3—4 minutes.
2. Stir in all the remaining ingredients and season. Bring to the boil, stirring, cover and simmer for 30 minutes, stirring occasionally and if necessary adding a little extra water.

FISH DISHES

In Britain we do not eat much fish and it is recommended that we eat more. White fish is a low-fat protein food and oily fish has a fatty acid profile which is particularly beneficial.

Herrings

Herrings are a nutritious and cheap food, which, in common with other cheap and nourishing foods like rhubarb and liver, is often not popular.

Sweet soused herrings

Ordinary soused herrings are often very vinegary. This recipe has a lovely flavour. It is a useful dish for a light meal and, providing there are no bones, young children like it.

4 herrings (fishmongers will usually clean and bone the fish ready for cooking)
1 onion, sliced thinly into rings
150 ml (¼ pt) cider or enough to cover herrings
1 tsp whole allspice
150 ml (¼ pt) water
1 tsp small pieces ginger
juice and rind of ½ orange
1 dill pickle, sliced
1 tsp brown sugar
1 bayleaf
made-up mustard

Serves 4

1. Lightly crush spices, cut orange rind into thin strips, and slice onion thinly. Simmer these with the ginger, bayleaf and dill in the liquids — orange juice, cider and water — for 5 minutes. Allow to cool.
2. Scale herrings, remove heads and clean (unless cleaned by the fishmonger).
3. Spread the filleted side of each fish with mustard and place a piece of dill and slices of onion at the head end of each fillet.

4. Roll up fillets from the head to the tail end. Secure each roll with a cocktail stick. Put into a casserole or pie dish with back fins uppermost. Place remaining onion rings on top.
5. Pour spiced liquid over and cover with lid or foil. Cook at 180°C, Gas Mark 4, for 20 minutes.
6. Allow to cool in the marinade before placing in the refrigerator to souse for 2 days.
7. Remove sticks and serve with tomatoes and green salad or vegetables and crusty bread.

Fresh mackerel or herring

The quickest and easiest way is to cook wrapped in foil in the oven, 180°C, Gas Mark 4, for about 30 minutes. Serve with salad or vegetables and fresh bread. There is little washing up and the fish has a good flavour.

Mackerel in foil

This is a more complicated recipe, which is very good.

4 fresh mackerel (mackerel deteriorates quickly and must be used on day of purchase or from frozen – ask the fishmonger to fillet the fish for you)
25 g (1 oz) butter or margarine
1 carrot
1 small onion or 4 spring onions
2 sticks celery
2 tbsp lemon juice
coriander or parsley
1 tbsp oil
2 tbsp fromage frais

Serves 4

1. Cut the carrots and celery into thin strips. Cut onion into very fine shreds.
2. Melt butter in a small pan. Add vegetables, cover with the lid and cook slowly for 5 minutes.
3. Cut foil into four squares 2″ (50 mm) longer than the mackerel. Brush foil with a little oil.
4. Put each fillet on sheet of foil. Divide vegetable filling between the fillets. Add a little coriander and sprinkle with lemon juice.
5. Fold up edges of foil and pour remainder of lemon juice over each piece of fish.
6. Wrap fish in foil, making parcels that are tightly sealed. Put on a baking tray and bake at 180°C, Gas Mark 4, for 25 minutes.

7. When cooked, open parcels carefully and pour juice into a small pan. Bring to the boil and simmer to reduce slightly. Add fromage frais and bring back to boil. Taste for seasoning. Keep mackerel in foil until ready to serve, with sauce separately.

Sardines, fresh

Sardines are good barbecued but otherwise the quickest and easiest way is to arrange on a plate, cover with cling-film and microwave for about 5 minutes. Serve with lemon juice, a salad, and fresh bread.

Sardines, canned

Surprisingly tasty as sardines on toast, as a sandwich filling (mash with a little vinegar or lemon juice).

Pilchards, canned

Use with a salad in the summer or as fish cakes in winter.

Easy fish cakes

I used to make these fish cakes when I was short of time and hadn't been shopping. They are very tasty, liked by children and adults and, with baked beans and canned tomatoes make a very economical meal. They are also nice served with salads or more interesting vegetables.

400 g (14 oz) can pilchards in tomato sauce
400 g (14 oz) cooked potatoes
1 egg (optional)

Serves 4

1. Mash the potatoes, add the can of pilchards and the egg if used and mix well.
2. Shape into fish cakes and either coat thinly with flour or brush with beaten egg and coat with breadcrumbs (easily made with stale bread whizzed in the food processor).
3. Fry in a little oil until golden brown.

Tuna, canned

Canned tuna is extremely useful. Young children often like tuna, rice and sweetcorn mixed together. Tuna, sweetcorn and mayonnaise or salad cream is a good filling for jacket potatoes, sandwiches, or with salad.

A very quick main meal is to serve pasta with a sauce made from a jar of ready-prepared tomato sauce mixed with a can of tuna or cooked chicken.

Rice with tuna and sweetcorn

This a more exciting dish.

½ green pepper
185 g (7 oz) can of tuna
½ red pepper
50 g (2 oz) salami
100 g (4 oz) peas
500 ml (1 pt) vegetable stock
50 g (2 oz) sweetcorn
225 g (8 oz) long-grain brown rice
4 tomatoes
1 clove garlic
1 tbsp oil
Watercress

Serves 4

1. Cut tomatoes into quarters and remove seeds. Cut long stalks from watercress. Remove seeds from pepper and cut into ¼" (6 mm) dice. Flake tuna with fork.
2. Heat oil in saucepan, add crushed garlic and rice. Sauté for a few minutes and add stock.
3. Bring to the boil, add peas and diced peppers. Reduce heat and simmer for about 15 minutes until rice has absorbed all the liquid and is tender.
4. Add flaked tuna, sweetcorn and salami. Stir well into the mixture and heat for 1 minute. Arrange in hot serving dish and garnish with tomatoes and watercress.

Tuna and pasta salad

This is very quick and easy. The oil from the tuna adds flavour, but it is not a low-fat dish. It is usually soya oil.

250 g (8 oz) dried pasta shells
185 g (7 oz) can tuna fish in oil
bunch spring onions
1 red pepper, sliced
125 g (5 oz) sweetcorn
juice 1 lemon
3–4 tbsp low-fat mayonnaise
black pepper

Serves 2–3

1. Cook the pasta in boiling water for 8–10 minutes.
2. Drain into a large bowl. Pour oil from tuna onto the pasta, mix well and leave until cold.
3. Add the rest of the ingredients and mix. Serve chilled with a green salad.

WHITE FISH, FRESH OR FROZEN

Most white fish (cod, haddock for example) is eaten fried in batter with chips. This is, unfortunately, a meal which is high in fat, although this does not mean that it can never be enjoyed. For example, the portion of chips need not be too large, it can be served with fresh bread and followed by a fruit salad. But there are other ways of cooking white fish. Both of the following are comforting foods which are easy to eat.

Poached white fish

Poach (cook in a little milk in the oven, in the microwave, or gently in a saucepan) and serve with a white sauce made with the liquid from the fish and flavoured with parsley, or with a few shrimps added, or chopped hard-boiled egg.

Kedgeree

350 g (12 oz) smoked haddock or any cooked fish
2 hard-boiled eggs
225 g (8 oz) long-grain brown rice
100 g (4 oz) frozen peas
1 tsp curry powder
½ tsp nutmeg
2 tbsp parsley
lemon juice
1 tbsp oil or butter

Serves 3–4

1. Wash and boil rice in stock or water till soft.
2. Poach fish in boiling water for 15 minutes with peas. Drain and remove any skin and bone. Separate fish into flakes. Halve eggs lengthwise and slice.
3. Heat fat in large pan. Stir in curry powder and heat very gently for 2 minutes. Add chopped peas, egg and fish. Lightly fold in rice.

4. Add nutmeg and lemon juice. Heat through gently and turn carefully without breaking up the ingredients. Sprinkle with chopped parsley.

Vegetables and salads   If we are to eat more vegetables, variety in the range and the methods of cooking is important. The value of steaming vegetables has already been mentioned (page 88). Here are a few other ideas.

Cabbage with juniper berries

This combines red and green cabbage, which are cooked with no added water, minimizing vitamin loss. The amount of fat used is very small.

100 g (4 oz) red cabbage
100 g (4 oz) green cabbage, both finely sliced
15 g (½ oz) margarine or oil
1 clove garlic
4–5 juniper berries
½ onion, finely chopped
pepper

Serves 4

1. Fry the onion, garlic and juniper berries in the fat for about 2 minutes.
2. Add the cabbages and stir. Put the lid on the pan and fry gently, stirring occasionally, for about 8–10 minutes, so the cabbage is still quite crunchy when served.

Cabbage with peas

This recipe is from Madhur Jaffrey's *Indian Cookery* (with the permission of BBC Worldwide Limited). Use the rest of the green cabbage for this tasty recipe.

100 g (1 lb) green cabbage, finely sliced
150 g (6 oz) frozen peas, separated under hot water
3 tbsp vegetable oil
2 tsp whole cumin seeds
2 bay leaves
¼ tsp ground turmeric
¼ tsp cayenne pepper
1 fresh green chilli, very finely chopped
¾ tsp sugar
¼ tsp garam masala

1. Heat the oil in a largish saucepan. When hot put in the cumin seeds and bay leaves.
2. After a few seconds add the cabbage and peas and stir them about. Add the turmeric and cayenne and stir to mix.
3. Cover, cook on a low heat for 5 minutes or until the vegetables are just tender. Add the green chilli and sugar. Stir.
4. Cover and cook for another 2–3 minutes. Sprinkle in the garam masala, remove the bay leaves and serve.

Red cabbage and apple

A recipe from Prue Leith's *Cookery Bible*. The rest of the red cabbage can be used for this recipe. Make half quantity for a small household or keep it in the fridge and serve it more than once. It will not be rich in vitamin C because of the long cooking, but it will contain the other nutrients.

1 small red cabbage
1 onion, sliced
25 g (1 oz) butter or oil
1 small cooking apple, peeled and sliced
1 small dessert apple, peeled and sliced
2 tsp brown sugar
2 tsp vinegar
pinch of ground cloves
salt and freshly ground black pepper

1. Shred the cabbage and discard hard stalks. Rinse well.
2. In a large saucepan, fry the onion in butter until it begins to soften.
3. Add the drained but still wet cabbage, and all the other ingredients.
4. Cover and cook very slowly, mixing well and stirring every 15 minutes or so. Cook for about 2 hours, or until it is soft and reduced in bulk. Add a little water if necessary during cooking.
5. Adjust seasoning.

Potato salad

455 g (1 lb) potatoes cooked and peeled
½ cup low-fat mayonnaise
1 tbsp lemon juice
1 tbsp olive oil
1 tbsp finely chopped chives
2 tbsp finely chopped leeks
freshly ground black pepper

1. Slice or dice potatoes according to size and place in a bowl.
2. Pour mayonnaise over and sprinkle with lemon juice, oil, pepper and half the chives. Carefully toss the potatoes until they are thoroughly coated with the mixture.
3. Put in a bowl and sprinkle the rest of the chives and leeks on top.
4. Cover and place in refrigerator to chill before serving.

Low-fat chips

From Rosemary Conley's *Hip and Thigh Diet Cookbook*.

1. Cut potatoes into chips.
2. Pour on boiling water to cover and leave for 5 minutes.
3. Heat 1 tablespoon of oil in oven, 200°C, Gas Mark 7.
4. Toss chips in hot oil.
5. Cook in oven 15–20 minutes.

Low-fat roast potatoes

These are cooked in the same way as low-fat chips, except that the potatoes are left in larger pieces and baked until tender.

Stir-fried spinach or Chinese leaves

700 g (1½ lb) fresh spinach
1 clove garlic, crushed
2 tbsp soy sauce
2 tbsp oil
1 level tsp caster sugar
30 g (1 oz) unsalted butter or margarine

1. Wash spinach thoroughly in several changes of clean water and drain very well.
2. Remove tough mid-ribs and any bruised parts from spinach or the leaves.
3. Heat oil in large pan, or wok. Add garlic and all the vegetable leaves into the pan, stirring constantly in the hot oil for 3 minutes. Stir in the soy sauce, sugar and butter and continue turning the leaves for another 2 minutes. Serve immediately.

Tomato and onion salad

6 tomatoes
1 tsp sugar
2 tbsp oil
1 dessertspoon white wine vinegar
1 level tbsp chopped chives or spring onions

1. Pour boiling water over the tomatoes and remove the skin. Slice thinly and place in a shallow dish. Sprinkle with sugar and season.
2. Mix oil and vinegar by shaking in a screw-top bottle. Sprinkle over the tomatoes.
3. Add chopped chives or onions. Chill in refrigerator before serving. Turn the tomato slices a few times.

Summer salad

225 ml (8 fl oz) crème fraiche or low-fat yoghurt
¼ cucumber
1 tsp lemon juice
1 lettuce
60 g (2 oz) button mushrooms
4 tomatoes
4 small new carrots
nutmeg
1 bunch watercress
pepper

1. Mix the crème fraiche or yoghurt with the lemon juice.
2. Wash mushrooms, carrots, watercress and lettuce and drain.
3. Slice mushrooms thinly, grate carrots into strips, peel cucumber and slice very thinly. Shred lettuce, cut away tough stems from watercress and separate into small bunches.
4. Fold prepared mushrooms and carrots into the cream mixture and season with a little nutmeg and pepper.
5. Serve the mushroom mixture in the centre of watercress, cucumber, tomato and lettuce.
6. Chill the salad in the refrigerator for 30 minutes before serving.

Waldorf salad

225 g (½ lb) red dessert apples
½ head celery
2 tbsp lemon juice
60 g (2 oz) shelled walnuts
1 level tsp caster sugar
1 lettuce
150 ml (¼ pt) low-fat mayonnaise

1. Wash lettuce leaves and chill in refrigerator. Wash and core apples. Cut into ½″ (12 mm) dice.
2. Prepare a dressing by mixing lemon juice, sugar and 1 tbsp mayonnaise.

3. Toss the diced apples in the dressing and let it stand for 30 minutes.
4. Wash and chop celery and chop walnuts. Add to the diced apple with the rest of the mayonnaise. Mix thoroughly.
5. Line a salad bowl with chilled lettuce leaves. Pile salad into centre and garnish with a few slices of apple brushed with lemon juice.

Serve with meat.

Coleslaw salad

½ small white cabbage, finely shredded
1 large carrot, peeled and grated
1 eating apple, cored and chopped
1 small green pepper, finely chopped
1 small onion, finely chopped
60 g (2 oz) walnuts, chopped
150 ml (¼ pt) low-fat mayonnaise or salad dressing

Mix all ingredients together in bowl. Pour the salad dressing over them and toss lightly together.

Salad dressing, low-fat

5 oz carton natural low-fat yoghurt
1 tbsp chives, chopped
¼ tsp dry mustard

Mix all ingredients well together. Add a little (½ tsp) curry powder or ½ clove of garlic to vary flavour.

Lemon and chive dressing

115 g (4 oz) cottage cheese
2 tsp lemon juice
2 tbsp French dressing
pepper
1 tbsp chives, chopped

Sieve the cheese. Add remaining ingredients and chill well before using.

French dressing

150 ml (¼ pt) oil
5 tbsp vinegar or lemon juice
¼ tsp pepper

¼ tsp mustard
¼ tsp salt

Place all ingredients in a screw-top jar. Shake well. Store in refrigerator.

Mixed bean salad

This is a pleasant addition to other fresh salads. It keeps well in the fridge for a few days. Mix some cooked (use canned for ease) beans, like red kidney beans, chick peas and haricot beans with finely chopped onion, pressed garlic and French dressing.

The recipes given here are either low-fat or use polyunsaturated fat.

Healthy baking

Fruit loaf

This is *very* easy to make, has no added fat, keeps well and can be eaten as it is or spread thinly with butter or margarine.

300 g (12 oz) mixed dried fruit
7½ fl. oz cold tea
100 g (4 oz) demerara sugar
200 g (8 oz) self-raising flour, half white, half wholemeal
1 egg

1. Soak the mixed fruit and sugar overnight (or at least for a few hours) in the cold tea.
2. Add the flour and egg to the fruit mixture and mix well.
3. Cook in a loaf tin, 180°C, Gas Mark 4, for 1¼ hours.

Chocolate cake

This is based on a recipe from Marks and Spencer's *Cakes, Pastries and Bread*. Everyone likes a chocolate cake and this one is very easy and quick to make. A polyunsaturated oil is used as the fat.

125 g (5 oz) plain flour
25 g (1 oz) cocoa powder
2 tsp baking powder
125 g (5 oz) brown sugar
2 eggs (size 2), separated
6 tbsp corn oil
5 tbsp milk
½ tsp vanilla essence

1. Well grease two 7–8″ (18–20 cm) sandwich tins and line the bases with greased greaseproof paper.

2. Sieve the flour, cocoa, baking powder into a bowl. Add the sugar.
3. Mix the egg yolks, oil, milk and vanilla essence and pour into the dry ingredients, beating well to form a smooth batter.
4. Whisk the egg whites to form stiff peaks and fold into the batter with a metal spoon.
5. Divide between the two tins, bake at 180°C, Gas Mark 4, for 20–30 minutes or until the tops spring back when lightly pressed.
6. Turn out to cool after about 2–3 minutes.
7. Sandwich together with apricot jam.

The flavours blend well together. For a treat, use a chocolate icing.

Flapjack

Flapjack is very easy to make, keeps well and is a high-energy food.

100 g (4 oz) polyunsaturated margarine
75 g (3 oz) soft brown sugar
75 g (3 oz) golden syrup (weigh the sugar first and then weigh the syrup on top of it, to avoid it sticking to the scale pan)
200 g (8 oz) rolled oats

1. Put the fat, syrup and sugar into a saucepan and melt over a low heat.
2. Stir in the oats and mix well.
3. Spread into a greased Swiss roll tin, approximately 8 × 12″ (20 × 30 cm), smoothing top with a knife.
4. Bake for 30 minutes at 180°C, Gas Mark 4.
5. Leave for 5 minutes and then cut into fingers. Remove from tin when cold.

Scones

Scones are low in fat and delicious when newly baked. Serve spread with strawberry jam and a rosette of cream from a pressurized container. It looks good and the cream is well aerated so that the actual amount eaten is very small. They need to be eaten quickly, though, or the cream shrinks to a smallish blob.

200 g (8 oz) plain flour
1 tsp bicarbonate of soda
2 tsp cream of tartar
45 g (1½ oz) margarine
About 125 ml (¼ pt) milk

1. Sieve the flour, bicarbonate of soda and cream of tartar into a bowl.

2. Rub in the margarine.
3. Add enough milk to form a soft but not sticky dough.
4. Turn onto a lightly floured surface and knead very lightly.
5. Roll out the dough to ½" (1. 5 cm) thick. Cut into rounds with a pastry cutter or make one large circle.
6. Place on lightly floured baking trays and bake at 220°C, Gas Mark 7, for 10 minutes or until risen and golden.

Makes about 8 scones.

Variations:
- Fruit scones: add 50 g (2 oz) sultanas or currants and 25 g (1 oz) sugar after rubbing in the fat.
- Cheese scones: sieve one teaspoon of dry mustard powder with the flour. Add 75 g (3 oz) finely-grated Cheddar cheese after rubbing in the fat.

Cheese and celery loaf

From Marks and Spencer's *Cakes, Pastries and Bread*. This bread can be served warm or cold and is excellent served with a vegetable soup.

250 g (10 oz) self-raising flour
½ tsp salt
50 g (2 oz) butter or margarine
2 sticks celery, finely chopped
100 g (4 oz) Cheshire cheese, grated
1 small clove garlic, crushed
1 egg, size 2
125 ml (¼ pt) milk

1. Well grease a 1 lb (400 g) loaf tin.
2. Sieve together the flour and salt.
3. Rub in the butter or margarine.
4. Add the celery, cheese and garlic and mix well.
5. Add the egg and milk and mix to a soft dough, kneading it lightly.
6. Bake in the tin at 190°C, Gas Mark 5, for 1 hour or until golden brown and well risen.
7. Turn out to cool after a few minutes.

Bread

Recipes for bread are given in most cookery books. I always halve the amount of salt and omit the fat. A mixture of half wholemeal and half white flour is often liked. For a large household, or one with hungry adolescent boys, it is useful to make a 1½ kg bag of flour into dough and divide this into four to make a pizza, some rolls, a fruit loaf and apple turnovers. For the fruit loaf, roll out the dough, after the first proving, sprinkle generously with sugar and dried fruit, roll up and put to prove in a 1 lb (400 g) loaf tin. For the apple turnovers, roll the dough out into thin circles after a first proving, and fill with raw cooking apple and sugar or cold, cooked, sweetened apple. Fold over to make a turnover, prove and bake. They are delicious eaten warm and have virtually no fat.

Muffins

A quick and easy recipe from Weight Watchers, low in fat, using oil, good for breakfast, snacks, etc.

2 cups flour
1–2 eggs
2 tsp baking powder
¼ cup oil
2 tbsp sugar
1 cup milk

1. Sieve the flour with the baking powder and stir all ingredients just to mix. Add apple, berries, nuts, cheese or chives, according to taste. Spoon into greased muffin tins.
2. Bake 30 minutes at 190°C, Gas Mark 6.

Puddings   ### Strawberry sponge

This quick and easy dish is always a favourite with children. It is a good way of including milk in the diet and evaporated milk is enriched with vitamin D. It can be made with jellies of different flavours.

1 packet strawberry jelly
½ pt water
1 (200 g) can evaporated milk

1. Dissolve strawberry jelly in ½ pt hot water. Leave in refrigerator until it begins to gel.
2. Pour evaporated milk into large basin. If the strawberry jelly is beginning to set, whisk milk until thick and fluffy. Whisk strawberry jelly into the evaporated milk.
3. Decorate with a few strawberries or grapes and chopped nuts.

Lemon sponge

This is a similar type of dish, soothing and easy to eat.

½ packet lemon jelly
¼ pt water

2 tbsp lemon juice
75 g (3 oz) Philadelphia cheese
50 g (2 oz) sugar
1 small can evaporated milk

1. Melt jelly in ¼ pt hot water and leave to cool.
2. Mix cheese and sugar in basin. Add lemon juice and mix in. Add cold jelly and mix in well.
3. Place in refrigerator and leave until it begins to gel.
4. Pour evaporated milk into large basin.
5. If lemon mixture is beginning to set, whisk milk until thick and fluffy. Add lemon mixture gradually and whisk into the evaporated milk.
6. Decorate with chopped nuts and sliced cherries.

Peach Rupert

This recipe combines fruit and rice pudding and so adds calcium and vitamin C to the diet.

1 can rice pudding
2 tbsp crème fraiche (optional)
vanilla essence
3 peach halves, canned or fresh
apricot glaze
chopped walnuts

1. Pour rice into a bowl. Add crème fraiche and fold in carefully. Add a little vanilla essence, to taste.
2. Divide mixture into four dishes or one large glass dish. Leave to chill.
3. Carefully place half a peach on top and glaze with apricot glaze. Decorate with chopped walnuts.

Apricot glaze:
4 tbsp apricot jam
3 tbsp water
little lemon juice

1. Mix together the jam and water. Bring to the boil in a small saucepan.
2. Boil for a few minutes.
3. Add a little lemon juice to flavour.

Fruit crumble

Fruit crumble and custard is popular, quick, easy and inexpensive.

500 g (1 lb) apples
100 g (4 oz) sugar

12 g (½ oz) demerara sugar

Crumble: 100 g (4 oz) flour; 38 g (1½ oz) caster sugar; 50 g (2 oz) margarine

1. Prepare fruit. Peel and core apples and slice thinly. Put into pie dish sprinkling in the sugar when half the fruit is in the dish. Press down well.
2. Sift flour. Cut up the margarine and rub lightly into the flour. Add the sugar and rub together until the mixture forms small soft 'crumbs'.
3. Spread this mixture over the apples and press down lightly. Sprinkle demerara sugar on top.
4. Place on a baking tray and cook in the centre of the oven at 190°C, Gas Mark 5, until brown and crisp and the fruit is soft.

Fruit salad

Any mixture of fruits in season, e.g.

2 oranges
1 pear
2 dessert apples
300 ml (½ pt) orange juice
50 g (2 oz) grapes
2 apricots or peaches
50 g (2 oz) nuts, chopped
50 g (2 oz) raisins or dates
1 kiwi fruit
2 bananas

1. Slice bananas. Cut apricots or peaches in half, remove stones and slice. Halve grapes and remove seeds. Slice kiwi fruit thinly. Separate orange into segments. Remove pips and pith. If orange is large, cut segments in half. Core and slice pears and apples.
2. Mix fruit, nuts and dates in a bowl. Pour the orange juice over and allow to stand in a cool place.

Spiced pears

A low calorie pudding, from Weight Watchers.

2 medium pears
16 whole cloves
1 tsp lemon juice
150 ml (¼ pt) water
1½ tsp brown sugar

Serves 2

1. Peel the pears leaving the stalks attached. Cut a very thin slice from the base so that the pears stand up. Press 8 cloves into each pear and stand in a small oven-proof dish. Mix together the lemon juice, water and sugar.
2. Cover and bake at 190°C, Gas Mark 5, for 50 minutes or until tender. Serve hot or cold.

Fruit swirl

A low-calorie recipe from Weight Watchers.

120 g (4 oz) young pink rhubarb, cut into 1″ (2.5 cm) lengths
120 g (4 oz) cooking apples, roughly chopped
juice of ½ medium orange
artificial sweetener or sugar to taste
good pinch of ground ginger
60 g (2 oz) fromage frais

Serves 1

1. Place the rhubarb, apple and orange juice in a saucepan and simmer very gently until the fruit is cooked and rather mushy, or cook in a microwave oven (on high for 4½ minutes). Purée in a food processor or blender. Sweeten and add ginger. Cool.
2. Reserve a little of the fromage frais, mix the remainder with the fruit purée, serve with the reserved fromage frais swirled on top.

Pancakes

Faced with hungry children who want a pudding, and with nothing in the house, pancakes are a good solution, even though the kitchen will smell of frying. They can be served with cooked or fresh fruit if liked.

4 heaped tbsp plain flour
1 egg
½ pt semi-skimmed or whole milk
a little oil
lemon juice, orange juice, sugar or maple syrup

1. Make a batter by adding the beaten egg and milk slowly to the flour. If it's lumpy, use an egg whisk.
2. The secret of good pancakes is to use a small frying pan, a very little oil and to get the oil really hot before pouring in enough batter to give a thin layer. Cook until the top is dry. Then turn over and quickly cook the other side.

3. Turn onto a plate, sprinkle with lemon or orange juice and a little sugar, roll up and serve.

Banana custard

Bananas sliced into warm custard make an old favourite for children.

Ice-cream

This is an old recipe but it is easy and good for calcium, protein and vitamin.

1 tsp powdered gelatine
½ (410 g) can evaporated milk
1 tsp vanilla essence
75 g (3 oz) caster sugar

1. Dissolve the gelatine in 2 tbsp near-boiling water.
2. Chill the evaporated milk and whisk until thick.
3. Whisk in the vanilla essence, caster sugar and gelatine. Pour into a container and freeze.

Packed lunches The difficulty with packed lunches is to provide variety, avoid the food being too dry and to achieve a nutritional balance.

Sandwiches are the mainstay, but variety can be achieved by using different types of bread (ordinary, rolls, pitta bread, granary) and sometimes providing something like a Cornish pasty or cheese and onion turnover.

Nutritional balance demands some protein food (cheese, cold meats, milk in the form of yoghurt or strawberry sponge (page 398)), energy from starch (bread, potato salad, fruit loaf), and fruit and vegetables. Vegetables can be added to sandwiches, mainly as lettuce, tomato and so on. Cherry tomatoes are useful. Rice salad can be packed easily, and so can fresh fruit or fruit salad in jelly. Carrot, pepper and celery sticks are useful.

IDEAS FOR SANDWICH FILLINGS

*   Tuna, sweetcorn and mayonnaise. Cover the bread with lettuce leave to stop it going soggy.
*   Peanut butter, Marmite and cucumber.
*   Corned beef and horseradish sauce and lettuce.
*   Sardines, tomato and cucumber.
*   Cottage cheese and pineapple.

- Peppered salami and tzatziki (not for those on a low-salt diet).
- Egg and watercress, mashed with mayonnaise if liked.

Nourishing drinks

A good combination of beverages can add considerably to the nutrient value of a diet. This is especially valuable for the young, the elderly and the sick.

Milk and **fruit juice** are both useful, milk for a number of nutrients, particularly protein and calcium and fruit juice for vitamin C.

There are a number of proprietary drinks which are very good.

- Horlicks is available as low-fat Instant Horlicks and as traditional Horlicks, which is made with milk. Both provide vitamins A, D, C, thiamin, riboflavin, niacin, folate, B6 and B12 at around 20% of the RDA. Calcium is also present.
- Ovaltine is similar in composition.
- Marmite is very good for the B-group vitamins and is sometimes liked when appetite is poor.
- Complan and similar products are also useful in some situations.

Malted honey whip

This attractive drink would be good for someone whose appetite is poor and who needs some calories.

1/8 pt milk
1 tbsp clear honey
2 tbsp vanilla ice-cream
1 heaped tsp Horlicks

Serves 2

Put all ingredients into a blender or food processor and whisk until frothy. A rotary whisk can also be used. Pour into glasses.

References and further reading

Chapter 1   Bell, J. (1994) *Doing Your Research Project*. Open University Press.

Bingham, S.A. (1987) The dietary assessment of individuals; methods, accuracy, new techniques and recommendations. *Nutrition Abstracts and Reviews (A)*, 57, 705–42.

Bingham, S. (1991) The Health of the Nation: Responses. *British Medical Journal*, 303, 353–5. (A useful and concise response.)

Burnett, J. (1989) *Plenty and Want*, 3rd edn, Routledge, London. (A fascinating book about the history of diet in the UK. Worth dipping into.)

Carey, G. and Hawkes, C. (1994) Good Questions. *Nursing Times*, 90(12), 23 March.

Department of Health (1991) *Dietary Reference Values for Food Energy and Nutrients for the United Kingdom*. HMSO, London. (Report on Health and Social Subjects 41.)

Department of Health (1994a) *Eat Well! An action plan from the Nutrition Task Force to achieve the Health of the Nation targets on diet and nutrition*. Available from BAPS, Health Publications Unit, DSS Distribution Centre, Heywood Stores, Manchester Road, Heywood, Lancs OL10 2PZ, UK.

Department of Health (1994b) *Nutrition. Core Curriculum for Nutrition in the Education of Health Professionals*, from The Nutrition Unit, Department of Health, Room 501A Skipton House, 80 London Road, London SE1 6LW, UK.

Jeliffe, D.B. (1966) *The Assessment of the Nutritional Status of the Community*. WHO, Geneva.

Kern, J.R. and Booth, D. (1992) *How to collect and use information for Planning, Monitoring and Evaluation*, HMSO, London.

MAFF *Household food consumption and expenditure*. Annual Reports of the National Food Survey Committee. HMSO, London.

Miles, M. and Huberman, M.A. (1994) *Qualitative Data Analysis*. Sage Publications.

Scotland's Health: A Challenge to Us All. A policy statement. (1993), HMSO, Scottish Office.

Skrabanek, P. (1994) *The Death of Humane Medicine and the Rise of Coercive Healthism*. Social Affairs Unit, London. (A work critical of present policies.)

The Health of the Nation (1992) A strategy for health in England, HMSO, London.

The Welsh Health Planning Forum (1990) *Protocols for Investment in Health Gain*. Welsh Office NHS Directorate. There are a number of such protocols.

Walker, A.F. (ed.) (1990) *Applied Human Nutrition for Food Scientists and Home Economists*. Ellis Horwood, London. (Contains some useful background material.)

Lamb, J.F., Ingram, C.G., Johnston, I.A. and Pitman, R.M. (1991) *Essentials of Physiology*, 3rd edn, Blackwell Scientific Publications, London. (Quite detailed physiology, but very clearly written.)

Thomas, B. (1994) *Manual of Dietetic Practice*, 2nd edn, Blackwell Scientific Publications, London. (Useful reference for common disorders, dietary treatment.)

Weller, B.F. (1989) *Baillière's Encyclopaedic Dictionary of Nursing and Health Care*, 2nd edn, Baillière Tindall, London.

Whitney, E.N., Cataldo, C.B. and Rolfes, S.R. (1993) *Understanding Normal and Clinical Nutrition*. West Publishing Company, St Paul. (An American book, very detailed, very user-friendly.)

British Nutrition Foundation (1990) *Complex Carbohydrates in Foods*. Chapman & Hall, London.

British Nutrition Foundation (1991) Briefing paper no. 22. *Non-Starch Polysaccharides*.

Davies, J. and Dickerson, J. (1991) *Nutrient Content of Food Portions*. The Royal Society of Chemistry.

Department of Health (1989) *Dietary Sugars and Human Disease*, HMSO, London. (Report on Health and Social Subjects 37.)

Department of Health (1991) *Dietary Reference Values for Food Energy and Nutrients for the United Kingdom*, HMSO, London. (Report on Health and Social Subjects 41.)

Department of Health (1994a) *An Oral Health Strategy for England*, Department of Health, London.

Department of Health (1994b) *Nutritional Aspects of Cardiovascular Disease*. (Report on Health and Social Subjects 46), HMSO, London.

Dutch Nutrition Council (1987) *The energy value of sugar alcohols*. Voedingsraad, The Hague.

Gregory, J., Foster, K., Tyler, H. and Wiseman, M. (1990) *Dietary Survey of British Adults*, HMSO, London.

Health Education Authority (1990) *A Handbook of Dental Health for Health Visitors*.

Nelson, N. (1983) *A dietary survey method for measuring family food purchases and individual nutrient intakes concurrently, and its use in dietary surveillance*. PhD Thesis, University of London.

Peterson, D.B., Lambert, J., Gerring, S. *et al.* (1986) Sucrose in the diabetic diet – just another carbohydrate? *Diabetic Medicine*, 2, 345–7.

Rapp, D.J. (1978) Does diet affect hyperactivity? *Journal of Learning Disabilities*, 11, 383–9.

Chapter 2

Chapter 3

Rugg-Gunn, A.J. (ed.) (1993) *Sugarless – the Way Forward*, Elsevier Science Publishers Ltd., London.

Schauss, A.G. (1980) *Crime and Delinquency*, Parker House, Berekely.

Thomas, B. (ed.) (1994) *Manual of Dietetic Practice*, 2nd edn, Blackwell Scientific Publications, London.

Todd, J. and Dodd, T. (1994) *Children's Dental Health in the United Kingdom, 1993*. A survey carried out on behalf of the United Kingdom health departments, in collaboration with the Dental Schools of the Universities of Birmingham and Newcastle. HMSO, London.

Trowell, H., Burkitt, D. and Heaton, K. (eds) (1985) *Dietary Fibre, Fibre-depleted Foods and Disease*, Academic Press, London.

Chapter 4   Davies, J. and Dickerson, J. (1991) *Nutrient Content of Food Portions*, Royal Society of Chemistry, London.

Department of Health (1991) *Dietary Reference Values for Food Energy and Nutrients for the UK*, HMSO, London. (Report on Health and Social Subjects 41.)

Garrow, J.S. and James, W.P.T. (eds) (1993) *Human Nutrition and Dietetics*, 9th edn, Churchill Livingstone, London.

Gregory, J., Foster, K., Tyler, H. and Wiseman, M. (1990) *The Dietary and Nutritional Survey of British Adults*. Office of Population Censuses and Surveys, HMSO, London.

Robinson, D.S. (1987) *Food Biochemistry and Nutritional Value*. Longmans Scientific and Technical, London.

Thomas, B. (ed.) (1994) *Manual of Dietetic Practice*, 2nd edn, Blackwell Scientific Publications, London.

World Health Organization (1985) *Energy and protein requirements*. Report of a Joint FAO/WHO/UNU Meeting. World Health Organization, Geneva (WHO Technical Report Series; 724).

Chapter 5   Davies, J. and Dickerson, J. (1991) *Nutrient Content of Food Portions*, Royal Society of Chemistry, London.

Department of Health (1991) *Dietary Reference Values for Food Energy and Nutrients for the United Kingdom*, HMSO, London. (Report on Health and Social Subjects 41.)

Department of Health (1994) *Nutritional Aspects of Cardiovascular Disease*, HMSO, London. (Report on Health and Social Subjects 46.)

Dreon, D.M. *et al.* (1984) Dietary fat: carbohydrate ratio and obesity in middle-aged men. *American Journal of Clinical Nutrition*, 47, 995–1000.

Garrow, J.S. and James, W.P.T. (eds) (1993) *Human Nutrition and Dietetics*, 9th edn, Churchill Livingstone, London.

Gregory, J., Foster, K., Tyler, H. and Wiseman, M. (1990) *The Dietary and Nutritional Survey of British Adults*. Office of Population Censuses and Surveys, HMSO, London.

Sinclair, H. (1953) The diet of Canadian Indians and Eskimos. *Proceedings of the Nutrition Society*, 12, 69–82.

Thomas, B. (ed.) (1994) *Manual of Dietetic Practice*, 2nd edn, Blackwell Scientific Publications, London.

VITAMIN A   **Chapter 6**

Thurnham, D.L. (1994) Beta-carotene, are we misreading the signals in risk groups? *Proceedings of the Nutrition Society*, 53, 251–62.

VITAMIN D

Poskitt, E.M.E., Cole, T.J. and Lawson, D.E.M. (1979) Diet, sunlight and 25-hydroxyvitamin D in healthy children and adults. *British Medical Journal*, 1, 221–3.

VITAMIN E

Burton, G.W. (1994) Vitamin E: molecular and biological function. *Proceedings of the Nutrition Society*, 53, 251–62.
Morrissey, P.A., Quinn, P.B. and Sheehy, J.A. (1994) Newer aspects of micronutrients in chronic disease. *Proceedings of the Nutrition Society*, 53, 571–82.

VITAMIN K

Barton, S.J., Tripp, J.H. and McNinch, A.W. (1995) Neonatal vitamin K prophylaxis in the British Isles: current practice and trends. *British Medical Journal*, 310, 632–3.
Golding, J., Greenwood, R., Birmingham, K. and Mott, M. (1992) Childhood cancer, intramuscular vitamin K and pethidine given during labour. *British Medical Journal*, 305, 341–6.

VITAMIN B6

Bender, D.A. (1994) Novel functions for vitamin B6. *Proceedings of the Nutrition Society*, 53, 625–30.
Department of Health (1991) *Dietary Reference Values for Food Energy and Nutrients for the United Kingdom*, HMSO, London. (Report on Health and Social Subjects 41.)

FOLATE

Scott, J. *et al.* (1994) The role of folate in neural tube defects. *Proceedings of the Nutrition Society*, 53, 631–6. (Also a good source of further references.)

VITAMIN C

Pauling, L. (1970) *Vitamin C and the Common Cold*, WH Freeman, San Francisco.

Schorma, S.C. *et al.* (1985) Blood ascorbic acid and histamine levels in patients with placental bleeding. *Human Nutrition and Clinical Nutrition*, 39C, 233–8.

ADDITIONAL GENERAL REFERENCES

Bender, A.E. and Bender, D.A. (1982) *Nutrition for Medical Students*, Wiley, Chichester.

Garrow, J.S. and James, W.P.T. (eds) (1993) *Human Nutrition and Dietetics*, 9th edn, Churchill Livingstone, London.

Ministry of Agriculture, Fisheries and Food (MAFF). *Household food consumption and expenditure. Annual report of the national food survey committee.* HMSO, London.

Nelson, *et al.* (1990) Nutrient intakes, vitamin-mineral supplementation, and intelligence in British schoolchildren. *British Journal of Nutrition*, 64, 13–22.

Oral contraceptives and vitamins. *Nutrition Reviews*, 30, 29, 1972.

Pietrzik, K. (ed.) (1991) *Modern Lifestyles, Lower Energy Intake and Micronutrient Status*, Springer-Verlag, London.

Which? (February 1990) Who needs vitamin pills? 77–81.

Chapter 7   CALCIUM

British Nutrition Foundation (1991) *Calcium*. Briefing paper 24, British Nutrition Foundation, London.

Children in Focus. Proceedings of a conference held in 1992. Available from the National Dairy Council, 5–7 John Princes St, London, WIM OAP, UK.

IRON

Bates, C.J., Powers, H.J. and Thurnham, D.I. (1989) Vitamins, iron and physical work. *Lancet*, ii, 313–14.

James, J. *et al.* (1989) Preventing iron deficiency anaemia in preschool children by implementing an educational and screening programme in an inner city practice. *British Medical Journal*, 299, 838–40.

Pollitt, E., Hathirat, P., Kotchabhakdi, N.J., Missell, L. and Valyasevi, A. (1986) Iron deficiency and behavioral development in infants and preschool-children. *American Journal of Clinical Nutrition*, 43, 555–65.

SODIUM

Law, M.R., Frost, C.D. and Wald, N.J. (1991) By how much does dietary salt reduction lower blood pressure? I. Analysis of observational data among populations. II. Analysis of observational data within populations. III. Analysis of data from trials of salt reduction. *British Medical Journal*, 302, 811–24.

POTASSIUM

Swales, J. (1991) Salt substitutes and potassium intake. *British Medical Journal*, 303, 1084–5.

Whalton, P. *et al.* (eds) (1986) *Potassium in Cardiovascular and Renal Disease*, Marcel Dekker, New York, pp. 411–16.

ZINC

Southon, S. *et al.* (1988) Trace element availability from the human diet. *Proceedings of the Nutrition Society*, 47, 27–35.

GENERAL REFERENCES

Davies, J. and Dickerson, J. (1991) *Nutrient Content of Food Portions*. The Royal Society of Chemistry, London.

Department of Health (1991) *Dietary Reference Values for Food Energy and Nutrients for the United Kingdom*, HMSO, London. (Report on Health and Social Subjects 41.)

Department of Health (1994) *Nutritional Aspects of Cardiovascular Disease*, HMSO, London. (Report on Health and Social Subjects 46.)

MAFF (1995a) *Manual of Nutrition*, HMSO, London.

MAFF, *Household Food Consumption and Expenditure: Annual Report of the National Food Survey Committee*, HMSO, London.

Pietrzik, K. (ed.) (1991) *Modern Lifestyles, Lower Energy Intake and Micro-nutrient Status*, Springer-Verlag, London.

Chapter 8

Anonymous (1994) Controversies in management: should obesity be treated? *British Medical Journal*, 309, 654–7.

Bruch, H. (1974) *Eating Disorders: Anorexia, Obesity and the Person Within*, Routledge and Kegan Paul, London.

Bush, A., Webster, J., Chalmers, G. *et al.* (1988) The Harrow Slimming Club: report on 10902 enrolments in 50 courses, 1977–1986. *Journal of Human Nutrition and Dietetics*, 1, 429–36.

Cahill, G.F. (1976) Starvation in man. *Clinical Endocrinology and Metabolism*, 5(2), 397–415.

Department of Health (1987) *The use of Very Low Calorie Diets in obesity*. HMSO, London. (Report on Health and Special Subjects 31.)

Department of Health (1991) *Dietary Reference Values for Food Energy and Nutrients for the United Kingdom*, HMSO, London. (Report on Health and Social Subjects 41.)

Garrow, J. (1988) *Obesity and Related Diseases*, Churchill Livingstone, London.

Garrow, J. (1991a) Importance of obesity. *British Medical Journal*, 303, 704–6.

Garrow, J. (1991b) Treating obesity. *British Medical Journal*, 302, 803–5.

Garrow, J.S. and James, W.P.T. (eds) (1993) *Human Nutrition and Dietetics*, 9th edn, Churchill Livingstone, London.

Holland, B., Welch, A.A., Unwin, D., Buss, D.H., Paul, A.A. and Southgate, D.A.T. (1991) *McCance and Widdowson's The Composition of Foods*, 5th edn, Royal Society of Chemistry, Cambridge.

Keys, A., Brozek, J., Henshel, A., Mickelson, O. and Taylor, H.L. (1950) *The Biology of Human Starvation*, University of Minnesota Press, Minnesota.

Lindberg, O. (ed.) (1970) *Brown Adipose Tissue*. Elsevier, New York.

Pentecost, B.L. (1991) *Medical Aspects of Exercise*, Royal College of Physicians, London.

Scott, D. (ed.) (1988) *Anorexia Nervosa and Bulimia: Practical Approaches*. Croom Helm, London.

Secretary of State for Health (1991) *The health of the nation*, HMSO, London.

Thomas, B. (ed.) (1994) *Manual of Dietetic Practice*, 2nd edn, Blackwell Scientific Publications, London.

Widdowson, E.M. (1936) A Study of English diets by the individual method. Part I. Men. *Journal of Hygiene (Cambridge)*, 36, 293–309.

Windsor, J.A. (1988) Wound healing response in surgical patients. *British Journal of Surgery*, 75, 135–7.

Chapter 9

Baron, J.A., Gleason, R., Crowe, B. and Mann, J.I. (1990) Preliminary results of general practice based nutritional advice. *Journal of the Royal College of General Practitioners*, 40, 137–41.

Burnett, J. (1989) *Plenty and Want*, 3rd edn, Routledge, London. A fascinating and detailed history of food and diet.

Department of Health (1994a) *The balance of good health*.

Department of Health (1994b) *Nutritional Aspects of Cardiovascular Disease*, HMSO, London. (Report on Health and Social Subjects 46.)

Douglas, T. (1976) *Groupwork Practice*, Tavistock.

Garrow, J.S. and James, W.P.T. (eds) (1993) *Human Nutrition and Dietetics*, 9th edn, Churchill Livingstone, London.

Gregory, J., Foster, K., Tyler, H. and Wiseman, M. (1990) *Dietary Survey of British Adults*, HMSO, London.

Health Education Authority. *Enjoy healthy eating*.

MAFF *Household Food Consumption and Expenditure*, Annual Report of the National Food Survey Committee, HMSO, London.

National Dairy Council Nutrition Service (1993) *Trends in patterns of disease and diet*. Fact file 10. Available from the National Dairy Council, 5–7 John Princes Street, London, W1M OAP, UK.

National Dairy Council. *Make a meal of it*. Available from the National Dairy Council, 5–7 John Princes Street, London, W1M OAP, UK.

Pietrzik, K. (ed.) (1991) *Modern Lifestyles, Lower Energy Intake and Micronutrient Status*, Springer-Verlag, London.

Prochaska, J.O. and DiClemente, C.C. (1986) Towards a comprehensive mode of change, in *Treating Addictive Behaviours: Process of Change*, (eds W.R. Miller and W. Heather), Plenum, New York.

Rollnick, S., Heather, N. and Bell, A. (1992) Negotiated behaviour in medical settings: the development of brief motivational interviewing. *Journal of Mental Health*, 1, 25–37.

Tesco Healthy Eating. *Get the balance right*.

Chapter 10

Bourne, G. (1989) *Pregnancy*, Pan Books, London.

Department of Health (1991) *Dietary Reference Values for Food Energy and Nutrients for the United Kingdom*, HMSO, London. (Report on Health and Social Subjects 41.)

Garrow, J.S. and James, W.P.T. (eds) (1993) *Human Nutrition and Dietetics*, 9th edn, Churchill Livingstone, London. (Good for physiological changes.)

Pietrzik, K. (ed.) (1991) *Modern Lifestyles, Lower Energy Intake and Micronutrient Status*, Springer-Verlag, London.

Scott, J. *et al.* (1994) The role of folate in neural tube defects. *Proceedings of the Nutrition Society*, 53, 631–6.

Sterr, P., Ash Alam, M., Wadsworth, J. and Welch, A. (1995) Relation between maternal haemoglobin concentration and birth weight in different ethnic groups. *British Medical Journal*, 310, 489–91.

Thomas, B. (ed.) (1994) *Manual of Dietetic Practice*, 2nd edn, Blackwell Scientific Publications, London. (Comprehensive and practical.)

Vines, G. (1995) Some of our sperm are missing. *New Scientist*, No. 1992, 26 August.

Winick, M. (1989) *Nutrition, Pregnancy and Early Infancy*. Williams and Wilkins, Baltimore, London. (American, excellent for scientific evidence.)

Worthington-Roberts, B. and Rodwell-Williams, S. (1994) *Nutrition in Pregnancy and Lactation*, 5th edn, Mosby, London.

Chapter 11

Armstrong, N. *et al.* (1990) Patterns of physical activity among 11–16-year-old British children. *British Medical Journal*, 301, 203–5.

Barker, D.J.P. (1995) *Mothers, Babies and Disease in Later Life*. British Medical Journal Publishing Group.

Barker, D.J.P., Bull, A.R., Osmond, C. and Simmonds, S.J. (1990) Fetal and placental size and risk of hypertension in adult life. *British Medical Journal*, 301, 259–62.

Barker, D.J.P., Winter, P.D., Osmond, C. *et al.* (1989) Weight in infancy and death from ischaemic heart disease. *Lancet*, ii, 577–80.

Bull, N.L. (1985) Dietary habits of 15–25-year-olds. *Human Nutrition and Applied Nutrition*, 39A (Suppl. 1), 1–68.

Department of Health (1994) *Weaning and the Weaning Diet*, HMSO, London. (Report on Health and Social Subjects 45.)

Department of Health and Social Security (1980) *Artificial Feeds for Young Infants*, HMSO, London. (Reports on Health and Social Subjects 18.)

Department of Health and Social Security (1989) *The diets of British School-children, Sub-committee on Nutritional Surveillance*, HMSO, London. (Report on Health and Social Subjects 36.)

Edsall Summaries for Health Professionals (1984) *Feeding children in the First Year*, Edsall, London. (Detailed, practical.)

Erhardt, P. (1986) Iron deficiency in young Bradford children from different ethnic groups. *British Medical Journal*, **292**, 90–3.

Hill, A. (1993) The Socio-cultural Context of Children's eating, in *Children in Focus*, National Dairy Council.

Hourihane, J. *et al.* (1995) Is water out of vogue? A survey of the drinking habits of 2–7 year olds. *Archives of Disease in Childhood*, **72**, 137–40.

Illingworth, R. (1986) *The Normal Child*, 9th edn, Churchill Livingstone, London. (Excellent on behavioural and developmental aspects.)

Lucas, A. *et al.* (1992) Breast milk and subsequent intelligence quotient in children born pre-term. *Lancet*, **339**, 261–4.

Mills, A. and Tyler, H. (1992) *Food and Nutrient Intakes of British Infants Aged 6–12 months*, HMSO, London.

National Diet and Nutrition Survey: Children Aged 1 to 4 Years (1995) HMSO, London. Volume 1 – Report of the Diet and Nutrition Survey; volume 2 – Report of the Dental Survey.

Sanders, T.A.B. (1986) Growth and development of British vegan children. *American Journal of Clinical Nutrition*, **48**, 822–5.

SMA Nutrition. *Iron – A Nutritional Guide for Babies from Six Months*. From SMA Nutrition, Huntercombe Lane South, Taplow, Maidenhead, Berks, SL6 OPH, UK.

Tanner, J. (1989) *Foetus into Man*, 2nd edn, Ware, Castlemead.

Thomas, B. (ed.) (1994) *Manual of Dietetic Practice*, 2nd edn, Blackwell Scientific Publications, London. (Comprehensive, clear, concise.)

Train, J.J.A., Yates, R.W. and Sury, M.R.J. (1995) Hypocalcaemic stridor and infantile nutritional rickets. *British Medical Journal*, **310**, 488–92.

UK height and weight standards are produced by The Child Growth Foundation and available from Harlow Publishing, Maxwell Street, South Shields, NE3 4PU, UK.

Walker, A. (ed) (1990) *Applied Human Nutrition*, Ellis Horwood. (Chapter 4 is academic and concise.)

Winick, M. (1989) *Nutrition, Pregnancy and Early Infancy*, Williams and Wilkins. (Detailed, easy to read.)

Woodward, D.R. (1985a) What sort of teenager has high intakes of energy and nutrients? *British Journal of Nutrition*, **54**, 325–33.

Woodward, D.R. (1985b) What sort of teenager has low intakes of energy and nutrients? *British Journal of Nutrition*, **53**, 241–9.

BOOKLETS

From first tastes to family meals – a nutritional guide. From the makers of Marmite Yeast Extract, Sylvia Meredith Health Education Advisory Service, 3 Elgin Road, Sutton, Surrey, SM1 3SN.

From milk to mixed feeding. Health Education Authority.

SMA nutrition. *Weaning – a step by step guide*. Available from SMA Nutrition, Huntercombe Lane South, Taplow, Maidenhead, Berks, SL6 OPH, UK.

Austoker, J. (1994) Cancer prevention in primary care. Diet and cancer. *British Medical Journal*, 308, 1610–14. (An excellent summary.)

Barker, J.D.P. (1994) *Mothers, Babies and Disease in Later life*. British Medical Journal Publishing, London.

Department of Health (1991) *Dietary Reference Values for Food Energy and Nutrients for the United Kingdom*, HMSO, London. (Report on Health and Social Subjects 41.)

Department of Health (1994) *Nutritional Aspects of Cardiovascular Disease*, HMSO, London. (Report on Health and Social Subjects 46.)

Department of Health (1995) *Sensible Drinking*, HMSO, London. (The Report of an Inter-Departmental Working Group.

Eastwood, M., Edwards, C. and Parry, D. (1992) *Human Nutrition, a Continuing Debate*, Chapman & Hall, London.

Garrow, J. and James, W.P.T. (eds) (1993) *Human Nutrition and Dietetics*, 9th edn, Churchill Livingstone, London. (A very good chapter on cancers.)

Keys, A., Menotti, A., Karvonen, M.J. *et al.* (1986) The diet and 15-year death rate in the Seven Countries Study. *American Journal of Epidemiology*, 124, 903–15.

Marmot, M.G., Rose, G., Shipley, M.J. and Thomas, B.J. (1981) Alcohol and mortality: a U-shaped curve. *Lancet*, 1, 580–3.

Multiple Risk Factor Intervention Trial Research Group (1982) Multiple Risk Factor Intervention Trial: risk factor changes and mortality results. *Journal of the American Medical Association*, 248, 1465–77.

Ornish, D. *et al.* (1990) Can lifestyle changes reverse coronary heart disease? *Lancet*, 336, 129–33.

Pietrzik, K. (ed.) (1991) *Modern Lifestyles, Lower Energy Intake and Micronutrient Status*, Springer-Verlag, London.

Royal College of Physicians (1987) *A Great and Growing Evil: the Medical Consequences of Alcohol Abuse*, Tavistock, London.

Survey of British Adults (1990) A survey carried out by the Social Survey Division of the OPCS with Dietary and Nutritional Evaluations by MAFF and the Department of Health, HMSO, London.

Sytkowski, P.A., Kannel, W.B. and D'Agostino, R.B. (1990) Changes in risk factors and the decline in mortality from cardiovascular disease. The Framingham heart study. *New England Journal of Medicine*, 322, 1635–41.

Chapter 12

Brown, J.J., Lever, A.F., Robertson, J.I.S. *et al.* (1984) Salt and Hypertension. *Lancet*, ii, 1333–4.

Chalmers, J. (1991) *British Medical Journal*, 303, 351 (Letter).

Davies, L. (1972) *Easy Cooking for One or Two*, Penguin Handbooks, London.

Davies, L. (1979) *More Easy Cooking for One or Two*, Penguin Handbooks, London.

Davies, L. (1981) *Three Score Years . . . and Then?* Heinemann Medical Books Ltd., London.

Davies, M., Mawer, E.B., Hann, J.T. and Taylor, J.L. (1976) Seasonal changes in the biochemical indices of vitamin D deficiency in the elderly: a comparison of people in residential homes, long stay wards and attending a day hospital. *Ageing*, 15, 77–83.

Chapter 13

Department of Health and Social Security (1979) *Nutrition and health in old age*, HMSO, London. (Report on Health and Social Subjects 16.)

Department of Health (1991) *Dietary Reference Values for Food Energy and Nutrients for the United Kingdom*, HMSO, London. (Report on Health and Social Subjects 41.)

Department of Health (1992) *The nutrition of elderly people*, HMSO, London.

Gerontology Nutrition Unit, slide lecture kit. *An emergency food store for the elderly.*

Gerontology Nutrition Unit, slide lecture kit. *What is a balanced diet?* (15 colour cartoon slides, lecture notes, 30 leaflets.)

Note: these lecture kits are available from the Gerontology Nutrition Unit, Royal Free Hospital School of Medicine, 21 Pond Street, London, NW3 2PN, UK.

Holmes, S. (1994) Nutrition and older people: a matter of concern. *Nursing Times*, 90(42), 31–3. (An excellent summary with useful references.)

Lawson, D.E.M., Paul, A.A., Black, A.E., Cole, T.J., Mandal, A.R. and Cavie, M. (1979) Relative contribution of diet and sunlight to vitamin D state of the elderly. *British Medical Journal*, 2, 303–8.

MAFF *Household Food Consumption and Expenditure*. Annual Report of the National Food Survey Committee. (Published annually.)

Scott, C.J. (1986) The ill elderly patient – is he dehydrated too? *Geriatric Medicine*, 16, 59–61.

Thomas, B. (ed.) (1994) *Manual of Dietetic Practice*, 2nd edn, Blackwell Scientific Publications, London.

Vousden, M. (1986) Problems with eating. *Geriatric Nursing and Home Care*, December.

Wilmshurst, P. (1994) Temperature and cardiovascular mortality. *British Medical Journal*, 309, 1029–30.

Chapter 14

British Diabetic Association. *Asian Information Pack*. From Diet Information Service, British Diabetic Association, 10 Queen Anne Street, London, W1M 0BD, UK.

Cruikshank, J.K. and Beevers, D.G. (1986) *Ethnic Factors in Health and Disease*, Butterworth, London.

Henley, A. (1979) *Asian Patients in Hospital and at Home*. King Edward's Hospital Fund for London. (An excellent guide to all aspects of life. Names of foods in Hindi-Urdu are given.)

Immigrant Foods (1992) Second supplement to McCance and Widdowson's *The Composition of Foods*, HMSO, London.

Kenn, J., Douglas, J., and Sylvester, V. (1986) Survey of infant feeding practices by Afro-Caribbean mothers in Birmingham. *Proceedings of the Nutrition Society*, 45(3), 87A.

Leeming, M. and Huang Man-hui, M. (1983) *Chinese Regional Cookery*, Rider, London. (Gives information on Chinese inheritance as well as contemporary influences on diet, and recipes.)

Rose, E. (1985) *The New Jewish Cuisine*, Robson Books Ltd, London.

Thomas, B. (ed.) (1994) *Manual of Dietetic Practice, 2nd edn*, Blackwell Scientific Publications, London.

Dwyer, J.T. (1991) Nutritional consequences of vegetarianism. *Annual Reviews of Nutrition*, 11, 61–91.

Kelsay, J.L. *et al.* (1988) Impact of variation in carbohydrate intake on mineral utilisation by vegetarians. *American Journal of Clinical Nutrition*, 48, 875–9.

Sanders, T.A.B. and Manning, J. (1992) The growth and development of vegan children. *Journal of Human Nutrition and Diet*, 5, 11–21.

Sanders, T.A.B. and Reddy, S. (1994) Nutritional implications of a meatless diet. *Proceedings of the Nutrition Society*, 53, 297–307.

Thomas, B. (ed.) (1994) *Manual of Dietetic Practice*, 2nd edn, Blackwell Scientific Publications, London.

Thorogood, M., Roe, L., McPherson, K. and Mann, J. (1990) Dietary intake and plasma lipid levels: lessons from a study of the diet of health conscious groups. *British Medical Journal*, 300, 1297–301.

Chapter 15

Health Education Authority (1989) *Diet, nutrition and healthy eating in low income groups*. Health Education Authority, London.

Lawrence, B. (1989) *How to Feed your Family for £4 a day*. Thorsons.

MAFF *Household Food Consumption and Expenditure: Annual Report of the National Food Survey Committee*, HMSO, London.

Malseed, J. (1990) *Bread Without Dough: Understanding Food Poverty*, Horton Publishing, Bradford.

National Children's Home (1991) *Poverty and Nutrition Survey*. From NCH, 85 Highbury Park, London N5 1UD.

Oppenheim, C. (1993) *Poverty: the facts*. Child Poverty Action Group Ltd.

Policy Studies Institute (1994) *Urban Trends 2: A Decade in Britain's Deprived Urban Areas*.

Stitt, S., Griffiths, G. and Grant, D. (1994) Homeless and hungry: the evidence from Liverpool. *Nutrition and Health*, 9, 275–87.

Thomas, B. (ed.) (1994) *Manual of Dietetic Practice*, 2nd edn, Blackwell Scientific Publications, London.

Chapter 16

Bridget Jones (1995) *The Dietetic Cookbook*, The Apple Press. (Good ordinary recipes, gives calories and carbohydrate values. Recipes are high in fibre and low in fat.)

Garrow, J.S. and James, W.P.T. (1993) *Human Nutrition and Dietetics*, 9th edn, Churchill Livingstone, London.

Lamb, J.F. *et al.* (1993) *Essentials of Physiology*, 3rd edn, Blackwell Scientific Publications, Oxford.

Department of Health (1991) *Dietary Reference Values for Food Energy and Nutrients for the United Kingdom*, HMSO, London. (Report on Health and Social Subjects 41.)

Thomas, B. (ed.) (1994) *Manual of Dietetic Practice*, 2nd edn, Blackwell Scientific Publications, London.

Chapter 17

USEFUL ADDRESS

British Diabetic Association, 10 Queen Anne Street, London W1M 0BD, UK.

Chapter 18   Arora, N.S. and Rochester, D.F. (1982) Respiratory muscle strength and maximal voluntary ventilation in undernourished patients. *American Review of Respiratory Diseases*, **126**, 5–8.

Basto, M.D., Rawlings, J. and Allison, S.P. (1983) Benefits of supplementary tube feeding after fractured neck of femur: a randomized controlled trial. *British Medical Journal*, **287**, 1589–92.

Bistrian, B.R., Blackburn, G.L., Hallowell, E. and Heddle, R. (1974) Protein status of general surgical patients. *Journal of the American Medical Association*, **253**, 1567–70.

Delmi, M., Rapin, C.-H., Bengoa, J.-M., Delmas, P.D., Vasey, H. and Bonjour, J.-P. (1990) Dietary supplementation in elderly patients with fractured neck of femur. *Lancet*, **335**, 1013–16.

Heymafiels, S.B., Bethel, R.A., Ansley, J.D., Gibbs, D.M., Felner, K.M. and Nutter, D.O. (1978) Cardiac abnormalities in cachetic patients before and during nutritional repletion. *American Heart Journal*, **95**, 584–94.

Holmes, R., MacChiano, K., Jhangiani, S.S., Agarwal, N.R. and Savino, J.A. (1987) *Combating pressure sores – nutritionally. American Journal of Nursing*, **87**, 1301–3.

Larsson, J., Unosson, M., Ek, A.-C., Nilsson, L., Thorsland, S. and Bjurulf, P. (1990) Effect of dietary supplement on nutritional status and clinical outcome in 501 geriatric patients – a randomised study. *Clinical Nutrition*, **9**, 179–84.

Lennard-Jones K.E. (1992) *A Positive Approach to Nutrition as Treatment.* The King's Fund Centre, 126 Albert Street, London, NW1 7NF. (£5.)

Lock, M. and Vald, V. (1994) Refer early to a dietician (Letter). *British Medical Journal*, **308**, 1370.

Mainous, M., Dazhing, X., Qi Lu, Berg, I.D. and Deitch, E.A. (1991) Oral-tpn-induced bacterial translocation and impaired immune defenses are reversed by re-feeding. *Surgery*, **110**(2), 277–84.

McWhirter, J.P. and Pennington, C.R. (1994) Incidence and recognition of malnutrition in hospital. *British Medical Journal*, **308**, 945–8.

Moy, R.J.D., Smallman, S. and Booth, I.W. (1990) Malnutrition in a UK children's hospital. *Journal of Human Nutrition and Dietetics*, **3**, 93–100.

Royce, C. and Taylor, M. (1994) Identifying malnutrition benefits everybody (Letter). *British Medical Journal*, **308**, 1370.

Thomas, B. (ed.) (1994) *Manual of Dietetic Practice*, 2nd edn, Blackwell Scientific Publications, London.

Zador, D.A. and Truswell, A.S. (1987) Nutritional status on admission to a general surgical ward in a Sydney hospital. *Australian and New Zealand Journal of Medicine*, **17**, 234–40.

Chapter 19   *Food Intolerance and Food Aversion* (1984) Joint Report of the Royal College of Physicians and the British Nutrition Foundation. Clear. (A concise report.)

Foodborne Illness (1991) A *Lancet* review, W.M. Waites and J.P. Arbuthnott (editorial advisers), Edward Arnold, London. (An excellent and detailed review of food-borne illness, covering bacterial, viral, protozoal illness as well as natural food-borne toxicants. An excellent chapter on BSE.)

Hide, D. (1993) Letter. *British Medical Journal*, **307**, 1427.

MAFF (1995) *Food Allergy and Other Unpleasant Reactions to Food*. Free from Foodsense, (PB1696), London, SE99 7TT, UK.

Sprenger, R.A. (1992) *The Food Hygiene Handbook*, 8th edn, Highfield Publications, Doncaster. (A brief, entertainingly-presented booklet, primarily for catering personnel.)

Young, E. *et al.* (1994) A population study of food intolerance. *Lancet*, 343, 1127–9.

Bender, A.E. and Bender, D.A. (1986) *Food tables*. Oxford University Press, Oxford.

Byrne, J. (1993) *Which? way to a healthier diet*. Consumers' Association and Hodder & Stoughton.

Davies, J. and Dickerson, J. (1991) *Nutrient Content of Food Portions*. The Royal Society of Chemistry.

Department of Health (1994) *The nutritional aspects of cardiovascular disease*, HMSO, London. (Report on Health and Social Subjects 46.)

Food Labelling Regulations 1984 (S.I. 1984 No. 1305). HMSO, London.

Foodborne Illness (1991) A *Lancet* review, Edward Arnold, London.

Foodsense. *About food additives*. MAFF. PB0552.

Foodsense. *Food protection*. MAFF. PB0554.

Foodsense. *Understanding food labels*. MAFF PB0553.

Note: the three 'Foodsense' brochures are available free of charge from Food Sense, London, SE99 7TT, UK. (They are written for the general public.)

Holland, B., Welch, A.A., Unwin, I.D., Buss, D.H., Paul, A.A. and Southgate, D.A.T. (1991) *McCance and Widdowson's The Composition of Foods*, 5th edn, Royal Society of Chemistry, Cambridge.

MAFF (1988) *Food Portion Sizes*, 2nd edn, HMSO, London.

MAFF (1993) *Dietary Intake of Food Additives in the UK: Initial Surveillance*. Food Surveillance Paper No. 37. HMSO, London.

Tan, S.P., Wenlock, R.W. and Buss, D.H. (1985) *Immigrant Foods*. Second supplement to *McCance and Widdowson's The Composition of Foods*. HMSO, London.

Thomas, B. (ed.) (1994) *Manual of Dietetic Practice*, 2nd edn, Blackwell Scientific Publications, London.

Which? (1995) *Cartons for kids* Which? way to health, Consumers' Association.

Which? report (1995)

WHO (1994) *Safety and Nutritional Adequacy of Irradiated Food*, Geneva.

Malnutrition, Learning and Behaviour, U.S. D.H.E.W. publication No. 76, 1036, April, 1976.

Morgan, K.J. and Zabik, M.E (1984) The influence of ready-to-eat cereal consumption at breakfast on nutrient intakes of individuals 62 years and older. *Journal of the American College of Nutrition*, 3, 27.

Morgan, K.J., Zabik, M.E. and Leveille, G.A. (1981) The role of breakfast in nutrient intake of 5- to 12-year-old children. *American Journal of Clinical Nutrition*, 34, 1418.

Chapter 20

Chapter 21

Sommerville, J. and O'Reagan, M. (1993) The contribution of breakfast to micronutrient adequacy of the Irish diet. *Journal of Human Nutrition and Dietetics*, 6, 223–8.

The Roper Organization, Inc.: Activities in Past 24 Hours. Roper Reports 86-3, 1986.

COOKBOOKS

There are so many good cookbooks that it is hard to choose between them. This is by no means a comprehensive list.

Lindsay, A. *The Everyday Light-Hearted Cookbook*. Grub Street. £10.99 Approved by the British Heart Foundation.

Madhur Jaffrey's *Indian Cookery*, BBC Publications. This gives excellent recipes including good ones for lentils and other pulses. I usually use less oil and salt than recommended.

Details of Louise Davies' books for cooking for one or two are given in Chapter 13.

Index